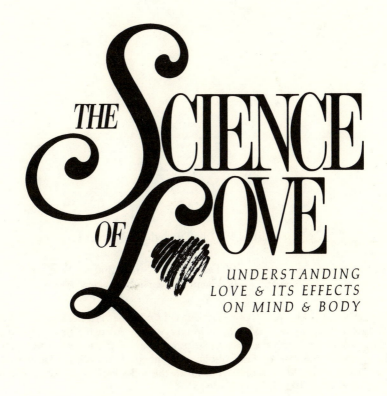

THE SCIENCE OF LOVE

UNDERSTANDING LOVE & ITS EFFECTS ON MIND & BODY

ANTHONY WALSH, Ph.D.

PROMETHEUS BOOKS
BUFFALO, NEW YORK

$$\frac{T}{G} = W^2$$

Published 1991 by Prometheus Books

With editorial offices located at 700 East Amherst Street, Buffalo, New York 14215, and distribution facilities at 59 John Glenn Drive, Amherst, New York 14228.

95 94 93 92 91   5 4 3 2 1

Library of Congress Cataloging-in-Publication Data

Walsh, Anthony, 1941–
    The science of love : understanding love and its effects on mind and body / Anthony Walsh.
        p.   cm.
    Includes bibliographical references and index.
    ISBN 0-87975-648-9
    1. Love. 2. Mind and body. I. Title.
BF575.L8W35   1991
152.4′1—dc20

90-2712
CIP

Printed in the United States of America on acid-free paper.

Contents

Foreword

Napoleon Bonaparte said that love was a "stupidity of two," while Henry David Thoreau held it was a "thirst that was never slaked." Love is blind, it makes the world go 'round, it can be a form of warfare, and it certainly breeds anxieties. Almost everyone has an opinion about love. But love is also something we can examine, analyze, and perhaps even begin to explain. It is not only poets who are the authorities on love. Scientists, too, of various sorts, from biologists to sociologists, from physicists to psychologists, have been interested in what attracts and what repels.

Anthony Walsh, while not ignoring the poet or the novelist, the romantic or the skeptic, has investigated what the current scientific research tells us about love, from infancy to old age. Though the nature of love changes as we pass through the different ages and stages of life, it is always recognizably *love*. The passions of first love might be only a lingering memory to the couple who has been together for fifty years, yet they can still be in love.

Physicians and psychiatrists have long recognized that love, or the lack of it, can have a significant effect on both physical and mental illness. Sociologists have devoted volumes to the study of alienation, the feeling of not belonging, in the attempt to explain all kinds of social malaise. And criminologists know that lovelessness is a key factor in lawlessness.

Love is also a major component of religion, from the "overwhelming love of God for the frail insufficient human," as St. Bernard put it in the twelfth century, to the "Jesus loves me" of today's evangelicals. But the same feeling of belonging, of being needed, of being loved, that helps tie religious people together, works for skeptics and agnostics as well through networks of friendships and organizations.

Obviously, love is also an important aspect of how we define ourselves sexually. Although in many ways love has little to do with sexuality, its association with sexuality has led to the inclusion of *The Science of Love* in Prometheus Books' general series on sex and gender issues. However, we should not be limited to seeing love only in that light. For love can range from the mother's caresses of a newborn infant to the sexual passion of two lovers, from the altruist's compassion for all humanity to the spurned lover's narrow hostility toward a former loved one.

Clearly, since it has such profound implications for individual and society, love is a subject about which we need to know much more than we now do. Though Anthony Walsh is a sociologist (criminologist), his approach in this book is interdisciplinary. Not only has he avoided the jargon that professionals sometimes use, but in the process of his exploration of love he has written a book that is fascinating and accessible to the general reader. Whether we feel friendless and unloved or deeply attached to a significant other, we can all learn by reading what Walsh has to say.

VERN L. BULLOUGH
Series Editor
New Concepts in
Human Sexuality

Preface

By wide acclaim, love is the noblest, most powerful, beautiful, exquisite, and meaningful experience of humanity. Because of it we are born, through it we are sustained, and for it we will sacrifice life itself. Love insulates the child, brings joy to youth, and comfort and sustenance to the aged. Love cures the sick, raises the fallen, comforts the tormented, and inspires the composer, painter, and poet. Love is "nature's second sun," it "springs eternal in the human breast," and it "moves the sun and other stars." Plato has called it the first creation of the gods, while Erich Fromm says it is the last hope for the problems of human existence. Philosophers as far apart in space, time, and outlook as the Iranian Zoroaster and the German-American Paul Tillich have declared love to be the ultimate universal law.

Love provides profitable grist for the mills of recording companies and publishing houses, which grind out unending formula songs and novels declaring the joys and the anguish of our perennial passion. Lusty love, love lost, love found, love requited and unrequited, secret love, shouted love, painful love, ecstatic love, neurotic love, perverted love, sacrificial love —the list goes on. Poets too (with nobler motives) milk this nectar of the gods to the final impassioned sigh. We are all of us, or so it seems, in love with love.

In 1956 the German-American psychoanalyst Erich Fromm published a phenomenally successful little book called *The Art of Loving*. It was a beautiful exploration of the philosophical, religious, and psychological aspects of love from a Freudian/Marxist perspective. One could not read this book without feeling uplifted, but it was lacking in hard scientific evidence to support Fromm's assertion that love "is the most fundamental passion, it is the force which keeps the human race together, the clan, the family, the society. The failure to achieve it means insanity or destruction —self-destruction or destruction of others. Without love humanity could not exist for a day."[1]

I hope that I have not been too arrogant in naming this book *The Science of Love*. To most people, the "art of love" is so much more appropriate than the "science of love." Love, as traditionally viewed, is one of those great intangibles like truth and beauty. We prefer to leave such subjects to the poet's pen lest they be somehow diminished by the cold stare of science. The romantic's response to having something beautiful explained in its particulars is exemplified by Wordsworth's lines (which drew upon Sir Isaac Newton's explanation of the prism):

> Our meddling intellect misshapes the beauteous form of things, we murder to dissect.

Perhaps there are those who enjoy the mystery of a phenomenon more than the phenomenon itself. But surely science enhances rather than diminishes the appreciation of any of the charms nature reveals. We need to understand love in its particulars, just as we need to enjoy its blessings. The confusions, contradictions, and misconceptions about the nature of love have cost humanity dearly. As long as we consider love to be some syrupy spiritual mystery that either strikes us or does not, we may search in vain for it. If we miss out on love, we miss one aspect of human existence that is truly essential. Love is not just the icing on the cake of human existence; in a very real sense it is existence itself. The human species might never have evolved countless ages ago had not evolution selected love into our biological inheritance. Families, bands, tribes, and nations have fractured under the unbearable weight of lovelessness. Individuals deprived of love become emotionally barren as they plod through dark lives. Many of the sciences, from anthropology to zoology, have documented and affirmed these statements.

So, what then is love? In response to this question, Sir Philip Sidney shouted, "Fool, look into thy heart, and write!" Sidney's agitated reply implies that somewhere in the deep recesses of the flesh we should all know the answer, and that it will be revealed to us if we will only engage in a little free-association poetry. Poetry has long been considered the only true language of love and thus the only medium that can answer this question. Poetry is a beautiful aid to human understanding, but love is too important a topic for it to be considered the exclusive realm of the poet— or novelist or priest. Love is so much more than the passionate fusion of two souls and four gonads. The poet Shelley, in an insight more scientific than poetic, defined love:

> That profound and complicated sentiment which we call love is the universal thirst for a communion not merely of the senses, but of our whole nature, intellectual, imaginative and sensitive. . . . The sexual impulse, which is only one, and often a small part of those claims, serves, from its obvious and

external nature, as a kind of expression of the rest, a common basis, an acknowledged and visible link.[2]

If I interpret Shelley correctly, he says that the romantic and sexual impulses commonly accepted as exhausting the meaning of love are merely felt manifestations of a more fundamental principle. These impulses are relatively concrete phenomena that point toward and participate in, but by no means exhaust, the richness of meaning contained in the verb "to love." There are those who would not agree with Shelley's definition of love, for anyone's definiton of love is open to criticism. Perhaps love is too profound, too expansive, to be contained in a single definition. Perhaps the reader will agree with Paul Tillich that love cannot be defined, because there is no higher principle by which it may be defined.

A Supreme Court Justice once admitted that he could not define pornography, but he was certain that he knew it when he saw it. Perhaps it is like this with love. We all know what love is until some philosophical curmudgeon comes along and demands that we define it. We do not need a comprehensive and universally agreed upon definition in order to explore the nature and effects of love, and its absence, any more than we need a hard and fast definition of pornography to study it. Nevertheless, we do need an operational definition of love, so that you and I are reading from the same sheet of music.

I define love as that which satisfies our need to receive and bestow affection and nurturance; to give and be given assurances of value, respect, acceptance, and appreciation; and to feel secure in our unity with, and belonging to, a particular family, as well as the human family.

This definition owes much to Shelley's, but it is couched in terms of love's manifestations rather than its sentiment. It is a broad definition of how we relate to others, which covers a wide range of subneeds, attitudes, and behaviors. It implies, most of all, an active concern for the well-being of others. Depending on what facet of this inexhaustible topic we are exploring, we will qualify, elaborate, and expand our definition at various points in the book, most especially when we explore the passion of romantic love.

My exploration of love presents the wisdom of many disciplines and the thoughts of many authors. These authors share a deep belief that love is indeed the glue of human existence. Unfortunately, love is infrequently studied by scientists who explore human behavior, for the word trips too uneasily on the tongue. We hesitate to introduce love into our work, preferring to leave this "mystical" and "unmeasurable" concept to the humanities. Social scientists prefer to focus on the negative face of humanity, on prejudice, war, crime, and hatred. (Defining hate, incidentally, doesn't seem to be much of a problem.) These are all manifestations of love's absence, deficiency, or betrayal, and are, of course, immensely important problems that demand our attention. They are also more amenable to the social scientist's methods of study because they represent concentrations of human energy, while love is an irradiation which, it is admitted, is more difficult to grasp.

Having made the point that most behavioral scientists seek professional nourishment by studying the decay of humanity, I shall devote this book to those who have found love to be a particularly rich pasture in which to graze. I have spent many years exploring the consequences of love's absence on criminality, hypertension, multiple sclerosis, self-esteem, and intellectual development. My own studies and those of others have convinced me that in our world of confusion and alarm we must probe the nature of love and learn how to generate and sustain it.

Humankind has always known that love was good for it. All great philosophers and religious leaders have preached the same message of love. What science has done is to verify and explain the particulars of these insights through a systematic examination of the mechanisms and processes by which love or its absence affects our physical, psychological, and spiritual being. This is what this book is about. If love is truly a human need (in the strictest sense of the word), it must be demonstrated that negative things happen to us if we don't get it and positive things happen to us when we do.

The Introduction offers an overview of love. It attempts to get to the heart of the concept by exploring what other cultures and traditions have had to say about this boundless topic. Is love an invention of the human intellect, or is it lodged in the very nature of our species? I also look at those traditions that have defined love as a gift from the gods. Many of these traditions view love as originating in a deep human desire to be connected with the primeval source of all existence. I take some of these fanciful myths and show that they are not as fanciful as they seem at first, for modern science is affirming an underlying truth that the ancients divined. We will find that we are connected to one another in deeper and more profound ways than we might imagine.

After this overview, the book is divided into three broad sections: skin love, kin love, and in love. Part One: Skin Love deals with the importance of love in early infancy. In chapter 1 I explore the magic of touch. Being touched in tender and loving ways is an infant's first message of love. We will see how these love messages affect the structure and function of the infant's developing brain. In chapter 2 we will see what science has to say about the difference between parental love from a male and from a female. Why is mother love so important? Are women by nature more loving than men? Is there an actual chemistry to mother love? Is there a maternal instinct? What is bonding? Chapter 3 deals with the impact of loving care on each of the three structures of what has been called the *triune, or "three-in-one" brain*. Early experiences, whether they are accompanied by love or are not, have a way of etching themselves into the very cells and neural pathways of the brain. What does "split-brain" research have to tell us about male and female differences, and is there a "love brain"?

Part Two: Kin Love explores the importance of loving ties with our fellow human beings and investigates the morass of psychological and physical problems associated with the absence or deprivation of love. Chapter 4 looks at love in terms of physical illness. What role does the absence of love play in developing chronic physical diseases such as hypertension and multiple sclerosis? On the other hand, can love prime the immunological system for a more efficient response to disease? What are the effects of love deprivation on the physical growth and development of children? Chapter 5 looks at mental illness. It explores the role played by love in schizophrenia, neurosis, depression, suicide, and substance abuse. Chapter 6 explores the dark and violent world of psychopathy and the impact of lovelessness on lawlessness.

I then turn to love "writ large." What have the great philosophers and social scientists had to say about social conditions as they relate to love? What relationship does love bear to work and to human authenticity? What social practices are inimical to love? Is there a relationship between sociopolitical systems, such as democracy and totalitarianism, and love? How was the coming of capitalism and democracy important to romantic love?

Part Three: In Love deals with romantic love. How is it generated and sustained? What is the importance of early skin love and kin love for an adult's successful romantic relationships? Is love different for men and women? What are the various styles of loving? Is there a definable chemistry of love? I explore monogamy and sexual license, jealousy and the objectification of love, the biological origins of homosexuality, and how we can become more loving beings.

Science has something to say about these topics. Science is the straightest and most reliable of the paths humanity has charted in its quest for truth. But is love rather than science most important in the final reckoning? When the French astronomer and mathematician Pierre Laplace lay dying, his friends tried to console him by reminding him of his discoveries and his books, but he turned them aside as unimportant. When asked by his friends what could be more important in the fullness of life, with his last breath Laplace replied, "Love."

A look at the Bibliography will reveal that the journal citations are more often from the natural sciences (general biology, physiology, neurology, medicine, etc.) than from the behavioral and social sciences. I do not mean to slight the latter. I am a medical sociologist and criminologist by training, but I have always had a strong biological orientation. The emphasis on the natural sciences in this book reveals my preference for reducing explanations to their most basic and concretely observable levels. In other words, I don't think it is sufficient to observe the relationship between what goes into an organism in the form of experiences and what comes out in terms of behavior. We have to open the box to try and fathom why a particular experience produces a particular effect.

But this is decidedly not a book pitting nature against nurture. Rather, I look at nature via nurture. Even the behaviorist John Watson believed that love was an innate emotional need that is fed by the tactile stimulation an infant receives as it snuggles in its mother's arms. Every animal, human or otherwise, arrives in this world with the genetically determined behavior patterns of its species. These behavioral patterns are as much a product of evolutionary selection as is the animal's physical appearance and biological structure. These basic behavioral patterns are molded, guided, and cultivated by experience. Some patterns of behavior are controlled more by nature, some controlled more by nurture, and some controlled equally by both.

I once attended a lecture by William Glasser, psychiatrist and father of reality therapy. He spoke to the issue of nature and/or nurture in terms of disease. Huntington's chorea, for instance, is totally a genetic—or "nature"—disease. If you have the gene for this disease, you will eventually get it regardless of how fit and healthy you may otherwise be. Cancer is more a genetic than environmental disease, but we can take certain steps to lessen our chances of falling afoul of it. Cardiovascular disease appears to be about equally under the control of genetics and the environment, in that a healthy lifestyle appears to reduce dramatically one's risk, even if a genetic predisposition exists. Finally, alcoholism would seem to be a disease that is preventable. There is evidence of a genetic predisposition to alcoholism, but if one learns how to resist the temptation to drink alcohol, the disease cannot materialize.

Healthy attributes, like disease states, are also a complex mixture of nature and nurture. I believe that the development of the human ability to give and to receive love is somewhere between cardiovascular disease and alcoholism, viewed in terms of Glasser's "nature-nurture hierarchy." That is to say, while love is an innate need of the human animal proper nurturing is required if the need is to be met. Unlike predispositions to particular disease states unfortunately inherited by a number of people, the need to love and be loved is a predisposition that exists in each and every one of us. We need love just as desperately as we don't need cancer and heart disease. This book is an attempt to demonstrate the truth of this statement.

NOTES

1. Erich Fromm, *The Art of Loving* (New York: Bantam, 1956), p. 15.
2. Cited in Karl Menninger, *Love Against Hate* (New York: Harcourt, Brace and World, 1942), p. 281.

Introduction

An Overview of the Many Faces of Love

> I tell thee, love is nature's second sun
> Causing a spring of virtue where he shines.
> —George Chapman

It is not the threat of death, illness, hardship, or poverty that crush the human spirit; it is the fear of being alone and unloved in the universe. Only when we are loved and can give love in return do we feel whole. We are incomplete beings without love, and we yearn to be connected. When we are incompletely connected we feel a deep emotional and spiritual emptiness. Apart from the purely survival needs dictated by our biological nature, love is important above all things to the human animal. The need for love envelops our personal, biological, sexual, social, and spiritual existence. When we have it we feel happy, complete, and fully alive. It beautifies our lives, it empowers our being, it ennobles us, it enriches us in every way, and it embues our minds and hearts with a sense of the fullness of life. It is indeed "nature's second sun," for all our needs, both the critical and the merely desirable, revolve around it.

For all our praise and desire for love, we find it difficult to obtain a firm notion of its nature. We are constrained by the attitudes and ideas our cultures bequeath us and by the language in which they are expressed. Each generation is impregnated by the intellectual seed of thinkers long gone to their reward or punishment. Like every other idea of importance, love has been strained through the sieve of received ideas. Each cultural perspective on love has something to tell us, so it is wrong to take any one part as the whole. It would seem desirable, therefore, to offer an overview of what love has meant to the inhabitants of times and places other than our own.

Wherever philosophers have put pen to paper to discuss love, they have seen it as coming from one of three sources: the human mind, the gods, or the deeply rooted nature of the species. The latter will be explored throughout this book; this chapter expounds the other two views. The first two views see love as something external to the essence of humanity, as something that is either discovered by the intellect and diffused throughout humanity by imitation or as something humanity receives, courtesy of supernatural beneficence. The position that love is a discovered idea has a certain relevance as far as romantic love is concerned, but we are not limiting ourselves to romantic love in this book. Love as a gift of the gods is not an idea that sits well with the sophisticated modern reader. Yet, that has been a way that men and women of many cultures, lacking science, have viewed it. Something so central to human life has to be explained for the curious in some fashion, and it has been only in the last century or so that science has poked around in love's nest. That love, our greatest sentiment, should be seen as a gift of the gods, our most awe-inspiring conception, attests to the importance and value that the ancients placed on love.

But let's first look at love as an invention of the human intellect.

LOVE AS A HUMAN INVENTION

When we speak of love as a human invention, we mean only romantic love. Our needs for nuturance, affiliation, and attachment have never, as far as I am aware, been considered anything but rooted in the biology of the species. Let us first, therefore, distinguish between romantic love and other forms of love.

Stripped to the barest essentials, romantic love is passion, the various other forms of love are compassion. The Greeks viewed romantic love as a combination of *erotike* (sexual passion) and *eros*, an ennobling feeling, which Euripides said could make "a poet even of a bumpkin." Here the needs and demands of the self and of the beloved are emphasized to the exclusion of all others. As I use the term here, *compassion* is a combination of the Greek terms *agape* (a selfless concern for the well-being of others) and *philia* (friendship, brotherhood and sisterhood, a warm feeling of we-ness). In compassionate love we acknowledge the needs and demands of others outside of any primary romantic love relationship we may enjoy. These forms of love can only be separated artificially, for the purpose of analysis. In actuality they are part of a coherent whole, each of the parts feeding the other, just as one hand washes the other. Passionate love and compassionate love are parts of a more general love principle that is rooted in our biology, a principle that moves us to exert physical and psychic energies to move toward unity and growth.

The philosopher Denis de Rougemont is among those who view romantic love as an invention of the Middle Ages.[1] Romantic love, he says, sprang from the soulful ballads of the troubadours sung in the drafty castles of medieval Europe. This so-called courtly love was a vulgarization of the ideals found in Plato's conception of love. It was also, in a sense, the humanization of European love, as devotion was transferred from God to men and women. Courtly love was most commonly identified as that which existed between a man and a woman who were married to other spouses; they were extramarital involvements. Its ideal, if we are to believe its chroniclers, was nonsexual. The deep idealization of and yearning for the loved one, coupled with physical restraint, was supposed to be ennobling and deeply spiritual. Physical consummation of any such love was considered to be destructive of both the characters of the participants and their relationship. This idea of love is still a preoccupation of the Japanese. Almost all of their contemporary love stories feature self-sacrificial men and women who love from afar, and with such nobility that if this love is consummated it results in death for one or both of the participants.

If romantic love has its origin in the human mind—that is, in human ideas—then love is a human invention that other humans can "disinvent." To believe this is to believe that the ecstasy of the heart and the trembling below is nothing more than a cultural invention, never to be experienced unless we are lucky enough to have heard about the remarkable intellectual "discovery" of these medieval singers. Surely the touching love stories of the Bible or the *Arabian Nights* provide ample evidence that romantic love is far older, and far more universal, than that. There was never a more sublimely romantic poem than the biblical Song of Solomon. Courtly love was a cultural re-creation, not an original creation.

There is truth of a kind in this view of love, however. Were we to ask for a single benchmark in the evolution of romantic love (as we view it in the contemporary Western world), then certainly the doctrine of courtly love is it. But it is a benchmark in the sense that Columbus's voyage was a benchmark for the diffusion of the knowledge of the roundness of the world. Men of education knew the world was round long before Columbus; Eratosthenes had even calculated its circumference with remarkable accuracy some 1,400 years earlier. Likewise, men and women ached for that one special person long before European balladeers set the ache to music.

Then why do some circles continue to insist that love is a cultural invention? The answer to this question probably lies in the profusion of field studies conducted by anthropologists in isolated, simple societies. Their members, anthropologists tell us, take their sex philosophically, with no more sentimental embellishment than is afforded the taking of food and drink. Missionaries, more concerned with the "native's" soul than his sex life, frequently remarked that a major problem in translating the Bible into native languages was that they had no equivalent for the word *love*.

This is not the place for a survey of the many exceptions to these observations. Let me rather make an appeal to authority to refute the idea that just because the anthropologist thinks he has observed casual sex or the priest has translation problems therefore love is nothing more than a cultural artifact. The anthropologist Bronislaw Malinowski has stated: "Love and marriage are closely associated in day-dreams and in fiction, in folklore and poetry, in the manners, morals and institutions of every human community."[2] In other words, Malinowski sees love as one of the cultural universals, perhaps not readily recognized sometimes but there nonetheless.

Let's look closer to home, at the native populations of North America. More is known about Native American tribes than any other aboriginal peoples in the world, for they are the natural targets for the yearly crop of new U.S. anthropologists. The American Indian recognized romantic love but considered it nothing to write poems about. Anthropologist Peter Farb tells us that the Indians liked to joke about young people's romantic enmeshments but believed that only an idiot would base something as important as marriage on love.[3] Compassion, not passion, was the emotion that kept family, band, and tribe united. Survival, both at the individual and at the group level, demanded unity, closeness, concern, altruism, and cooperation to a greater extent than is required in modern society. Indeed, among early white settlers, Indians had such a reputation for compassionate love that many whites went to live with them. The number of whites marrying Indians and going to live with them was so serious that the Virginia colony enacted laws against such a practice.[4]

When Farb says that the Indians like to joke about romantic entanglements, he has stated a generality as broad as the attribution of some other characteristic to Europeans. Just as there are a great variety of cultures in Europe, there are a great variety of peoples we call Native American. More than one of these cultures had romantic notions that we would recognize. The Cheyenne of the Great Plains are perhaps the best example. Courtship and marriage among the Cheyenne was a very romantic and protracted affair, often lasting four or five years. Cheyenne women were extremely coy, and they made their hapless swains sweat blood and tears to win their hand in marriage. The brave had to shower her with presents and words of endearment. If this proved inadequate, he might resort to serenading her on a special "love flute" or enlist the powers of the medicine man. In other words, the Cheyenne male felt and behaved in a way that the most ardent suitors of Western culture's most romantic periods would recognize.[5]

But why is romantic love not as readily recognized and valued among preliterate cultures as it is in ours? Let me approach this question via an analogy. The German poet and philosopher Schiller wrote that "hunger and love move the world." Love and hunger are drives, and drives are the physiological experiencing of a need to rectify some biologically important deprivation. Hunger is a drive to eat so that the individual may survive. Love is a drive to unite so that the species may survive. The pains of hunger remind us that we must eat, the pains of romance that we must love.

Wartime stories coming out of prisoner-of-war camps tell of human reactions to extreme hunger. Prisoners thought of little else but food; they dreamed about it, fantasized about it, and covered pinups of Betty Grable's legs with pictures of steak and eggs. Food took on an inestimable value and was gilded with an aura of almost holy desirability. When we are severely deprived of something vital to our biological survival, nature demands that we direct all our energies toward correcting the deprivation.

Have you ever rhapsodized about food like a hungry POW? Neither have I. Those of us who eat whenever we please don't expend much energy idealizing our breakfast—we take it "philosophically and without sentimental embellishment." This doesn't mean that these food-intoxicated POW's invented hunger; we too would be passionate about our steak and eggs were they not so readily at hand.

The reason that the aboriginal takes his sex as philosophically as we take our breakfast is because, generally speaking, sex is as available to him as food is to us. Among the Eskimos, for instance, a man will loan out his wife to a fellow hunter almost as nonchalantly as we loan a cup of sugar to our neighbors. Because prenuptial, nuptial, and extramarital sexual relations are relatively abundant in many preliterate cultures, passion is not dammed up to a breaking point by denial. The urge to copulate and its fulfillment follow with as little delay for the aboriginal as hunger and eating follow for us. This being so, the native sees little reason to brood over or idealize his passion.

This idealization, brooding, and longing, generated by the barriers of denial erected by custom and morality in our society, are a good part of the reason why our passion is romanticized in poetry and song. Think back to the syrupy sweet adjectives used to describe one's lover in the songs of the sexually restrictive 1950s and early 1960s, and compare them with the earthy, and often obscene, descriptions in today's songs. In the metalic cacophany that passes for music today, we are just as likely to hear casual sex, or even brutal sex, extolled as we are to hear whispers of endearment. History and anthropology provide ample evidence that permissive sexuality subverts the exquisite joys of romantic love, and also all the tenderness, friendship, and caring that accompany it, just as surely as indiscriminately stuffing one's face makes one fat, unappealing, and unappreciative of the place of food in one's life.

In case you are wondering if this is the case among our fellow romantics, the Cheyenne, the answer is yes. Their code of sexual conduct would have met even Queen Victoria's stern approval. After her first menses, each Cheyenne girl was fitted with a chastity belt, which she wore until married. Any form of sexual impropriety on the part of a man or women was severely punished by the tribe. We are told that premarital or extramarital sex were practically unknown within the Cheyenne culture.[6] If preliterate man was as constrained by sexual propriety as Westerners or the repressed Cheyenne, he too would feel a biological yearning from the depths of his being.

This does not mean that romantic attachments never occur among preliterate peoples, who do not view love as the best motivation for marriage. Even in the Trobriand Islands, where Malinowski tells us that sexual freedom is "considerable," he found many instances of romantic involvement. This was especially true if a man was attracted to a woman placed beyond his reach by social standing or taboos of kinship. He would go to great lengths to win the love of the one toward whom he felt affections, even employing special "love magic." No amount of sexual excess with other fair maidens would assuage the yearning he had for the love of this one very special woman.

Culture molds the idea of romantic love in ways that fit it into an overall cultural pattern. Sometimes it is molded in such a way that outsiders, despite their learning, fail to recognize it. However, whatever way it is molded, bent, and shaped, it no more loses its essence than water loses its inherent properties as it is molded by the various containers into which it is poured. Let me remind the reader that I am talking about passionate love and not compassionate love here. Affectionate bonds between family members and others within preliterate cultures tend to be remarkably strong. They have to be, for no culture has ever survived the loss of compassion. In chapter 7 we will see what happened to the Iks of Uganda when, because of a tragic set of circumstances, they lost compassionate love.

What about romantic love in premodern Western society? Love as a motivation for marriage is relatively new, being no more than one or two centuries old among the great majority of people. Throughout much of human history, as we scratched out a bare existence in harsh environments, marriage was for the European as it was for most American Indians, a practical and commercial transaction and little more. Marrying for love was a luxury that had to await certain cultural changes: a greater respect for the dignity of the individual, a view of women as equal to the male, and a general rise in wealth and leisure are prerequisites. We have realized these to a great extent in modern society, so we can indulge ourselves in romance. Our distant ancestors were too ill-considered and too poor to be romantic. This train of thought must await our discussion of love and society in chapter 7. Let us now turn our thoughts heavenwards to view the idea that love is a gift of the gods.

The human animal, in his or her more philosophical moments, has always somehow known of the importance of love in the scheme of things. It has been expressed in a variety of languages and modes of thought from the time that we first began to ponder ourselves and our place in the universe. The earliest writings that have come down to us on love and on our deep yearning for connectedness have been in the form of myths and legends. Myths are the stories we have used to explain our ultimate concerns: "What is the nature of the universe? Who am I? Where do I come from, and where am I going? What is the meaning of life, and how do I lead a good one?"

The answers given in myth and legends to these concerns express the collective mentality of a given age. Myths are not allegories or misleading stories; they are projections of our hunger to know. They are metaphors, not lies. Myths reflect the mentality of an age rather than just a culture, for anthropology and history show us that myths seeking to explain our most urgent concerns are remarkably similar across cultures and across historical epochs. This is hardly surprising, for ultimate concerns would not be ultimate unless they were independent of culture. Myths encompass the species experience and make it comprehensible. They organize our perceptions, tell us what is true and reasonable, collect our diverse thoughts, and package them into that coherent whole we call reality.

Science, along with a smattering of religion, accomplishes this task for us today. Although science and mythology employ different words and different methods, both are ways of organizing experience and answering questions. The answers emerging from modern science regarding the human need for love and connectedness, both in the passionate and compassionate sense, are remarkably similar to those provided by ancient mythology. Myths about love attest to the ageless importance of the topic. Whether we seek to explain it as a gift of the gods or by the methods of modern science, the fact remains that we yearn for it and seek to understand it.[7]

Many of the prototypes of the ideas that comprise the reality of our modern Western culture originated in ancient Greece. Our religious concepts of the soul, Purgatory, and Hell, our political ideals of democracy and republicanism, our ideas of education, sport, truth, beauty, justice, and much more have their origins in Greek thought. Likewise, the various types of love—love of self, sexual and romantic love (both homo- and heterosexual), God as love, love as desire for possession of the good, love as "the good" itself, love as the desire for inclusion—all have their philosophical origins in Plato's *Symposium*. If we are to understand the nature of love, said Voltaire, "meditate on Plato's *Symposium*."[8]

Although Plato's conceptions of love constitute the major Greek contribution to many of our present-day notions of love, it would be a mistake to take his ideas as representing anything more than his own interpretations. After all, it is hardly likely that a genius such as Plato simply reflected in his philosophy what was taken for granted in his time. What is a philosopher if he merely plays the role of a pollster? It was Plato's idea of ennobling love, cleansed of the procreative instinct and free from the bounds of matrimony that resurfaced as courtly love in the twelfth century. It was his idea of love as pure goodness (*agape*) that found a home in Christianity. Plato's "true" *eros*, as that which exists between man and man, has appeal for the warriors of Gay Liberation, and his love of unrestrained sexuality curries favor among hedonists of all sexual persuasions. When we speak of love we knowingly or unknowingly reveal the influence of Plato. Let us now see how Plato attempted to explain the origin, nature, and purpose of love.

In the *Symposium*, through the medium of Aristophanes, Plato recounted an ancient myth about a time when love did not exist and in which the "human" race was physically very different. Plato's protohumans were rolly-polly spherical creatures, with two appendages and organs for every one we have today. (Everyone was literally "two-faced" back then.) To make things even more complicated, there were three sexes—male, female, and hermaphodite. Despite this bounty of organs, reproduction was asexual, being joylessly accomplished by "emission onto the ground, as is the case with grasshoppers." Terrible was the pride of these creatures, for they dared to storm the heavens to challenge the power and authority of the gods. The lesser gods wanted to destroy these rotund upstarts, but the compassionate Zeus merely punished them by cutting them in half lengthwise, "like a sorb-apple which is halved for pickling."

With this primal partitioning, our human ancestors became incomplete beings, literally "split personalities," as it were. This was not a desirable state of affairs. Each incomplete person began to yearn for its alter ego. Whenever the parts encountered one another, "the two parts of man, each desiring the other half, came together and threw their arms about one another, eager to grow in union." So strong was this desire for reunion that once reunited the parts would not separate, even to take care of basic survival needs. Zeus reasoned that if he was to continue to receive the honors and sacrifices that were his due, he had to devise a way to assure the survival of humanity. He decided that it would be wise to move the reproductive organs of his creatures around to the front so that they could beget other creatures while still in one another's fond embrace. Here then is the beginning of love. It lies in the expression of the ancient need for unity, the reason being that "human nature was originally one and we were a whole, and the desire and the pursuit of the whole is called love." Otherwise interpreted, "true" love is a way of loving oneself through loving others, and we are only happy and whole(some) when we love and are loved.

We may be excused a little smug amusement upon reading Plato's version of the origin of love. But remember, it is metaphor that he is using, and let us not forget that science itself tells us that we are all descended from little, round, unicellular organisms that slithered and floated about in the primordial mud, reproducing themselves as asexually and as joylessly as Zeus's spheres. Sexual specialization occurred some countless millions of years ago with a chance mutation that separated complementary halves (cells containing nuclei) of what was a whole. This chance mutation precipitated the eternal search for our "better half." Those sexually specialized halves that obeyed the nascent urging to complement themselves by union passed on that urge to the products of that union. As Ashley Montagu, English anthropologist and perhaps science's foremost expositor of love, puts it: "I see the need—or urge, or drive—of organisms to be with one another as originating in the reproductive process itself. It is not only that every cell originates from another cell but also that every cell has for some time been a part of another cell."[9] Thus—or so the scientific speculation goes—the origin of love lies in the reproductive process that accompanies the union of complementary parts. Same story, different terminology.

The similarity between the Platonic myth and the myth of the biblical Adam and Eve is evident. The God of Genesis, you will recall, created Adam from the dust of the earth. God loved his creation, and his creation loved him. But recognizing Adam's need for a more corporeal love, for "it was not good that man should be alone," God created Eve from Adam's rib. Adam and Eve were thus complementary parts of what was once a whole. Even though our "first parents" were separate beings, their maker knew reunity to be imperative: "Therefore shall a man . . . cleave unto his wife, and they shall be one flesh."

Judeo-Christian mythology had to explain humanity's estrangement from its Creator just as Greek mythology had to. By having the first couple commit the sin of pride by eating from the tree of knowledge of good and evil and having to endure God's wrath and punishment, the estrangement was plausibly explained. Since all great gods presumably think alike, the Judeo-Christian God also found it desirable to invent sex after expelling his creations from his presence. Sex was necessary so that our first parents could "be fruitful and multiply," albeit "in sorrow"—thus assuring humankind would continue to offer God the love and homage he desired. God's sending of the Man/God, Jesus Christ, to atone for our sins provides a nice twist to the story that speaks of the mutuality of love between God and humanity. Christ's sacrifice expresses the healing power of love, and the word we use to describe his sacrifice—atonement—is etymologically derived in early modern English from "at-one-ment," the polar opposite of estrangement.

The Hindu myth of the Primal Being, or Brahman, is another indication of the universality of the desire to love and be loved. In this version of the human expression of a need for unity, we have a formless power substituting for an anthropomorphic god. For untold eons Brahman had existed without self-consciousness. Brahman's first conscious thought was that he/she/it was alone in the universe and wished that it was otherwise. This thought caused Brahman to split into two (yet another ancient rending of a whole) to become the male and female parents from whom sprang all life in the universe.

It is obvious from the creation myths of these three cultures that the fear of being alone, and the desire not to be, is at the heart of all our motivations to move toward union with others. By projecting those motivations onto some higher primal being, we affirm the truth of our feelings and are somehow admitted to a sense of oneness with all of creation. Mahatma Gandhi expressed this yearning for union and inclusion when he wrote: "Love is basically not an emotion but an ontological power, it is the essence of life itself, namely, the dynamic reunion of that which is separated."[10]

These myths of love contain many insights that are in concert with some modern scientific assumptions. A century before the birth of Christ, the Chinese philosopher Huai-nan Tzu talked about the great, empty Oneness: "All things issued from this Oneness but all became different." Modern cosmology and the theory of evolution tell of an increasing heterogeneity arising from a primeval homogeneity. We, and all the rest of creation, were formed from the hot gases of the Big Bang and the empty "Oneness" that preceded it. In a very real sense we are integral parts of the cosmic Oneness and the distant relatives of even Aristophane's lowly sorb-apple.

The intimacy and interconnectedness of all creation, even beyond human creation, is made clear in studies that follow the comings and goings of atoms in the human body. Studies using tracer elements reveal that we exchange the trillions of atoms in our bodies with other humans, jungle insects, Idaho potatoes, and even the stars, at a dizzying rate. The body contains only about 2 per cent of the atoms that were spinning in it one year ago.[11] Research physicist George Harrison tells us that we can be fairly certain that at one time or another we have coursing through our bodies some of the atoms, perhaps even some of the actual molecules, that once were part of Julius Caesar, George Washington, or Omar Khayyam![12] What ancient and unconscious wisdom was contained in the age-old myths that speak of our desire for union and inclusion, for love!

On a less esoteric level, it has been calculated by geneticists that the family trees of each and every one of us must merge into a single human genetic tree by the time we go back just 30 generations.[13] Assuming 25 years for a generation, 30 generations take us back 750 years to about the year 1241 A.D. If we trace our personal ancestry back just 30 generations by taking the 30th power of 2 (2 parents, 4 grandparents, 8 great-grandparents, and so on), we reach a number that is much larger (1,073,741,824) than the number of people who were alive in 1200 A.D.

This calculation assures us that we would encounter a common ancestor of both our parents, even if they happen to be of quite different races and nationalities, long before reaching the 30th generation. The more generations we go back, the more certain we are to find common ancestors on both sides of our parental lineage, regardless of our race, color, creed, or any other attribute by which we differentiate and set ourselves apart from other members of the human family.

This information may be as discomforting to racial purists and Mayflower aristocrats as it is comforting to humanists. Nevertheless, Guy Murchie, to whom I am indebted for the above calculations, assures us that a single sexual contact between an Asian and an African during a thousand-year period means that every African alive today is closer than 50th cousin to every Chinese.[14] Simple mathematics and a knowledge of genetics assert the unity of all humankind.

Some exciting new evidence supporting the notion of the interrelatedness of the entire human family comes from a team of geneticists at the University of California at Berkley. Led by Rebecca Cann, the Berkley team really shook up the human family tree by claiming the discovery of a female ancestor common to us all, whom they (naturally) called Eve. The Berkley team was able to do this with the aid of placental material from 147 women from Europe, Australia, Asia, and Africa. Placentas carry a kind of DNA called mitochondrial DNA, which is inherited only from the mother and is not subject to the constant cutting, sorting, and shuffling that nuclear DNA in genetic material from the male undergoes. Since mitochondrial DNA is subject to mutations with a fairly well-known rate of occurrence, it is ideal for tracing the family tree. To make a long and complicated story very short and simple, despite the racial and cultural diversity of the women who supplied placental material to the research, it was concluded that they were all part of a common family tree that originated above 200,000 years ago with Eve as the common ancestor. Another team of geneticists, led by Douglas Wallace of Emory University, came to a similar conclusion, based on blood samples of 700 people on four continents.

Unintended images are conjured up by the appropriation of the biblical name Eve. These geneticists are not saying that their primeval mom suddenly appeared on the scene in an act of divine creation, or even that she was the first woman. Thousands of generations of hominid creatures preceded her. Nor was this "mitochondrial supermum" the first female member of the species Homo sapiens. What is apparently unique about the geneticists' Eve is that she alone among her sisters had an unbroken line of daughters to pass on her mitochondrial DNA. Other females alive at the same time as Eve contributed to our lineage via nuclear DNA, but somewhere along the way the lineage of these other females was broken by the failure to produce a daughter to transmit the mitochondrial DNA.

This research has its detractors and skeptics among geneticists and anthropologists, and some flatly reject it. But if it is correct, the philosophical implications are profound. Harvard paleontologist Stephen Jay Gould, a man who has become something of a household name in science, is among those who support the theory. Gould feels that the most important philosophical implication of this work is that it admits all human beings into a "single biological brotherhood" (perhaps "sisterhood" is more appropriate), despite our often fiercely maintained external differences. I wonder if the diffusion of this knowledge might somehow persuade us all to love the larger human family without discrimination.[15]

We have seen that a deeply felt urge to be reunited with a loving creator-being appears to underlie many of the creation myths of a variety of religious traditions. In a more contemporary mode, paleontologist and Jesuit priest Teilard de Chardin sees humanity as evolving toward a mystical reunion with the universe through a growing "hyperpersonal consciousness." This hyperpersonal consciousness is viewed as a sort of collective consciousness that will in time superimpose itself above the biosphere. Teilhard calls it a "noosphere." Humanity simply must evolve its intellectual and ethical attributes further, merging them into love, which Teilhard saw as "a universal psychic energy," and it will reach "Point Omega." Point Omega is humanity's destiny—a return to the source of all and a vast outpouring of love. The Persian, Indian, Turkish, and Arabic Sufis wrote in a like vein.

Teilhard's philosophical concepts are rather fanciful (some would say bizarre) for a man schooled in science. His religion clearly guides his speculations more than his paleontology does. Nevertheless, it is ennobling in its enunciation, and it once again reminds us of our ultimate concerns and of the part love plays in them. Yet should we be such unabashed materialists as to dismiss Teilhard's speculations in toto, even if we feel we must dismiss them in their particulars? Teilhard wanted to make the human spirit the basis of an evolutionary cosmology, asking "Why not construct a physics whose starting point is spirit? . . . an evolution with a basis of spirit preserves all the laws noted by physics . . ."[16] Should we not, with modern physicists, start to think in terms of relative and multiple realities, rather than imprisoning our thoughts in the world of appearance?

In what sense can we view Teilhard's "spirit" as preserving "all the laws noted by physics"? If spirit is indeed something that is identifiable, what else can it be if not energy? What is energy? For the physicists, all is energy; the atom reduces to the electron, and the electron to lesser particles with queer-sounding names like quarks, leptons, and neutrinos. The whole menagerie dissolves into some sort of guiding energy that Henri Bergson called *elan vitale* and which Teilhard is free to call love. Think of it: we are living organisms composed of molecules that are visible only under the microscope. Those molecules are made of atoms, the atoms of electrons, protons, and neutrons, and they themselves of still smaller particles. There appears to be an almost infinite divisibility of matter. In fact, the term *matter* really has no meaning at this level, such particles being *organizations of behavioral properties* rather than specks of physical matter. Solidity and mass are properties they attain only in aggregates of trillions. To borrow J. B. S. Haldane's quaint remark, "the universe is not only queerer than we suppose, it is queerer than we can suppose."

In the final analysis, what is the stuff of the universe? Theoretical physicist Allen D. Allen, commenting on the apparent infinite divisibility of matter, states that he and his colleagues are on their way to agreeing in principle with the opening line of the Gospel of St. John: "In the beginning was the Word."[17] If Bergson chooses to call Allen's "word" *elan vitale*, or Teilhard chooses to call it a psychic love force or spirit energy, how do we compose arguments to tell them they are wrong? So, the hard-nosed physicist and the mystical theologian sometimes speak to one another in mutually intelligible terms.

THE ORIGIN OF ROMANTIC LOVE IN PLATO

The origin of romantic/sexual love is obvious in Plato's myth. The realization among human beings that they were not whole without their complementary halves gave rise to the romantic imperative, which thinkers from Aristotle to Freud have considered a way of loving oneself through loving other people. Sexual coupling is both a celebrating and cementing of the union, as well as a most delightful way of perpetuating the species. But Plato would heap scorn upon modern notions of monogamous romance. He advocated promiscuity as a means of liberation from the empirical world. Love is really the search for what is good and beautiful in oneself, and this search cannot be realized through the medium of just one other person.

In the Platonic myth, the perpetuation of the species is accomplished only by the unity of the former hermaphrodite spheres, since one of the halves had male organs and the other female organs. In the reunion of halves having identical male or female organs lies the origin of homosexual love. Although, as was common in his age, Plato was frankly homosexual, this was not, promiscuous or otherwise, the ideal form of love. "True love" was not physical at all: "Copulation lowered a man to the frenzied passions characteristic of beasts."[18] Love is desiring the Good—truth, beauty, knowledge, rationality—and, therefore, only the philosopher can "truly" love. Love is not the sparkle in the eye or the shudder in the loins; it is an idealization of the intellect. Lovers beg to differ!

But which came first, sex or love? Plato puts love first in that the yearning for one's other half came before Zeus's rearrangement of the sex organs to make reproduction possible. One might almost say that in Plato's scheme of things sex is irrelevant to love. Remember, Platonic love is the search for a previous state of self-wholeness in which sex did not exist. For Plato, then, sex is a derivative of love.

Later thinkers turned Plato's ideas upside down to make love a derivative of sex: "Love is a snare set by sex to ensure the survival of the race," exclaimed Schopenhauer. He, and many others, seem to feel that in a brute sense love is not necessary to ensure the survival of the race. But as we shall see, some modern anthropologists and demographers assert that during the early days of the history of our species, sex was not a sufficient condition to "ensure the survival of the race." It is true in modern times that the pleasures derived from sexual intercourse are quite sufficient for that task. But who would deny that sexual intercourse accompanied by deep love is far more a spiritual communion than a simple biological imperative? The oneness felt by entwined lovers is infinitely superior to the grunting urgency of the casual hump.

It is almost universally accepted among biologists today that evolutionary pressures, as well as being responsible for the original halving of the whole, also undertook Zeus's task of shifting the human genitalia to the fore as we evolved into upright, bipedal creatures. While the ancient method of rear-entry intercourse was doubtless more pleasurable than the grasshopper's emission onto the ground, the uniquely human face-to-face position adopted by upright bipedal creatures is more conducive to the stirrings of love. Face-to-face copulation allows for the simultaneous stimulation of the lips, ears, and nipples, all richly endowed with pleasure-bearing nerve endings. We will develop this theme more fully in chapter 8. Suffice it for now to recognize once again the reverberation of ancient myth in modern science.

I believe it is the spiritual superiority of the oneness felt by lovers in sexual embrace over unemotional and impersonal sex that Plato tried to convey in his myth of the primal cutting. In joining together in love, lovers recapitulate the oneness they once felt in their mothers' arms. Many psychologists agree that mother/child love is the template for later adult love. If mother love is the cradle of adult love and if adult love is necessary for (apologies to Dr. Ruth) "really good sex," then love, not sex, would appear to be primary in a very real, if not literal sense.

Although Western culture and Christian philosophy have borrowed much from Plato, the church appropriated only agapic love for its theology. It accepted, and even emphasized, the Platonic division of body and soul. However, in the church's view the body was the seat of sin. This profoundly asexual and ascetic religion consigned the body to Hell, and eros along with it. While the Greeks and many of the Oriental religions glorified eros with codes of love and sexual rites, both sacred and profane, traditional Christianity has nothing to say about eros except to demean it.

The denial and enunciation of erotic love in Christianity has at times reached ridiculous proportions. Origen, one of the early church fathers, went so far as to emasculate himself to avoid "sinful" thoughts, and many a saint of the church went to other extremes to avoid the same. Recall that in some Christian traditions passionate love is the "original sin" of man and woman. St. Augustine, after enjoying a rather lusty early life himself ("Lord, lead me out of temptation—but not just yet"), wrote about Adam's fear at viewing the "shameless novelty" of his erect penis. It did not bode well for wanton eros that the church fathers viewed the rising penis as the symbol of the Fall of man.

Apparently it did not occur to doctrinaire Christian leaders that by denying the sensuality and sentimentality of erotic love they were denying the greatest gift of their God. In a very real sense, by elevating agape as the only worthwhile form of love and denying eros they missed much of the very essence and vitality of love. By spiritualizing love they set it apart from ordinary human life, a sin that Karl Marx was to make much of. As I previously indicated, passion (eros) and compassion (agape) are two sides of a coin of the same mint. Eros is egocentric, desiring, and "caused." Agape is theocentric, altruistic, and "uncaused." Eros strives for perfection of the self, and is caused by the recognition of value in the love object and by the desire to possess it. Agape is pure selfless love, which is "uncaused" because it does not depend on the attributes of the object loved. In both forms of love the individual is wrenched out of preoccupation with the self to consider the wants and needs of the other. The individual grows and recognizes a better self than he or she ever thought possible.

Love must be sought, cultivated, and developed by people if we are to make a better world. Agape, the generous and unselfish giving of oneself, is a noble ideal, but it must be augmented by eros if it is to stand any hope of being realized. In the sacred sense, agape is the love that God pours down upon humanity, while eros is the vehicle through which humanity ascends to God. In the secular sense, agape creates value in the object loved by bestowing love upon it. In the act of creating value in the beloved we simultaneously create more joy for ourselves (eros), and in the act of creating joy for ourselves we create joy for the loved one. The merging of eros and agape is the essence of ethical goodness. Few of us ever achieve such a lofty goal, yet no nobler goal has ever been set. Love is goodness, and goodness is love; through it and by it we achieve completeness and unity with the universe outside of ourselves.

LOVE AS AN ONTOLOGICAL FORCE

I earlier quoted Gandhi as saying that above all love is an ontological force. Ontology is the study of the Nature and relations of being. An exploration of the "ontology of love" means that one is studying love as something that is a primary force akin to Teilhard's concept of it as universal psychic energy. Within the christian tradition, the love force became God, the source of all things, and God is love itself. One might say that the Christian God is the apotheosis of love, a divine projection upon which humanity can concentrate its heartfelt need to love, to be loved, and to be reassured of its participation in the cosmic wholeness. When the Christian theologian Paul Tillich, evidently surrendering his earlier position that love is not definable, defines love as "the dynamic reunion of that which is separated,"[19] he is echoing the yearning in our bones that has reverberated down through the ages. Is it merely an accident that so many diverse religions share myths with Plato that speak of a dark time in prehistory when humanity was cut off from its primal source?

Much of religion's appeal is the prospect of reunion with this source. The very term *religion* means "to bind," or "to link" (with others and with the source). It matters not whether we consider ourselves to be identical in essence with the source—as in Buddhism or Hinduism—or of a vastly different nature—as in Islam or Christianity; the urge for unity fuels the faith of billions. St. Bernard of Clairvaux recognized the yearning for unity-cum-love when he wrote that God and man can be unified, not by a fusion of natures as in the Oriental tradition, but by the "glue of love." This glue of love, the need to give it and receive it, to no longer be alone in the universe, is at the very heart of the essence of what it means to be human.

Gandhi was not the first thinker to describe love as an ontological force. Empedocles, a pre-Platonic Greek philosopher, saw the whole cosmos as being driven along its various paths by the forces of love and strife. Love was seen as a great unifying life-force functioning to bond all things, both animate and inanimate. It is important to note that Empedocles was not using metaphor. He saw love literally as being an integrative, creative energy or power. According to the Russian sociologist Pitirim Sorokin, thinkers subsequent to Empedocles came to view all kinds of natural phenomenon, such as magnetism, gravitation, and chemical affinities, as a form of love energy operating on the physical world just as altruism, passion, gregariousness, and so forth were manifestations of the love force in the psychological and social world.[20]

In those animistic ages in which all objects were invested with spirits or souls, we see many examples of natural attractions explained in terms of love and desire for union and inclusion. The Chinese called the magnetic lodestone "the stone that loves" because it attracted metal. The Indians described the rising of smoke as the smoke's desire for intercourse with beautiful clouds, and, naturally, the death of the fire was attributed to suicidal jealousy over the loss of its smoke to its nebulous competitor. Aristotle, erroneously believing that falling objects fell with increasing speed as they approached the ground, explained the increasing velocity by referring to the "jubilance" felt by the falling object at the impending reunification with the ground from which it came.

Opposing this life-force and repelling all things was strife. These opposing forces were transmuted within various cultures into Venus and Mars (Rome), Light and Darkness (Zoroaster), Eros and Thanatos (Freud), and God and Satan, who are, in Christian lore, the "embodiments" of love and strife. There is, then, a continuity of thought, at least in the Western and Near Eastern traditions, which views the unitary structure of love and strife as constituting the fundamental mechanism of existence.

All of these traditions view strife, or its various transmutations, as being necessary to give meaning to love. Empedocles, in fact, saw no possibility of love without strife. Interestingly, Konrad Lorenz, Nobel Prize-winning ethologist, who once described love as "the most wonderful product of ten million years of evolution," makes much the same point on a more mundane level. Noting that indications of love and altruism are only found in aggressive species of animals, he asserts that while aggression can exist without love, there can be no love in species lacking aggression.[21] The existence of aggression makes the evolution of love imperative if aggressive species are to live peacefully among themselves and work for common ends. Psychiatrist Smiley Blanton agrees, stating: "From the very beginning of our lives, the two primitive drives of love and aggression meet and become inextricably entangled with one another. Each of these forces is an indispensable source of energy, and human life would be impossible if either were to be eliminated."[22]

I think that we can safely dismiss love as an organizing force at the inanimate level. But a good case can be made for the existence of a biological "love energy" driving Homo sapiens along the paths of altruism, cooperation, and caring when no tangible rewards are evident. It does seem evident that as the dependency period of the young of a species becomes longer, the greater is the necessity for a form of bonding attachment to evolve. There must exist strong bonds of loving attachment between the caregiver and the dependent care-taker for the latter to survive. Love is the mother's only reward for the painful sacrifices she is called upon to make. To render tender, loving care to her infant and to perceive the faint beginnings of love returned is sufficient reward for most. There may be eons of evolutionary sense in Lord Byron's famous lines: "Man's love is of man's life a thing apart; / 'tis woman's whole existence." To the infant, the mother is the fountainhead of all satisfactions. The mother/infant bond is the template for all other bonds. In a concrete sense, the infant's mother "programs" its brain in ways that will determine how it will live the rest of its life. To this subject we now turn.

NOTES

1. Dennis de Rougemont, "Love," in *Dictionary of the History of Ideas*, ed. P. Weiner (New York: Charles Scribner's Sons, 1973), pp. 94–108.

2. Bronislaw Malinowski, *Sex, Culture, and Myth* (New York: Harcourt, Brace & World, 1962), p. 4. Also see Malinowski's *The Sexual Life of Savages* (New York: Eugenics Press, 1929) for love among the Trobriand Islanders.

3. Peter Farb, *Man's Rise to Civilization* (New York: Avon, 1969), pp. 44–45.

4. Ibid., pp. 313–315.

5. E. Hoebel, *The Cheyennes: Indians of the Great Plains* (New York: Holt, Rinehart and Winston, 1960), chapter 2.

6. Ibid., p. 95.

7. For connections between mythology and science, see E. McCormac, *Metaphor and Myth in Science and Religion* (Durham, N.C.: Duke University Press, 1976).

8. Plato, "The Symposium," in *The Republic and Other Works*, trans. B. Jowett (Garden City, N.Y.: Dolphin, 1960).

9. Ashley Montagu, "My Conception of Human Nature," in *Explorers of Humankind*, ed. T. Hanna (New York: Harper & Row, 1979), p. 92.

10. Mahatma Gandhi, *Self-Restraint versus Self-Indulgence* (Ahmedabad, 1928), p. 102.

11. George Harrison, *The Role of Science in Our Modern World* (New York: William Morrow, 1965), p. 95.

12. Ibid., p. 95.

13. Guy Murchie, *The Seven Mysteries of Life* (Boston: Houghton Mifflin, 1978), p. 346.

14. Ibid., pp. 348–349.

15. Much has been written on the "mitochondrial supermum," both in the popular press and in the scientific literature. For popular synopses, see: A Kozlov, "Woman of the Year: The Old Girl Network," *Discover* (January 1988): pp. 30–31, or J. Tierney, L. Wright, and K. Springen, "In Search of Adam and Eve," *Newsweek* (January 11, 1988): pp. 46–52. For scientific critiques, see R. Lewin, "Africa: Cradle of Modern Humans," *Science* 237(1987): pp. 1292–1295, and R. Lewin, "The Unmasking of the Mitochondrial Eve," *Science* 238 (1987): pp. 24–26. For a balanced pro-and-con argument, see J. Shreeve, "Argument over a Woman: Science Searches for the Mother of Us All." *Discover* (August 1990): pp. 52–59.

16. Teilhard de Chardin, *How I Believe* (New York: Harper & Row, 1969): pp. 31–33.

17. Allen Allen, "Does Matter Exist?" *Intellectual Digest* 4(1974): p. 60.

18. Quoted in Vern Bullough, *Sexual Variance in Society and History* (Chicago: University of Chicago Press, 1976), p. 165.

19. Quoted in Irving Singer, *The Nature of Love from Plato to Luther* (New York: Random House, 1966), p. 67.

20. Pitirim Sorokin, *The Ways and Power of Love* (Boston: Beacon Press, 1954), p. 6.

21. Konrad Lorenz, *On Aggression* (New York: Oxford University Press, 1973), p. 209.

22. Smiley Blanton, *Love or Perish* (New York: Simon and Schuster, 1956), p. 38.

Part One

Skin Love

1

The Neurophysiology of Touch and Love

The greatest gift I can conceive of having from anyone is to be seen
by them, heard by them, to be understood and touched by them.
—Virginia Satir

"God," wrote the poet Edwin Arnold, "can't be always everywhere: and,
so, invented mothers." Arnold's tribute to motherhood is a poetic expression of a scientific proposition growing in momentum and certitude among
anthropologists, endocrinologists, physiologists, psychiatrists, psychologists,
neurophysiologists, and many other kinds of scientist. More is being learned
every day about the tremendous importance of love in human development and about the vital role of mothers in awakening and developing this
most human of human qualities. Although *mothering* and *motherhood* are
considered old-fashioned words in some circles, their task of nurturing the
human potential for love and trust in a lifetime of human relationships
is as timeless as life itself. Romantic notions of motherhood aside, in the
critical task of humanizing the species, of teaching it to love, biologically
and psychologically, nature has placed women at the center of the universe.
No sexual politics are played here; anatomy may not be destiny, but modern neurophysiology is reaffirming Freud's belief of the centrality of the
mother's role in making us human.

THE PLASTIC BRAIN

In the Introduction I defined love as an inherent need to receive and bestow affection and nurturance; to be given and to give assurances of value,
respect, acceptance, and appreciation; and to feel secure in our unity with,
and belongingness in, the human family. Implicit in this definition are two
points of central importance: (1) love is not merely theologically or philosophically desirable but is also a biological and psychological necessity;
and (2) love does not reside in the object loved but is a developed quality

in the lover that is actualized by the object loved. Love is not ineffable spirit that is just "out there" awaiting discovery; it exists in a fully corporeal sense in the neural lattices of the brain in variable conditions of development depending on how the lattices were structured by early experience.

All living organisms, from the lowly amoebae to the stately primates, carry on the various functions of living driven by electrochemical processes governed by their genetic endowment. Some of these processes are fixed and relatively unchanging, others are extremely malleable. If you were an organism belonging to a species with high fecundity, going about the business of living, feeding, and reproducing in a relatively static environment, you might think it rather nice to have genes that fix it so that you will do the right thing at the right time. The evolution of your species has produced genes that "hard-wired" much of your central nervous system to produce appropriate responses to the relatively limited range of stimuli you confront.

This kind of genetic hard-wiring would be disadvantageous, even disastrous, to organisms with low fecundity inhabiting highly variable environments. The more variable the environment, the more frequently creatures living in them must adapt. This means that some sort of decision-making program would have to be incorporated into the nervous system so that the organism can evaluate stimuli before responding. The genetic endowment of such organisms must be less specialized, less rigid, and less fixed. In fact, the genes must surrender much of their control of behavioral traits to a more open, plastic, and complex system of control. As we go up the phylogenetic scale to human beings, we observe greater and greater freedom from the fixed patterns of responses that dominate organisms at the lower end of the scale. The system that allows us this freedom is the "plastic" human brain.[1]

It is this brain plasticity that makes for the almost limitless variability in human beings, of the uniqueness and irreplaceability of each and every one of us. Each of us has different experiences and learns different things, giving us all a unique set of characteristics and emotions with which to confront the world. Human beings have operated successfully in a bewildering variety of physical and cultural environments, from the simple caves of the Stone Age to the immense complexity of urban life in the nuclear age. The plastic brain allows us not only to adapt to changing conditions but also to create the very conditions to which we must adapt. Certainly, the brain has a specificity about it that determines the common characteristics of the species. It is the combination of the specificity and plasticity of the brain that simultaneously makes every person like every other person, like some other persons, and like no other person. The important thing for our present discussion is that experience, especially during infancy and early childhood, can produce long-lasting effects in the brain's chemistry and function.

Let's take a brief look at this marvelously pliable organ and the environmental influences that may radically alter its chemistry and function. Before we do, I want to make sure that we don't use the terms *environmental influences* or *experience* too loosely when speaking of their effect on the developmental process. There are different kinds of developmental processes that are influenced in different ways by experience. Neurophysiologists differentiate between *experience-expectant* and *experience-dependent* processes.[2]

Experience-expectant processes have evolved as neural preparedness to incorporate environmental information that is vital, ubiquitous, and common to all members of the species. These processes are maturational and are genetically predetermined. What this means is that nature has recognized that certain processes—speech, depth perception, sexual maturation, and so on—are vital, and has provided for neuronal mechanisms designed to take advantage of experiences that occur naturally in the organism's normal environment. These maturational processes can be retarded if the experiences do not occur at certain sensitive junctures. For instance, children totally deprived of human contact (the so-called "feral" children discovered from time to time) suffer serious impairment of their genetically programmed speech abilities, which is reflected in the atrophy of the parts of the cortex that involve speech. Similarly, animals deprived of light from the moment of birth show apparently permanent damage to the visual cortex with as little as six weeks of deprivation. It appears that not only the nature of the experiential input but also the timing of the input determines the developmental outcome of experience-expectant processes. The "sensitive" period for most of these processes is early infancy.

Experience-dependent processes are facilitative; they serve to maintain experience-expectant processes and to store information derived from the individual's specific experiences. Infants who are stimulated and exercised a lot tend to walk earlier, and infants who are spoken to a lot tend to verbalize earlier. While the process of learning to speak is an experience-expectant process, how we speak and in what language is experience-dependent. Mozart undoubtedly had genes that destined him to be a great composer, but his early exposure to music and his training expedited his precocity. Had Mozart been adopted during infancy by a family with neither the time nor inclination for music, his musical abilities might have remained dormant.

Keeping the distinction between experience-expectant and experience-dependent processes in mind, we may explore the influence of love or its absence on infant neural development. It is my belief that love is so vital to the species that its development is an experience-expectant process, but not to the same extent that, say, speech is. In a very real sense, the development of love is an experience-dependent process also.

The human infant greets the world overflowing with slumbering potentialities. The awakening, development, and actualization of these potentialities depends considerably on experience. These experiences that make us what we are and may become are perceived, processed, and acted upon via an intricate electrochemical maze of interactions among roughly 10 billion brain cells (neurons). There may be a few billion more or a few billion less—no one has yet heard from God how many there actually are. Neurons, the complex building blocks of the nervous system, are units of communication and are surrounded by the more numerous but noncommunicating glial ("glue") cells that function to insulate, support, and nourish the neurons. Projecting out from the body of the neuron are axons, which transmit information from one cell to another in the form of electrical signals of constant strength but varying frequencies, at infinitesimal junctions or gaps called synapses ("to clasp").

The information is transmitted across the neuronal synapses by chemical "handshakes" in the form of tiny squirts of chemicals called neurotransmitters. Neuroscientists have identified approximately 60 different kinds of neurotransmitters thus far, and new ones are being discovered at a steady rate. Among the most recently discovered neurotransmitters are the peptides. These peptides are as much as 10 times larger than the earlier discovered transmitters such as serotonin and norepinepherine. Peptides are proteins consisting of strings of the various amino acids (the stuff of DNA); they have immense information-carrying capacity. So great is this capacity thought to be that some scientists have honored them by considering them only one step removed from genes.[3] The most interesting of these peptides are the endorphins, so named because they are "endogenous, morphinelike substances."

These peptides are largely concentrated in the limbic system, the emotional center of the brain. At the molecular level, neurotransmitters are what make us happy or sad, enraged or quiescent, anxious or relaxed. When a normal person is under emotional stress, for instance, his endorphins act to keep him on something of an even keel by providing a perfectly legal opiate tonic, so to speak. When an infant is lovingly snuggled in its mother's arms, endorphins keep it contented. If separated from its mother, its endorphin level falls and its level of the stress hormone cortisol rises, triggering separation anxiety and distress crying. In experiments with animals, it has been found that, among a wide variety of drugs tried, only endorphins mollify a baby animal separated from its mother in the same way that actual reunion of mother and infant will.[4] Mothers are good for us. They make us happy, they ease our anxiety, they make us feel warm and secure, they keep our endorphins at pleasant levels, and make us "high" on life.

Dendrites receive the transmitted information and pass it on to the next cell for further processing. This neuron-axon-dendrite-neuron progression can be viewed simplistically (all analogies with the brain break down quickly because of the brain's awesome complexity) as a kind of communication relay-system of the brain. Each piece of communicated information is received only by the neurons for which it was intended. This fine-information differentiation is accomplished by neuroreceptors. There are thousands of receptors, each specialized for chemically receiving particular transmitters. For instance, the endorphin peptide can kill pain, cause euphoria, or sedate the individual. The varying but related effects of endorphins depend on where in the brain circuitry they are operating and on the type of receptor they bind with. Somehow the brain marvelously knows where to secrete the substance in response to the immediate needs of the organism. All this activity takes place at a dazzling pace. The number of potential connections that our brains could make are as numerous as the stars. Each one of our billions of neurons can perhaps make as many as 3,000 connections with other neurons. That's about 100 times more potential connections than are made by all the telephone systems in all the countries of the world combined!

The neurons in the infant's brain, with their attendant structures, are to a certain extent unorganized and undifferentiated at birth. To be sure, the architecture of the brain follows the genetic blueprint of the species, but like everything that develops organically, the environment influences the final form. We can view the infant brain as a kind of gigantic erector set piled willy-nilly in a barrel being painstakingly assembled during the first few months of life into a fully integrated mechanism, partly by chemically coded genetic specifications and partly by the guiding hand of the environment. The intimacy of gene/environment interaction is a central feature of brain development, governing cortical thickness, the amount of neurotransmitter chemicals, and most importantly, the brain's neuronal pathways.

Except for those connections governing reflexive behavior, the human infant brain at birth is not "ready-wired" to function independently in its environment almost immediately, as are the brains of lower animals. The human infant cannot within hours or days start to walk or swing from trees. It is true that the potential to do all the things that human beings do is contained in the infant's genes at birth but the genes are "switched on" at appropriate developmental junctures and in response to environmental experiences. Within hours or days of birth most nonhuman mammals are developmentally at the stage that it will take human infants about one year to reach.

This developmental lag, and hence protracted dependency in human infants, is the reason that love is so crucial a part of the human emotional-behavioral repertory. Mammals in general, and humans in particular, *must* be more caring creatures because they must nurture their young. They do not "lay 'em and leave 'em" like the reptiles. For instance, an oyster produces 500,000 eggs a year, a fish 8,000, and a frog 200. A species with such high fecundity can afford to "waste" the vast majority of its offspring and still survive. The human species, producing at most one offspring per female per year, must assiduously cultivate the development of each and every precious new member. If no one feeds a human infant it will starve; if no one moves it, it will stay put; if no one shelters and protects it, it will die. The human infant is at the mercy of the adults of its species far longer than any other newborn. Only a strong biologically based tendency on the part of the mother to care for the infant unconditionally will see it successfully through its period of dependency. The human adult's willingness to invest time and energy in someone else's goals, even at the expense of one's own, is called love—an active concern for the well-being of another.

Intelligence and adaptability are also crucial parts of the human repertory, requiring a cortex much larger relative to body size than is necessary for other animals. By the end of the first year of life the human infant's brain will have almost tripled its birth weight. If humans were developmentally equal to nonhuman mammals at birth, the size of the human head would be too large to pass through the birth canal. One evolutionary strategy to accommodate the increasing human cranium would have been increasing the size of the female pelvis. Evolution may have tried this tactic at one time, but had to discard it. The disadvantage of such a strategy would be that the mobility of the female would be considerably constrained. The loss of the ability to move fairly speedily across the open savanna would have proved disastrous in the presence of so many predators. The strategy that evolution finally settled upon was that human infants would be born at an earlier and earlier stage of brain development.

The evolutionary compromise reached to accommodate both the increasing brain size of the human infant and the continuing need for the speedy mobility of their mothers leads many authorities to believe that humans are born with only the first half of the gestation period completed. The first half of human gestation is called *uterogestation* (gestation in the womb), and the second half is called *exterogestation* (gestation after birth). The period of exterogestation encompasses the period between birth and the beginning of crawling—about ten months.

Although interuterine experiences can have an influence on the infant's subsequent development, the experiences it has during the ten months or so after its birth are of greater importance. The infant is safe and secure in its sac of amniotic fluid during uterogestation, and one infant's experience during this period is very much like every other infant's unless the mother is in particularly poor health, is malnourished, takes drugs, uses alcohol and tobacco to excess, or is extremely stressed. Exterogestation is a very different matter. As Ashley Montagu points out, "a continuing symbiotic relationship between mother and child in the exterogestative period is designed to endure in an unbroken continuum until the infant's brain weight has more than doubled."[5] Montagu goes on to expand on this by stating that love is the cement of this relationship:

> It is, in a very real and not in the least paradoxical sense, even more necessary to love than it is to live, for without love there can be no healthy growth or development, no real life. The neotenous principle for human beings—indeed, the evolutionary imperative—is to live as if to live and love were one.[6]

Life and love are indeed so intertwined as to be almost synonymous. Anthropologist Sydney Mellen speculates that if a sense of love, bonding, and attachment between men and women had not evolved during the Plio -Pleistocene age (about 500,000 years ago), our species would have died out. Mellen bases his speculation on the work of evolutionary demographers who estimate an infant mortality rate of between 53 and 65 per cent during that period. Our sexual appetites assure plentiful pregnancies with or without love. But without long-term attachments between men and women during which the men provide food and protection for their women and children, this already high infant-mortality rate would have risen to levels spelling extinction for the species. "This," says Mellen, "is why most of us today have strong tendencies to love as well as make love."[7] Mellen's work lends substance to the old saying that the purpose of woman is to serve the species, and the purpose of man is to serve woman. We will develop the topic of male/female attachments more fully in chapter 8.

It is most pleasant to realize that the selection for intelligence and plasticity in humans made the selection for love so necessary: we're smart because we love and love because we're smart. Both love and intelligence are necessary for humans to be the kind of beings we are. Without love, intelligence would make for the never-ending oppression of the dull by the bright. We only have to recall the twisted genius of Hitler to realize the tyranny of intelligence unleavened by love. Love without intelligence would be less a concern, but intelligence allows us to guide our love in ways that better the lot of the human family. Luckily, evolution has selected for both love and intelligence, each feeding the other in mutually beneficial ways.

The negative side to this pleasant thought is that because we are so plastic, so subject to environmental influences, our programming can go awry. What if infants do not experience Montagu's "continuing symbiotic relationship?" The human infant can be molded and cultivated into a decent and caring adult, or its development can be distorted horribly in a way that no nonhuman animal can have its nature altered by experiences that occur within its species. If animals exhibit psychotic, neurotic, or psychopathic-like behavior, it is because they have experienced the influence of human beings. Their instinct-driven behavior protects them from extreme deviations in a normal habitat. Human beings do not have strong instincts that can override their experiences and protect their development into adjusted adulthood. A good part of this book is devoted to exploring the consequences of the lack of loving relationships throughout the entire life-cycle. For now, though, we will concentrate on the "ideal" process for the development of love. As philosopher George Santayana once noted, "Everything ideal has a natural basis, and everything natural has an ideal development."

Applying Montagu's neotenous principle to the infant at the neurophysiological level, it means that the neonate's plastic, undifferentiated brain must be organized for love—quite literally, a "wiring" of the neuronal pathways. Whether she is aware of it or not, the infant's mother is the major organizer during this critical period of exterogestation. This is both her existential burden and her crowning glory. To describe motherhood as "slavery," as some radical feminists have been wont to do, is absurd and destructive, and indicative of a deep alienation from the self as nature ordained it to be.

An analogy to show what I mean by the process of neuronal wiring may prove useful here. Imagine a small circle of newly planted rose bushes. If we could peer through the surface soil and observe their roots we would see that they are sparse and widely separated. This is roughly the spatial patterning of the axons and dendrites (the "roots") within the neonate's brain. Viewing the same cluster of bushes ten months later (assuming adequate nurturing), we would discover that the roots had branched out like hundreds of tiny fingers to contact the roots of neighboring bushes. Further time would reveal an even greater mass of intertwined roots, their number and density varying positively with the quality of environmental conditions. The patterning of neuronal growth in an infant newly placed on this earth takes place like this and is similarly dependent on the quality of environmental conditions.

Unlike the roots of the rose bushes, the touchings of the neuronal "roots" are of great importance. As we have already seen, these synaptic "touchings" establish functional connections between neurons. Intelligence, for example, can be viewed neurophysiologically as a function of the density and complexity of the synaptic connections, the strength of these connections, and the speed with which they are made. Studies using EEGs verify the connection between intellectual performance and speed of neuronal activity. This density and complexity of structure and interconnective speed is governed by both our genetic inheritance and our experiences, especially early experiences of being stimulated positively and nurtured.

During the period of intensely active development, the human infant's brain makes many more neuronal connections than it will ultimately use—there is much competition going on in the brain for synaptic space. Many connections will be pruned because of disuse, others will be firmly established because of frequent use (experience-dependency). Interneuronal communication becomes habitual the more often the electrochemical synapses governing a particular response are activated. The process is rather like the establishment of a trail in the wilderness. The more often the trail is trodden, the more distinct it becomes from its surroundings, and the more functional it becomes.

In a series of brilliant experiments for which he received the prestigious Laskar Award in 1983, neurobiologist Eric Kandel demonstrated this process of synaptic habituation in his laboratory.[8] He used four-pound marine snails called Aplysia because of the exceptionally large size of their neurons and because their synapses are virtually identical with those of human beings. He subjected his snails to a variety of stimuli and was able to observe and photograph the changes at the synapse produced by the stimuli. Kandel's work unequivocally demonstrated how environmental input regulates gene expression in the brain, even in instinct-driven organisms like snails and how it modifies brain function by altering synaptic strength. Kandel's work also strengthened the notion held by many neuroscientists that emotions, such as love and hate, are related to specific areas of the brain rather than being diffused across the entire brain.

From similar research, psychophysiologist Gary Lynch has developed a neurophysiological theory of long-term memory.[9] He theorizes that an experience with strong emotional content is accompanied by especially strong neuronal stimulation. The strength of the stimulation results in the neurons involved becoming more sensitive and responsive to similar stimuli for weeks or months. If the emotional experience is repeated, the synapses become more receptive and further sensitized. Lynch calls this phenomenon long-term potentiation. His work suggests that in the process of long-term potentiaton, an enzyme (complex substances that bring about or accelerate chemical reactions) called *calpain* works on the neuronal membrane to expose additional receptors at the synapse.

More active receptors mean more information transfer and a possible reshaping of the dendritic branching and the creation of new synapses. If the information being transmitted is negative—"you're not worthwhile or lovable," "the world is a cold, harsh, and abusive place"—the developmental consequences are obvious. Later communications, even if they are positive, will tend to be relayed along the same negative track as though some mischievous switchman were stationed at a critical neurological junction ready to derail any train of pleasurable thought or feeling.[10]

As I have said, synaptic connections can also be pruned by disuse, just as a trail can disappear if no longer trodden. Well-trodden pathways laid down during the sensitive periods of infancy and childhood tend to be more resistant to pruning than pathways laid down later in life.[11] This is both good and bad, depending on whether the trail leads to love or to some pathology. To give an example of the strength of early learning in contrast with later learning, it is well known that very young children can learn two languages simultaneously with very little effort. They can continue to be comfortable with both languages throughout their lives, with neither language being contaminated by the accent of the other. Anyone who has tried to learn a foreign language in adulthood knows how difficult it is and how it is almost impossible to speak it without an accent. Children have this ability because their young brains are physiologically more receptive, and because children tend to accept information unquestioningly, lacking the mental maturity to do otherwise.

The information communicated to children during the critical early years of life regarding their self-worth and lovableness contributes strongly to their later evaluations of their own worthiness or unworthiness. One study of self-esteem showed that early parental nurturance completely overshadowed all other factors examined in explaining levels of self-esteem among college students. [12] If love is so tremendously important to us throughout the life-span, it is imperative that the brain's "love trails" be well and truly trodden during this period. Deeply etched love trails in the brain will strongly predispose the infant in later life to respond to the world with caring, compassion, and confidence.

Responses, of course, require stimuli, and stimuli for the infant originate in a very limited environment. The more stimuli experienced by the infant, the greater the number, complexity, and speed of the interneuronal connections. The less stimuli experienced, the fewer will be the functional neuronal connections and the weaker they will be. It has been repeatedly shown in animal studies that organisms raised in stimuli-enriched environments develop greater cortical density and generate greater quantities of essential neurotransmitters than organisms raised in less stimulating conditions. For instance, physiologists Rosenzweig, Bennett, and Diamond conducted a series of 16 experiments over a period of 9 years assessing neurological consequences of raising rats in stimuli-enriched and stimuli-impoverished environments.[13] In 14 of the 16 experiments they found that rats raised in stimuli-enriched environments had significantly greater cortex weight and significantly greater quantities of a number of neurotransmitters than rats raised in stimuli-impoverished environments.

The experimental evidence is not restricted to rats. One interesting study with human infants was carried out by a team of health professionals in Dallas, Texas, led by psychologist Ruth Rice.[14] Knowing that premature infants, because of relatively long periods of neonatal mother/infant separation, are at risk for physical, neurological, and social handicaps, as well as at risk for parental abuse, the team decided to see what effects a daily dose of tactile stimulation would have on such infants. Fifteen premature infants were assigned to an experimental group and fourteen premature infants were assigned to a control group. The experimental infants were given a full-body nude massage by their mothers for 15 minutes four times a day for one month. Following the massage, the infants were rocked and cuddled for an additional five minutes. The infants in the control group were just provided with the usual hospital care, the massage being the only difference in otherwise identical treatments for the two groups.

Comparing the two groups after a period of four months, Rice found that the experimental infants were significantly superior to the control infants in weight gain, mental development, and most markedly, in neurological development. (There were no differences between the groups prior to the beginning of the experiment.) Rice and her colleagues also provided evidence that the mothers and infants in the experimental group became more attached to one another than did the mothers and infants in the control group. Plentiful tactile stimuli, a behavioral manifestation of love, is thus reflected in neural structure and chemistry, as well as a more secure love bond between mother and infant.

Another important study pointing to the importance of environmental stimulation in conjunction with adequate nutrition for neural development during the critical period of brain growth was conducted by neuropsychologist R. Lewin.[15] He studied a number of very young children whom he classified into four groups on the basis of the amount of nutrition and stimuli they received. These groupings were: (1) malnourished children from stimuli-enriched environments, (2) malnourished children from stimuli-deprived environments, (3) well-nourished children from stimuli-enriched environments, and (4) well-nourished children from stimuli-deprived environments. Lewin then administered various tests of intellectual development to each child. His results clearly showed that both malnourishment and stimulation-deprivation have deleterious effects on intellectual development. Well-nourished children growing up in stimulating environments averaged 71.4 points on Lewin's tests, while well-nourished children from stimuli-deprived homes averaged 60.5. This latter group of children actually averaged less on the tests than malnourished children who were fortunate enough to live in stimuli-enriched homes, whose group average was 62.7. Predictably, the children who scored lowest on the tests, an average of only 52.9, were children suffering a combination of malnutrition and a stimuli-poor environment.

Adequate nourishment and adequate stimulation are not mutually exclusive variables in terms of brain development. Malnourishment results in lethargic and apathetic behavior in the infant, which in turn results in diminished interest in the child on the part of the caregiver, meaning that he or she will be less disposed to providing the infant with the vital stimuli it needs. The synergistic effects of malnourishment and deprivation of stimuli are aptly demonstrated in Lewin's study.

If a condition of malnourishment occurs in an adult, very little brain damage results because the body will take nourishment from other organs to satisfy the voracious appetite of the brain. For an infant, however, a protein-deficient diet has terrible consequences. Protein is essential for the myelination of the neuronal pathways. Myelin is a fatty substance that coats the axons. Myelin insulation acts like the rubber insulation around an electrical wire in that it prevents the nerve impulses from "short-circuiting" and paying attention to irrelevant stimuli. Myelin also prevents neuronal fatigue, maximizes conduction velocity, and maximizes the possible rate of neuronal firing. Nerves can function with less than adequate myelin, but their efficiency is severely retarded. In fact, multiple sclerosis is a disease characterized by progressive demyelination of the axons.

The infant's brain at birth is relatively low in myelin, the vast proportion being laid down in the first two years of life. The lethargic and apathetic behaviors characteristic of unfortunate individuals suffering from pellagra and kwashiorkor, diseases of malnutrition, are traced at the neural level to the inadequate myelination of the brain. We see manifestations of this condition when viewing the starving children of Ethiopia and the Sudan on our television screens. They stand around with eyes staring and mouths agape, as though transfixed, while flies feed on the sweat of their tiny brows and the tears in their sad little eyes. The lower IQ levels of children from poverty-stricken homes are probably attributable in large part to the inadequate, protein-deficient diets during infancy and early childhood, as well as to the lack of stimulation, which may be secondary to inadequate nutrition.

The single best method of assuring adequate infant nutrition is supplied by the wisdom of nature—breastfeeding. Breast milk is truly an elixir of life for the human infant. It confers many immunological benefits on the infant and is rich—far richer than any other kind of milk—in *cystine*, an amino acid which many researchers feel may be essential to an infant's developing brain physiology. Breastfeeding, of course, carries other benefits beyond the infant's ingestion of the most nutritious food it will ever experience. It increases the period of time which the infant and mother interact with one another and in which the infant is experiencing vital stimuli. It has been determined that lower-class mothers are least likely to breastfeed their children in the United States. Lower-class infants are thus at once deprived more than their higher-class counterparts of mother's milk and the benefits of the tactile stimulation accompanying this feeding method. There might be a causal connection here between lower-class feeding methods and the greater incidence of child abuse and neglect among the lower classes.[16]

The particular stimuli with which we are concerned are acts of tactile stimulation—affectionate touching, kissing, cuddling—tactile assurances for the infant that it is loved and secure. These manifestations of mother love are not merely mutually satisfying psychological experiences; they are neurophysiologically *critical* during the sensitive period in which the neural pathways are being laid down. The importance of tactile stimulation to infant development has been aptly put by Anna Freud, daughter of the great Sigmund Freud:

> In the beginning, being stroked, cuddled, and soothed by touch libidinizes the various parts of the child's body, helps to build up a healthy body image and body ego, increases its cathexis with narcissistic libido, and simultaneously promotes the development of object love by cementing the bond between child and mother. There is no doubt that, at this period, the surface of the skin in its role as erotogenic zone fulfills a mutliple function in the child's growth.[17]

The effect of tactile stimulation on the structure of the brain can be appreciated in the understanding that the skin is almost an extension of the brain, formed as it is from the same layer of tissue during the embryonic stage of life.[18] It has been established that the nerve fibers connecting the skin to the central nervous system are better developed than are the fibers of any other organ. The intimate connection between the skin and the brain is attested to by many neuroscientists who have found that even minimal levels of stimuli deprivation during the stage of active cell growth results in reduced neural metabolism, reduced dendritic growth, and the atrophy of neuron-nourishing glial cells.[19] It is therefore of the utmost importance that infants be exposed to plentiful stimulation, especially loving tactile stimulation, during this critical experience-dependent period. The brain doesn't get another chance.

Apart from its effect on dendritic growth, stimuli also appear to influence the rate of myelination. It has been shown experimentally that animals who are petted and loved have significantly greater amounts of the material necessary for myelin formation than animals who are not. The more the nerve fibers of the brain are used, the more rapidly they become myelinated. Breastfeeding thus provides the raw nutrients for myelination, and the natural tactile stimulation accompanying this feeding method may act as a sort of sculpting hand that takes hold of the raw material and fixes it firmly in its proper place. The "proper place" for us means the myelination of the pathways to the love centers of the brain.

From the research of neuropsychologist James Prescott, it appears that yet another brain structure, the cerebellum ("little brain"), may be involved in developing the human ability to love.[20] The cerebellum is responsible for an organism's balance and its coordination of muscular movement. At the heart of Prescott's research is the notion that the cerebellum is intimately connected with the limbic system, the brain's emotional center. This connection, says Prescott, is the reason we feel exhilaration when we engage in hard physical movement, as in running and various kinds of sports. The baby's lack of movement, massage, rocking, cuddling, being whirled around, and so forth, Prescott calls "somatosensory (body sense) deprivation." Somatosensory deprivation results in inadequate wiring of the pathways between the cerebellum and the limbic system. Inadequately developed pathways to the pleasure centers of the brain during infancy result in a later inability to fully experience love and pleasure. Prescott views this lack of early manifestations of love as a basic cause of many physical and psychological disturbances such as autism, depression, hyperactivity, substance abuse, sexual aberrations, and violence.

Predictably, Dr. Prescott avoids the use of the word *love*, although he does say that he uses, "somatosensory stimuli" as a synonym for what "psychologists call 'tender loving care.' " He can, of course, use any term he chooses to describe the deprivation resulting in the stunting of neuronal growth along the "love pathways." "Somatosensory" sounds more acceptably scientific, and it denotes observable and quantifiable behavior. *Love*, on the other hand, still has a mystical ring to it for many scientists, and it denotes an attitude not easily measured. However, the amount of somatosensory stimulation afforded the infant by its mother (and others) is a direct function of the love she or they have for it. We would not expect a mother deficient in the love of her child to expend much energy kissing, cuddling, and stroking it. Love is a motivator that exists prior to its manifestation as somatosensory stimulation. Replacing that singularly beautiful word *love* with a cold and technical one implies that love is solely a function of the dendritic branching in the cerebellum-limbic system. It is this, of course, but it is also much more.

Nevertheless, it remains plain that the infant can only experience and express love or its absence through its body. It has no psychological referents by which to interpret the multitude of emotional states it is experiencing. A lack of intimate bodily contact between mother and child has to be interpreted as abandonment, since, in a very real sense, the infant can only "think" with its skin. The infant's contact-comfort experienced during times of duress from its mother's sensitive responses tells it that everything's O.K., "She's there for me," "I'm safe," "All's right in my world."

Ashley Montagu summarizes the relationship between tactile stimulation and human development for us when he writes: "The kind of tactuality experienced during infancy and childhood not only produces the appropriate changes in the brain, but also affects the growth and development of the end-organs in the skin. The tactually deprived individual will suffer from a feedback deficiency between skin and brain that may seriously affect his development as a human being." [21]

From the work of Kandel, Lynch, Prescott, Montagu, and others, we can now be fairly certain that the kind of physical stimulation an infant receives during this sensitive period strongly predisposes the synaptic connections associated with that stimulation to be dominant. If the infant's experiences are positive and loving, the neural pathways to its pleasure centers will be well laid down. These firmly entrenched neural circuits will strongly predispose the individual, in later life, to perceive many of his or her experiences with others as positive and loving. In the terminology of psychiatrist Eric Berne's transactional analysis therapy, the individual will interact with life from an "I'm O.K., you're O.K." position. [22] The loved individual will know that he or she is "O.K." because the taproot of self-esteem or personal "OKness," as we have seen, is love.

On the other hand, if the infant's experiences were of a cold, abusive, and neglectful kind, its neural circuitry will be "wired" to its displeasure centers. Such unfortunate infants will have storehouses of personal memories—even if stored in the unconscious—that reflect their early negative experiences. They will tend to interpret subsequent experiences negatively, pessimistically, and possibly react to them with violence. They will probably confront the world from an "I'm not O.K., you're not O.K." position. Their self-esteem will have been seriously compromised, and, since so many early experiences with significant others were negative, they will most likely generalize that negativity to the outside world. They will have difficulty establishing positive peer relationships in childhood and romantic and sexual relationships in adulthood. This link, "from skin love, to kin love, to in love," is a tight one. (I am indebted to psychologist Lawrence Casler for this delightfully alliterative phrase.)[23]

The results of a remarkable long-term study sums up for us the positive start in life offered by early love relationships and the negative effects of the lack of same. Harvard psychiatrist George Vaillant followed a representative sample of 94 males over a period of 35 years from childhood to early mid-adulthood.[24] He found that those men who had enjoyed a happy childhood were happy adults and that those who had unhappy childhoods were also unhappy in adulthood. Some of the unhappy men had attained the outward trappings of the "American dream" but were failures in the only thing that seems to confer happiness beyond the moment: secure, loving interpersonal relationships. Vaillant summarizes his study by quoting Joseph Conrad: "Woe to the man who has not learned while young to hope, to love, to put his trust in life."

WHAT CAN BE DONE?

What might we be able to do as a society to improve loving relationships among our citizens, based on the evidence presented? As a society we recognize the need for food and shelter as basic, and there are poorly funded agencies charged with assuring a minimal level of these commodities for most, but not all, citizens. There are no similar institutions monitoring the nation's love needs, nor is there likely to be any time soon. The establishment of a "Ministry of Love" sounds, at best, Pollyannish and, at worst, Orwellian. On second thought, we do have ministries of war that deal in the development of hate, so perhaps it's not such an outrageous idea. (Freud once toyed with the idea of an "Academy of Love.")

But we can do more than we currently are. For instance, prenatal care and education among the poor in this country is primitive compared with what is available in other industrialized democracies. Malnutrition of the mother, and hence of the fetus, can leave the fetus vulnerable to poor brain development and many kinds of childhood ailments. The failure of the United States to provide all its citizens with free and comprehensive prenatal care is reflected in our high rates of infant and maternal deaths. The 1986 U.N. Demographic Yearbook figures show the U.S. to have the highest rates of both infant and maternal mortality among all modern democracies.[25] The rectification of such a disgrace should be among the highest priorities of our society.

A change in the practices of some hospitals also appears to be called for to make those practices compatible with accumulating evidence relating to early neurological growth. We need to do more to promote the maternal attachment (bonding) of mother and child during the immediate post-partum period, even if it means the temporary disruption of the hospital's smooth routine. We need to educate parents about the role of loving stimulation in the development of the child's personality, and we need to support this learning by making it possible for mothers to be with their infants as much as possible during the stage of active neuronal growth. Surely it would be socially advantageous (and fiscally sound) to assist the continuance of mother-child contact during the period of maximal neuronal growth by making paid maternal leave a right guaranteed to all mothers. No less than 117 other nations afford women such a guarantee, in many cases with full pay and assurances that their jobs will be waiting for them at the end of their leave, so it cannot be considered "radical" or "utopian." When the military draft was still part of American life, we gave such a guarantee to draftees while we taught them how to kill. Why not offer the same guarantees to mothers while they teach their infants to love? *American women cannot consider themselves "liberated" until they enjoy the same maternal-leave rights granted to so many of their sisters around the world.*

It is not simply desirable that the United States take this step; it is *morally* and *legally* obligated to do so. The United States is a signatory to the *United Nations Convention on the Elimination of All Forms of Discrimination Against Women.* The nations involved agreed to "introduce maternity leave with pay or comparable social benefits without loss of former employment, seniority, or social allowances."[26] The U.N. manifesto evolved out of the neurological evidence attesting to the importance of mother/child interaction during the important neo- and post-natal periods of brain development. Most of the evidence came from American research, but we alone choose to ignore it.

Where governments fail, loving and caring individuals often step in to fill the void. A recent AP news story told of a remarkable volunteer program at New York's St. Luke's-Roosevelt Medical Center.[27] This hospital caters to infants who are abandoned, neglected, or born drug-addicted or with AIDS. Lacking the staff to do much more than care for the physical needs of infants for food and hygienic conditions, the infants received almost no vital skin-to-skin stimulation. It was reported that these poor victims of the sins of their parents would simply lie sullen and listless in their cribs. It was remarked that after a while they did not even react to sound. When caring volunteers provided the human contact that was lacking, a dramatic change was noted in the behavior of the infants. The volunteers had no special skills or magic potions. They came armed only with an active concern for the well-being of the infants—in other words, a love for them. Their task was simply to pick up the infants, cuddle them, stroke them, and generally to "love them up." After a number of these "love sessions," the infants became more frisky and alive. They smiled, cooed, became reactive to all kinds of stimuli, and they began to thrive physically. Commenting on the remarkable changes noted in the infants, Virginia Crosby, director of volunteers at the hospital, said: "They began to react to the love, and you could see a real difference." A truly uplifting demonstration of the power of love.

NOTES

1. For the plastic human brain, see generally Steven Rose, *The Conscious Brain* (New York: Vintage, 1978).

2. W. Greenough, J. Black, and C. Wallace, "Experience and Brain Development," *Child Development* 58 (1987): pp. 539–59.

3. Melvin Konner, *The Tangled Wing: Biological Constraints on the Human Spirit* (New York: Holt, Rinehart and Winston, 1982), p. 256.

4. Michael Liebowitz, *The Chemistry of Love* (New York: Berkley Books, 1982), p. 107.

5. Ashley Montagu, *Growing Young* (New York: McGraw-Hill, 1981), p. 92.

6. Ibid., p. 93.

7. Sydney Mellen, *The Evolution of Love* (San Francisco: W. H. Freeman, 1981), p. 141.

8. Eric Kandel, "From Metapsychology to Molecular Biology: Explorations into the Nature of Anxiety," *American Journal of Psychiatry* 140 (1983): pp. 1277–93.

9. Lynch's work cited in Y. Baskin, "The Way We Act: More Than We Thought, Our Biochemistry Helps Determine Our Behavior," *Science* 85 (November 1985): pp. 94–101.

10. Rhawn Joseph, "The Neuropsychology of Development: Hemispheric Laterality, Limbic Language, and the Origin of Thought," *Journal of Clinical Psychology* 38 (1982): pp. 4–33.

11. For a brief review of the literature on brain development and environmental stimuli, see Anthony Walsh, "Neurophysiology, Motherhood, and the Growth of Love," *Human Mosaic* 17 (1983): pp. 512–62.

12. John Buri, Peggy Kirchner, and Jane Walsh, "Familial Correlates of Self-Esteem in Young American Adults," *The Journal of Social Psychology* 127 (1987), pp. 583–88.

13. M. Rosenzweig, E. Bennett, and M. Diamond,"Brain Changes in Response to Experience," in *The Nature and Nurture of Behavior: Developmental Psychobiology* (readings from *Scientific American*), ed. W. Greenough (San Francisco: W. H. Freeman, 1973).

14. Ruth Rice, "Neurological Development in Premature Infants following Stimulation," *Developmental Psychology* 13 (1977): pp. 69–76.

15. Roger Lewin, "Starved Brains," *Psychology Today* 9 (1975): pp. 29–33.

16. According to 1988 census data, college-educated women are most likely

to breastfeed (72 percent), and black mothers are least likely (22 percent). Guy LeFrancois, *The Lifespan* (Belmont, Calif.: Wadsworth, 1990), p. 167.

17. Anna Freud, *Normality and Pathology in Childhood* (New York: International Universities Press, 1965), p. 199.

18. Gordon Taylor, *The Natural History of the Mind* (New York: E. P. Dutton, 1979), p. 136.

19. Michael Rutter, *Maternal Deprivation Reassessed* (Middlesex, England: Penguin, 1972), p. 57.

20. James Prescott, "Body Pleasure and the Origins of Violence," *Bulletin of the Atomic Scientists* 31 (1975): pp. 10–20.

21. Ashley Montagu, *Touching: The Human Significance of the Skin* (New York: Harper & Row, 1978), p. 208.

22. Eric Berne, *Games People Play* (New York: Grove Press, 1964).

23. Lawrence Casler, "Toward a Re-evaluation of Love," in *Symposium on Love*, ed. M. Curtin (New York: Behavioral Publications, 1973).

24. George Vaillant, *Adaptation in Life* (Boston: Little, Brown, 1977), p. 284.

25. United Nations, *U.N. Demographic Yearbook* (New York: United Nations, 1986), pp. 364–70.

26. Quoted in Anthony Walsh, " 'The People Who Own the Country Ought to Govern It:' The Supreme Court, Hegemony, and Its Consequences," *Law and Inequality* 5 (1988): p. 445.

27. AP News Service, "Wanted: Someone to Love Babies, If Only for an Hour," *Idaho Press-Tribune*, Caldwell, Idaho (September 18, 1988): p. D1.

2

The Chemistry of Mother Love

Love is the increase of self by means of others.—Spinoza

IS THERE A MATERNAL INSTINCT?

Friedrich Wilhelm Nietzsche, a brilliant but quite mad German philosopher, once said that a woman is a riddle whose solution is a child. Such a statement is guaranteed to raise the ire of modern feminists, the more radical of whom consider motherhood to be a crafty method devised by males to keep women in servitude. For Nietzsche, motherhood is a biological imperative; for the radical feminist, it is a male-imposed impediment. Both positions are silly extremes knocking heads with one another. Motherhood is without doubt the fulfillment of natural purposes and functions, as Nietzsche asserted. Just as surely, we are happy and fulfilled, almost by definition, when we conform to natural purposes. But is maternity an imperative? Will nature bear with a woman who finds some other purpose to absorb her energy and fulfill her life? Although the happiest women I know are engaged in meaningful work as well as being mothers, therefore refuting both extremes, it is not necessary for a woman to reproduce to be happy. If you disagree with my position, you are among the many who believe in the existence of a maternal instinct.

An instinct is a response to environmental stimuli; it is genetically determined and unalterable. It is a somatic "itch" that simply has to be scratched—an unconscious tension that has to be removed by some species-specific behavior. There is no reasoning process mediating between stimuli and response where instinctual behavior is concerned, and instinct-driven behavior will occur even in the face of inevitable death. From this brief definition of instinct, it is clear that a maternal instinct, as such, cannot exist in human beings. Women do not experience some overwhelming, unalterable, and unreasoned tension which is only relieved by reproducing and pouring love and attention on their offspring. I am not aware of any scientist, however biologically oriented, who believes that women do have a maternal instinct in this "must do" sense. But this does not mean to say that maternalism is solely culturally determined behavior shorn of biological underpinnings, as the claim is often made.

The wholesale rejection of biological underpinnings to maternal behavior by many behavioral scientists today is, in part, an overreaction to an uncritical acceptance of the role of instinct in human behavior by earlier behavioral scientists. This early acceptance stemmed from an unfortunate translation of the writings of Sigmund Freud, who had a tremendous influence on our thinking about all aspects of human behavior. In his writings about the engines of human behavior, Freud used the German term *Trieb*, a word that can be translated into English as either *instinct* or *drive*. While this distinction is of little importance in German, it has great importance in English. With the translation being rendered as *instinct*, early behavioral scientists began to posit instincts for everything from religious worship to biting one's nails. The concept became a catchall term used by lazy thinkers to avoid further exploration. It is no wonder that the more sophisticated dropped the term altogether. Unfortunately, when they dropped the concept of instinct, they dropped any kind of biological explanation whatsoever.

To deny a maternal instinct is not the same as denying an underlying biological sensitivity toward maternal behavior in women. If women are biologically primed for motherhood, calling motherhood an instinct appears to me to be less a scientific sin than to deny biological sensitivity altogether. The use of the term *maternal instinct* is a mistake in the use of language, analogous to the use of the term *need* to describe a want. A need is something that one must have, based on the survival requirements of the species; a want is a culturally generated desire (achievement, success, power, etc.). A want is not a need, but we want just the same. A biologically based maternal sensitivity or tendency is not an instinct, but the tendency is there nonetheless.

The idea of maternal tendency, while appearing to be a given in the minds of lay people, has been assiduously denied by psychologists and sociologists for the past 50 years or so. Sociologists in particular are notorious for denying innate individual differences. For most sociologists, the only factor responsible for the variations we observe among people is variation in the environment. The strong expression of the sociological position is that genetically normal people are all born with roughly equal potential. What a given individual becomes (the phenotype) is solely the product of variable environmental forces operating on a constant genotype. The weak expression of the sociological position admits to variation in genotypes, but it downplays the role of genetic variation in producing the finished human being and his or her behavior.

The strong sociological position has led to the writing of a lot of unsupportable theorizing regarding gender roles, especially as they apply to motherhood. For sociologists holding the strong sociological position, men and women differ only in terms of the obvious physical characteristics. To them the motherhood role is simply that—a socially learned role devoid of biological input other than in the obvious reproductive sense governed by physical make-up. Randall Collins, a much respected sociologist, offers a typical sociological explanation for why women are the ones who do the mothering. (To be fair, this is based more on what other sociologists have written than on his own ideas or opinions.) He says:

> The reason that women do the mothering, then, is because the maternal personality is simply a typical female personality. A woman's personality needs are to be close to other people and submerge herself in the group. She surrounds herself with her husband and children because she herself remains underseparated from her own mother. Because she never broke her unconscious erotic ties with her mother, she continues to need this kind of close and nurturant relation with others. Women become mothers because their experience with their own mother has given them the kind of personality that needs to mother. Mothering thus reproduces itself in a chain across the generations.[1]

Notice that Collins does say that the maternal personality is "a typical female one," and that females need to be "close to other people." He doesn't beg the question of how such personalities were formed in the first place but explains these observations in terms of some residual "unconscious erotic ties with her mother." Nary a thought is given to eons of evolutionary selection for this kind of behavior. Biology is immaterial and is ignored in favor of untestable psychoanalytical speculation. Certainly, women have to learn the specifics of the mother role, but this learning is superimposed on a strong biological foundation. Women also have to learn to love, but their biology makes this learning easier for women than for men. To deny that these attributes have a biological basis because we observe poor and unloving mothers is analogous to denying that sexual impulses have a biological basis because Catholic priests and nuns apparently live asexual lives. Motherhood is no more an arbitrary social behavior than is sexual intercourse. Exceptions to the rule in the form of uncaring, cruel, abusive, and even murderous mothers simply point out the wide range of human potential and the relative freedom from genetic determinism enjoyed by humans.

The strong sociological position may be in decline. Alice Rossi, a sociologist and a feminist, and also a scientist in the deepest sense of the word, is among those who realize the importance of biology in motherliness and nurturing behavior. In her 1983 Presidential Address to the American Sociological Association, she berated her sociological colleagues for refusal to integrate knowledge from the biological sciences into their theories of gender and parenthood. She reminded them that differences between males and females have emerged from countless ages of mammalian and primate evolution, and were not simply matters of socialization, male chauvinism, or "modes of production." Gender differences, she says, have arisen because of the fundamentally different roles males and females play in reproducing the species. Before we are anything, we are primates with genes, glands, and hormones that have been finely tuned by evolutionary pressures to carry out the sex-differentiated task of reproducing ourselves. Viewing motherhood as nothing more than a set of socially defined roles diverts attention from the importance of biological factors. She goes on to say that theories that neglect the fundamental differences between the sexes "carry a high risk of eventual irrelevance against the mounting evidence of sexual dimorphism from the biological and neurosciences."[2]

Some may accuse Rossi of dirtying her own doorstep, but sometimes additional dirt provides the impetus for a thorough housecleaning. There is absolutely nothing remiss in examining the effects of socialization experiences, roles, groups, and other sociological variables in the exploration of gender and motherhood. But what Rossi sharply points out is that social scientists must integrate the hard data of the more basic sciences into their theories if they are to be viable; they cannot ignore or contradict such data. The integration of basic biological data can only sharpen theories involving social behavior. The environment has profoundly important effects on our behavior, and so does our biology. Our environment *and* our biology are locked tightly together, each influencing the other, the whole making us the kind of beings we are.

MOTHER LOVE AND FATHER LOVE

It should be clear from the preceding discussion that not everyone who has written on the importance of early love experiences attaches the same importance to the role of mothers as I do. For instance, anthropologist Ronald Rohner, while asserting that love is of the utmost importance for the infant, feels that some of us have an unwarranted, even "fictionalized" view of motherhood. For Rohner, "Mother can be anybody."[3] This is, of course, a statement of possibility—anybody can be mother. The important point is how *probable* is it that just anybody can or will encapsulate the infant's total social and emotional life the way mothers do? Anyone can minister to the physical wants of the infant for food, clothing, and shelter, but that is not enough. A mother is "primed" by her physiology to perform all those tasks that go beyond considerations of brute survival in ways that mother substitutes are not.

What about fathers as alternative caregivers? In a book based on a work session of the Neurosciences Research Program, researchers Robert Goy and Bruce McEwan concluded that the literature does not support the view that fathers can function just as easily as mothers as primary caregivers. They go on to inform us that no known society replaces the mother as the primary caregiver and that while the research findings seem to indicate that female attachment to an infant is probably innate, male attachment is probably socially learned.[4]

However, let us not slight the role of fathers in the parenting of their offspring. Father love is of great importance, but it is different from mother love. The best mother love is rather like the theologian's agape—selfless, sacrificial, and complete. A mother loves her child indiscriminately just because it is her child, just like God is said to love us all simply because we exist. A typical mother's love for her child is all but unconditional and independent of the attributes of the beloved. Her love survives the morning sickness, the distended belly, the swollen breasts, and the pains of childbirth. Sleepless nights, interminable crying, and soiled diapers are usually forgotten as she basks in the warmth of the smell and the smile of her creation. By all the laws of operant psychology, the ratio of tangible rewards to punishments attending the period from conception to the child's first "Momma," she should loathe the "selfish monster." But she does not, for this issue of her womb is both an extension and affirmation of herself. This is a love relationship that generally cannot be broken, and it needs no nuptial oaths or legal commitments to keep it together until death's parting.

If we liken mother love to unconditional agape, we can liken father love to conditional eros. Father love is love earned, it is conditional on the desirable qualities of the beloved: "I love you because you are sweet, you are brave, you do the right things, and because you are like me." Many students of parenthood have commented upon the different styles of parental love exhibited by mothers and fathers. This should not offend fathers. There is a strong component of agape love in fathers, just as there is a strong component of eros love in mothers. These love types are "pure types" that are more characteristic of one sex than of the other. These two styles of loving are not superior and inferior but simply different and complementary.

We observe this difference between fathers and mothers across many mammalian species. Among nonhuman primates fatherhood is unknown, in the sense of a set of role behaviors analogous to motherhood, an observation that supports those who believe that the fatherhood role is a uniquely human cultural invention. Even among the highest nonhuman primates, an adult male's protective function is little more than a generalized responsibility for all the young in the troop with no special emphasis observed for the protection of his own offspring. Human fathers, of course, have a deeper bond with their offspring, derived from the intellectual knowledge of their paternity. This human paternal bond, like the maternal bond, depends on the prior establishment of affectional ties to others of the species during the father's own infancy and childhood. We can roughly quantify the difference in male and female attachment to their children, for it remains a sad fact that about 20 times more fathers than mothers desert their children before the children have fully grown. Almost all of these deserting fathers have histories showing a lack of affection in their own childhood.

An evolutionary explanation is offered for differences in male and female parental behavior by anthropologist Sydney Mellen.[5] Mother love had to be selected very early in the history of the species because of the long dependency period of the human infant. Father love has a shorter and different evolutionary history. Mellen speculates that the beginnings of male parental affection as we know it today probably occurred about 500,000 years ago. It would have been counterproductive, he says, if fatherly love had been as strong and as immediately compelling as that of the mother. Had father love been identical to mother love, fathers might have been led to neglect their hunting roles, thereby providing their dependents with less food. So even the feeble immediacy of the male's love for his offspring confers survival benefits for the offspring. Lacking the tireless solicitude for the child that mothers show, fathers were freed to concentrate on feeding and protecting the family—a different kind of love to be sure but just as vital in its own way.

In more recent times, studies of the transition to parenthood have shown that new fathers tend to distance themselves from the parental role during the infancy stage but take increasing interest as the child becomes older. New fathers see the infant rather like a "thing" rather than a new person who needs interaction. Only when the child becomes more autonomous and is able to react meaningfully, in the sense that the father understands the reaction, does the father take pleasure in his parental role. In other words, the child begins to "earn" the father's interest and love by displaying various skills and attributes of which the father approves.[6]

Fathers do not generally improve their infant nurturing skills with second and subsequent children, as one might expect. The same pattern of behaviors—that is, distancing themselves from infants but becoming more and more involved as the children get older, is observed in second-time fathers. This is not just an American phenomenon, for it is observed cross-culturally.[7] The male pattern of relating to infants is even seen among non-human primates. Females in monkey colonies insist on proximity to the newborn infants of even other females, while males exhibit little or no interest.[8]

Psychologists have studied the phenomenon of male and female differences in interest in babies by analyzing pupilary responses. In one such study males and females were shown pictures of babies while researchers measured pupilary response. Females, regardless of age, marital status, or whether or not they had given birth, showed pupilary dilation, an unambiguous physiological indicator of emotional arousal and interest. When the same pictures were shown to males, their pupilary response was one of constriction, indicating a lack of any kind of interest. The exception was married men who had children. The lesson of studies such as these is that while women seem to be genetically prepared for maternal reactions, men have to learn to be interested in children and appear to do so only after having had their own.[9]

While fathers tend to distance themselves from the parenting role during the child's infancy, mothers embrace and submerge themselves in the mother role. Demonstrated competence on the part of the infant also obviously pleases the mother, but unlike the father she takes intense pleasure at the pure being and presence of the infant. She values interaction with the child that consists simply of holding, stroking, rocking, kissing, and cuddling, the very behaviors that infants need for optimal brain development. She takes consistent pleasure in the simple smile and gurgling responses of her infant that many fathers soon become bored with. She relates to the infant with a high degree of physical and emotional intimacy because it is in her nature to do so. Nature is wise indeed in its selection for those behaviors that contribute to our survival.

We should not make judgments as to the superiority of one type of love over the other. Both types of love are necessary and desirable for the optimal social and psychological growth of the child. Mother love is that which makes the child *capable* of love; father love takes that capability and cultivates it through the inculcation of the ideals of humanity and makes the child *worthy* of love. If you think of it for a moment, a socialization that included only unconditional and uncritical love would breed some pretty sad human beings. Individuals assured of love no matter what their behavior forgive themselves for anything. A mother that loves, cherishes, and excuses her offspring right up to the electric chair may have helped to put him there. "My offspring, right or wrong" can be as dangerous as the patriot who has the same sentiments about his country. This is the unhealthy side of agape, and it is not overly exaggerated.

This is why it might be better, in the final analysis, to talk about "parental" love rather than "mother" or "father" love. In a stable family the two types of love tend to converge as the loving styles of mother and father influence one another. In two-parent families the incidence of child abuse tends to be much less than in single-parent familes. Some studies have found a rate of maternal abuse almost twice as high among single-parent families than among two-parent families.[10] Women need to have time free from their maternal duties to pursue other interests if they are to have the energy to love and enjoy their children as nature intended. The presence of a male in the household who can assume some of these duties can facilitate the mother's pursuit of interests outside the home. A series of studies reviewed by Jessie Bernard showed that it is the mother who freely chooses motherhood and who enjoys other avenues of self-affirmation who is more the mother "God invented."[11]

Nevertheless, mother love at the stage of infancy is more important than father love. Eons of evolutionary time have made women the more naturally loving of the two sexes. A mountain of psychological studies attest that women tend to be more caring, sacrificial, and giving than men. The logic of evolution demands this. The nurturing behavior of women is a naturally selected pattern of behavior necessary for the survival of the species. The long period of dependency of human infants renders it imperative that another human being will be motivated to administer to another's— the infant's—needs unconditionally. Any motivational system that confers survival benefits is favored by pressures for selection. Nothing could be more important to the human infant's chances of surviving to pass on its genes than the evolutionary selection of mother love. Man's only *necessary* biological contribution to the survival of the species is limited to a few pelvic thrusts, after which he can be on his way. Thankfully, the evolution of a love bond between man and woman added a sense of responsibility to the pleasures of the flesh.

CHEMICAL MOTHERHOOD

A mother's endocrinal system is geared for her loving task. During the various stages of pregnancy she experiences profound hormonal changes that prepare her for the bonds of affection between her and her child. An expectant mother experiences a slow rise in the levels of progesterone and estradiol over the period of her pregnancy, a rapid fall in the levels of both just prior to delivery of the child, and a rise in prolactin after delivery.

Progesterone and estradiol are the female sex hormones (from the Greek, "to arouse"). What is being aroused by these hormones during pregnancy is an intensification of a woman's natural femaleness. She is becoming chemically more feminine and nurturing. These female hormones have other functions, such as enhancing or damping sexual receptiveness, which need not concern us here. The rapid decrease in progesterone and estradiol after childbirth is accompanied by increased prolactin and oxytocin, which are themselves stimulated to production by the nursing infant's suckling at its mother's breast.

There is an extensive literature attesting to the profound importance of these chemical changes in producing nurturing behavior. Across a wide variety of mammalian species, it has been shown that a course of hormonal treatment duplicating the conditions of pregnancy induces virgin animals to respond maternally to neonates as if they were their own.[12] These findings emphasize the independent influence of maternal chemical changes and processes. Of course, women are also culturally "primed" for nurturances and motherhood, but culture appears only to be reinforcing the natural order of things. There are also cultural expectations attending fatherhood, but men undergo no hormonal changes preparing them for that role. High levels of the male sex hormone testosterone have, in fact, been shown to inhibit nurturing behavior in both males and females.[13]

Progesterone/estradiol and testosterone, the hormones that intensify the female and male attributes, are present in both sexes, but in different balances. Males do have more testosterone, but apparently it takes less of it to produce an effect in females than in males. For instance, women who undergo androgen treatments report dramatic increases in sexual desire, but the same treatment for men has no effect unless their androgen level was seriously below the norm prior to treatment.[14] Similarly, depletion of androgen has more of an effect on female sexuality than on male sexuality.

The sex hormones appear to interact differentially with male and female brains in areas sensitized to be receptive to them. Both act on the limbic system, the brain's emotional center, *in areas known to be structurally different* in males and females. Estradiol promotes maternal behavior by lowering the threshold for the firing nerve fibers in the media preoptic area. This area has been shown to be essential to maternal behavior in a variety of animal studies.[15] Testosterone, on the other hand, lowers the firing threshold of the amygdala, the area of the brain most involved with violence and aggression.[16]

Given these important differences in the male and female sex hormones and how they react with different areas of the brain, it should not surprise you to learn that males constitute about 85 per cent of all felony arrests for violent offenses in the United States. The gender differential for violent offenses is even more pronounced in most other countries. Criminologists Simon and Sharma's crosscultural study of gender differences in arrest rates for all crimes showed that the percentage of total arrests accounted for by females ranged from a low of 2.02 in Brunei to 20.9 in the West Indies.[17] Such large differences between cultures means that clearly we cannot ignore cultural variables when trying to account for male/female differentials in violence. Biological processes unfold and are influenced in a cultural context just as surely as culture unfolds and is influenced by human biology. But even more striking is the consistency of the male/female arrest ratio *across cultures* that range from highly urban and industrialized nations to rural third-world countries. Men are by their nature simply more disposed to crime, especially violent crime, the very antithesis of love, than are women. Stated more positively, women are by their biological (hormonal) nature simply more disposed to be supportive, nurturant, and loving than are men.

When women commit violent crimes, it appears that they are much more likely to do so during periods when the ratio of estradiol to testosterone circulating in the body is skewed in favor of testosterone. It has been estimated that approximately 62 per cent of the violent crimes committed by women are committed in what is called the paramenstruum period. This period begins about three days prior to the onset of menstruation and lasts about four days into menstruation. If the monthly cycle had no affect on the commission of crime among women, we would expect to find their crimes evenly distributed throughout the cycle. That is, 25 per cent of violent crimes would be committed during each seven-day period rather than being highly concentrated in the paramenstruum period.[18]

Many females whose violent outbursts appear to be concentrated during this period have been diagnosed as suffering from premenstrual syndrome (PMS), a disorder related to cyclical hormonal imbalances. In the paramenstruum period, estradiol falls to 50 per cent of baseline (midcycle) measures, while testosterone remains relatively high at 82 per cent of baseline. During this period, then, a woman's ratio of male to female hormones is closer to that of a man's, and remember, it takes *lower levels* of the hormone for it to affect women than it does to affect men. It appears, further, that PMS sufferers experience a more drastic change in sex hormone ratios than women who do not suffer from PMS. But PMS is not simply a matter of hormonal imbalance, since some women get complete relief from symptoms by taking medication and others do not. According to one theory, persistent sufferers of PMS are abnormally sensitive to the brain's opiates (the endorphins). These comforting opiates also decline just before menstruation, leading researchers to speculate the PMS victims may actually be suffering drug-withdrawal pains and all the tension, anxiety, and irritability that go with them.[19]

PMS affects about 20 per cent of the female population, but the symptoms can range from a mild irritability to raging violence. Thankfully, only a small fraction of those women affected by PMS ever experience extreme symptoms. Thousands of PMS women suffer these monthly discomforts without becoming the least bit violent. It may be that a social/psychological predisposition coupled with extreme physical symptomology (such as opiate sensitivity) and the use of alcohol, which exacerbates the symptoms, are required to produce extreme behavioral outcomes.

Given our present knowledge of the behavioral correlates of sex hormones, it is tempting to view them as biochemical analogues to Empedocles's love and strife. There is an antagonism between the androgens and estrogens, in that the biological effects of one can be inhibited or neutralized by the other. Some biochemists would exercise more caution in making such an analogy, because the androgens and estrogens actually represent different stages of biosynthesis in the gonads and adrenals. But then, Empedocles also viewed love and strife as different manifestations of an irreducible whole. He might be right. It has been reported that women taking progesterone-dominant contraceptive pills report strong feelings of nurturance and affiliation but feel irritable and hostile when they stop taking them.[20]

It must be pointed out that hormonal explanations of behavior are not as simple as one might suppose. There is certainly no one-to-one "push-pull-click-click" relationship between hormonal levels and behavior. Further compounding any definitive statements about a causal relationship is the fact that hormones are secreted in episodic bursts, so it is often difficult to perform accurate hormonal assays. Many different samples have to be taken at various times of the day and month for valid assessments. Unfortunately, this is not typically done.

I don't want to leave this section without once again emphasizing that anatomy is not irreconcilably destiny. Men can, and should be, more nurturing. It is not that nurturing is unlikely in males, only that it is less readily evoked in males than in females. John Money, a professor of pediatrics and a prominent researcher in the area of sexual dimorphism, points out that even in rats, a species far more under the control of hormone-induced, sex-dimorphic behavior than humans, nurturing behavior will eventually be released in males with repeated exposure to a litter of helpless pups. He goes on to add that by way of contrast such behavior is released almost instantaneously in females.[21]

IS THERE A "CRITICAL PERIOD" FOR
MOTHER/INFANT BONDING?

Some scientists have hypothesized a "critical period" during which the mother/infant bond is cemented. Rather than using the term *critical*, other scientists prefer the term *sensitive* or *facilitative*. These latter terms imply that there is a phase of infant development during which a bonding process may be more readily accomplished than at some other phase.[22] The stronger term *critical*, on the other hand, implies a discrete period of development when the bond *must* occur. Nevertheless, considering the profound physiological changes preparing a woman for motherhood, coupled with the cultural expectations surrounding the role. It is not unreasonable to suppose that mothers experience maximum sensitivity to their infants, and infants to their mothers, during the immediate postpartum period. This intriguing "critical-period hypothesis" states that there is an optimum time for organisms to experience certain things that are important to them, such as a bird's first flight. In a state of nature these things almost invariably occur when they are biologically "supposed to."

The arguments for a critical or sensitive period in human development rely on three consistent findings in the literature: (1) the roots of many disorders can be traced to early childhood; (2) disorders that do have their roots in early childhood are notoriously resistant to therapeutic intervention; and (3) the correlation of measures of such attributes as IQ and personality taken at childhood and then again during adulthood are much stronger in the first half of childhood than in the second half.[23] These findings mesh well with what we also know about the brain's sensitivity to environmental input during infancy and early childhood.

One of the earliest studies in the area of postpartum bonding was conducted by Nobel Prize-winning ethologist Konrad Lorenz. Lorenz observed that geese will follow the first moving object they see within the first 16 to 24 hours after hatching. Except when human hands intervene to change the normal course of things, the moving object will be the gosling's mother. When this occurs the gosling is said to have been "imprinted," and a strong bond exists thereafter between the gosling and its mother. Imprinting is thought to be some sort of genetically controlled, chemical releaser mechanism that is triggered by an environmental stimulus, in this case, movement.[24]

Lorenz experimented with his geese by presenting them with objects, such as a rolling basketball or himself, during this critical period. The poor goslings thereafter dutifully followed the rolling basketball or Lorenz and could not easily be trained to stay with their real mothers. This experiment played havoc with the biological directives of these unfortunate birds. When they became sexually mature, the objects of their amorous efforts turned out to be the objects on which they imprinted. Films depicting their attempts to copulate with the embarrassed Lorenz or a basketball produce great hilarity in the usually sober business of scientific investigation.

We do not know for certain if any such critical period exists for human infants. If there is, it certainly is not as time-restrictive (hours or days) as it is among lower species, nor are the consequences anywhere near as dramatic. Nevertheless, almost all textbooks on child development cite one study or another in which it was determined that about one hour of nude contact between mother and infant immediately after delivery, plus extra contact beyond hospital norms, has a markedly positive influence on the degree of maternal attachment. Additionally, this skin contact supplies the tactile stimulation seemingly so neurophysiologically important for the infant. Such nude contact immediately after birth, we should remind ourselves, has been the experience of human infants for the vast proportion of human evolutionary history. It has only been the advent of modern hospital technology and procedures that has significantly altered this ancient birthing experience.

BREASTFEEDING

Ashley Montagu lends his considerable scientific stature to the proposition that there is indeed a mother/infant bonding process and he views breastfeeding as a vital component of it. He writes in his book *Touching: The Human Significance of the Skin*:

> Physiologically, the nursing of her babe at her breast produces in the mother an intensification of her motherliness, the pleasurable care of her child. Psychologically, this intensification serves further to consolidate the symbiotic bond between herself and her child. In this bonding between mother and child, the first few minutes after birth are crucial.[25]

What is it about breastfeeding that appears to intensify motherliness? The sheer sensual pleasure experienced by the breastfeeding mother—the panoply of sight, sound, smell, touch, and the tangible evidence in her arms that affirms her womanhood—may be sufficient explanation. Chemical changes going on in the breastfeeding mothers may also play an important role. A series of studies by zoologist Peter Klopfer has led him to believe that the hormone oxytocin plays an important part in initiating maternal care in animals.[26] In human mothers, oxytocin, involved in the onset of labor and in the birth process, is secreted in response to the crying of their infants. The secretion of oxytocin prepares a mother for nursing by contracting her uterus and erecting her nipples. Further oxytocin is released in the mother's system in great quantities by the suckling of her infant. Even artificially stimulating the release of oxytocin has been shown to induce maternal behavior in goats, so it is a most important maternal hormone. Psychophysiologist Niles Nelson is so impressed by various studies involving oxytocin and maternalism that he is prompted to honor it by calling it "the hormone of love."[27] Bottlefeeding mothers, lacking the suckling action of their infants, do not stimulate the release of oxytocin so readily.

All this does not mean that bottlefeeding mothers cannot be excellent mothers or that breastfeeding mothers are necessarily superior mothers. Nevertheless, the feeding of the newborn infant at the mother's breast is a phylogenetic trait of all mammals. Phylogenetic traits are traits that somehow contribute to the inclusive fitness of the species. Humans are no exception to this rule. We delude ourselves if we think that we improve on nature by propping up a bottle as a substitute for the breast. And its encouragement in third-world countries borders on the criminal. Breast milk is the most nutritious food a human being will ever ingest. In addition to its well-known immunological qualities, human milk is rich in cystine, an amino acid that some biochemists think may be essential to an infant's developing brain physiology. Cow's milk or formula milks are not rich in cystine, nor do these substitutes confer the immunological benefits of breast milk.

The same hormones that are hypothesized to enhance motherliness also benefit the mother physically. The oxytocin released by suckling contracts the uterus. These contractions have the effect of quickly arresting uterine bleeding and the detachment of the placenta. Summarizing the benefits of breastfeeding for the mother in another of Montagu's many works on love, he writes: "By suckling at the mother's breast the baby confers survival benefits upon her in a creatively enlarging manner—the definition of love."[28] Recent neurological and endocrinological evidence points strongly to the connectedness and embeddedness in each other of mother and infant that fully supports Montagu's belief. It appears that closeness and attachment serve the function of maintaining and regulating biological homeostasis (chemical and physiological balance) in both. Upset this balance by separation, and physiological and behavioral pathologies will appear.[29]

The benefits accruing to breastfed children in later life have been known for a long time. One of the earliest comparative studies was done by Hoefer and Hardy in 1929. Their study showed that breastfed children were superior to bottlefed children in all mental and physical tests. Furthermore, the longer the child was breastfed the more superior he or she tended to be.[30] More recently, a 1979 article in *Science Digest,* appropriately entitled "Human Milk Aids Health, Fosters Love," cites a study involving 1,000 infants whose histories were monitored for a number of years. This study found that infants who were breastfed were dramatically less likely to be victims of child abuse, accidents, and retarded growth than were children who were bottle-fed. The same article quotes Dr. John Kenell of Case Western, who somewhat extravagantly speculated that many of the social problems of our time may have something to do with the decline in breastfeeding.[31]

Love is more than a warm feeling; it is also a *heightened sensitivity* to its love object. Breastfeeding may release certain chemicals, such as oxytocin, for instance, that may account for this sensitivity. It has been reliably shown that lactation in nonhuman mammals is associated with a reduced sensitivity to environmental stressors, thus allowing for greater sensitivity to the infant. There is less evidence available for human mothers, but a recent study by Alan Weisenfeld and his associates lent general support to these findings. In comparing breastfeeding and bottlefeeding mothers they found differential physiological responsivity between lactating and non-lactating mothers. Skin conductance and cardiac-response measures showed significantly less stress responses to infant stimuli in women who were breastfeeding than in women using artificial feeding. Lactating mothers also showed significantly more desire to pick up their babies (a greater sensitivity) under all stimulus conditions presented to them (baby smiling, crying and remaining quiescent) than did nonlactating mothers.[32]

We have to be considerably more careful in evaluating human studies than in evaluating animal studies, however. Animal experimenters can randomly assign their subjects to experimental and control conditions. Random assignment means that any differences observed between the experimental and control groups can be validly ascribed to the experimental variable. Scientists using human subjects must accept their subjects' decisions regarding such matters as feeding method. They simply cannot take 100 women and randomly tell 50 of them that they will breastfeed their babies and 50 that they will not. Given this restraint, it is always possible with human research that some variable other than the experiment alone can account for observed differences between groups.

In the above study, for instance, lactating and nonlactating mothers gave different reasons for their decisions about feeding methods. Bottlefeeders gave more self-centered reasons for their decision, such as convenience and the freedom to travel and work afforded by bottlefeeding. Breastfeeders gave more infant-centered reasons for their decision, such as the emotional and physical benefits to the infant. Thus, the greater relaxation and higher sensitivity of the breastfeeding mothers could be attributable to preexisting personality and attitudinal differences between the two groups of mothers.

It seems to me that one way out of this impasse would be to repeat the study including a group of mothers who had made the choice to breast-feed prior to the birth of their infants but who for some reason or another were not able to. Comparisons between such a group of mothers and lactating mothers should remove some of the uncertainty caused by preexisting personality and attitudinal differences. Any significant differences found between these two groups could then be more reliably attributed to the method of feeding.

The process of breastfeeding offers us some evidence that human infants do "imprint" in the sense that they can recognize their mothers by scent alone. Infants will, even when sleeping, instinctively turn their heads and start sucking motions if a researcher places their mothers' breast pads in the crib. This response is not elicited from infants if the breast pads of other women are placed in their cribs. Rather, infants will either ignore the pad or become fussy and start crying. Clearly infants can discriminate between their very own protectors and other mothers long before conscious connections of any kind can possibly be made. It has also been shown that mothers too have the ability to recognize their offspring from among others by smell alone, and even from the sound of their cries disguised among the cries of other infants. One study in Glasgow, Scotland, found that about 80 per cent of mothers can discriminate between the crying of their own babies and that of other babies after only 15 seconds of listening. Fathers cannot do this regardles of how involved they are with baby's care. Mother and child seem to be almost totally "at one" with each other during this period.[33]

If there is a sensitive period for the organization and consolidation of the maternal bond, the disruption of this period should have adverse consequences. It has long been recognized that premature infants, separated immediately at birth and placed in incubators, are the unfortunate recipients of more than their share of child abuse, and they have a much higher retardation rate than full-term babies. Not only are premature babies deprived of immediate contact bonding with their mothers; they are also subjected during the first crucial weeks or months of their lives to an environment lacking in stimulation, particularly tactile stimulation from mother. Unfortunately, premature birth disproportionately occurs in settings of poverty and illegitimacy. Such a permutation of regrettable events renders it difficult to be unequivocal as to whether we can attribute the later consequences of premature birth to the perinatal environment or to later stressors.

What about shorter periods of mother/infant separation caused by illness, work, or some other problem? Among the many studies of this phenomenon is that of Gail Peterson and Lewis Mehl of the Center for Research on Birth and Human Development at Berkeley. Looking at the variables of period of mother/infant separation, birth experience, length of labor, and prenatal maternal attitude, they found that over 50 per cent of the variability in maternal attachment was uniquely attributable to the amount of mother/infant separation.[34] This means that after the effects of the other three variables had been mathematically factored out, more than half of the difference in levels of attachment mothers had for their offspring could be accounted for by differences in length of mother/infant separation. In the human sciences it is extremely rare to find one isolated variable exerting such a powerful influence on another.

Peterson and Mehl go on to cite case studies of four of their mothers, two of which are shortened and paraphrased here. The first is of a mother who gave birth without analgesia/anesthesia and hence was not separated from her infant. "She was emotionally closer to this baby than she had been to her first child at the same age. She felt no postpartum depression with this delivery, although she had with her first. She attributed the sense of attachment to this second child to the fact that she could hold, nurse, and sleep with her baby immediately after she was born."[35]

The second case was one of a mother who had her child under anesthesia and was separated from it for about 18 hours for the first three days after delivery. This woman felt "distant" from her child, felt that she did not feel that it was "truly hers," and felt that the baby was "a stranger in the house." Peterson and Mehl conclude their study by stating:

> Maternal attachment is dependent on many factors. We hypothesize that the factors operative prenatally along with hormonal influences aid in the development of maternal behavior, which is organized by the birth experience and then consolidated by the presence of the infant and the interaction of mother and infant during the immediate postpartum period.[36]

What can we conclude about this loving togetherness of mother and child during the critical period of infancy? Being neither a poet or a priest, I do not wish to posit the existence of any metaphysical or spiritual property for that incipient human quality being infused into the infant by its mother that we will later call love. While love in its mature sense encompasses the conscious feelings of respect, understanding, appreciation, acceptance, sympathy, empathy, compassion, involvement, and tenderness, in its infantile state it is primarily a physiological process. If the infant is not adequately mothered during this period, the infant's neuronal pathways may not be structured to experience those beautiful feelings just enumerated. Otherwise stated, beneath the manifestations of mother/infant attachment, neurochemical processes provide a facilitating substratum, but social experience can distort its proper functioning.

Although we have always somehow known that nature has equipped mothers for love, we are only now beginning to understand the precise mechanisms. Culture merely has to remove the barriers so that the wisdom of nature can take its course. I do not think it too great a liberty to claim that love is the mechanism that forges the synergistic bond between biology and culture. The tactile sensations we received snuggled in our mother's arms, closing our lips around a nipple to drink in the milk of her human kindness, sent electrochemical impulses along our neuronal pathways to create the mind that experiences our noblest emotions. Spinoza would be delighted to hear that modern science has substantiated his claim: "Love is the increase of self by means of other."

NOTES

1. Randall Collins, *Sociology of Marriage & the Family: Gender, Love, and Property* (Chicago: Nelson-Hall, 1986), p. 271.

2. Alice Rossi, "Gender and Parenthood: American Sociological Association, 1983 Presidential Address," *American Sociological Review* 49 (1984): p. 4.

3. Ronald Rohner, *They Love Me, They Love Me Not: A Worldwide Study of the Effects of Parental Acceptance and Rejection* (New York: Hraf Press, 1975), pp. 60–61.

4. Robert Goy and Bruce McEwen, *Sexual Differentiation of the Brain* (Cambridge, Mass.: MIT Press, 1980), p. 60.

5. Sydney Mellen, *The Evolution of Love* (San Francisco: W. H. Freeman, 1983), p. 133.

6. R. LaRosa and M. LaRosa, *Transition to Parenthood* (Beverly Hills, Calif.: Sage, 1981).

7. T. Weisner, "Sibling Interdependence and Child Caretaking: A Cross-Cultural View," in *Sibling Relationships: Their Nature and Significance Across the Lifespan*, ed. M. Lamg and B. Sutton-Smith (Hillsdale, N.J.: Lawrence Erlbaum, 1984).

8. Stephen Suomi, "Sibling Relationships in Nonhuman Primates," in *Sibling Relationships: Their Nature and Significance Across the Lifespan.*

9. Glenn Wilson, *Love and Instinct* (New York: Quill, 1981), pp. 103–104.

10. W. Sack, R. Mason, and J. Higgins, "The Single-Parent Family and Abusive Child Punishment," *American Journal of Orthopsychiatry* 55 (1985): pp. 252–259.

11. Jesse Bernard, *The Future of Motherhood* (New York: Penguin, 1974).

12. Joseph Terkel and Jay Rosenblatt, "Hormonal Factors Underlying Maternal Behavior at Parturition: Cross Transfusion Between Freely Moving Rats," *Journal of Comparative and Physiological Psychology* 80 (1972): pp. 365–371.

13. M. Zarrow, V. Denenberg, and B. Sachs. "Hormones and Maternal Behavior in Mammals," in *Hormones and Behavior*, ed. S. Levine (New York: Academic Press, 1972).

14. Alice Rossi, "A Biosocial Perspective on Parenting," *Daedalus* 106 (1977):

pp. 1–31.

15. Melvin Konner, *The Tangled Wing: Biological Constraints on the Human Spirit* (New York: Holt, Rinehart and Winston, 1982), p. 318.

16. Ibid., p. 117.

17. R. Simon and N. Sharma, "Women and Crime: Does the American Experience Generalize?" in *Criminology of Deviant Women*, ed. F. Adler and R. Simon (Boston: Houghton Mifflin, 1979), p. 394.

18. L. Taylor, *Born to Crime* (Westport, Conn.: Greenwood Press, 1984), p. 87.

19. M. Clark and D. Gellman, "A User's Guide to Hormones," *Newsweek* (January 1987): pp. 50–59.

20. D. Asso, *The Real Menstrual Cycle* (New York: John Wiley, 1983), p. 64.

21. John Money, *Love and Lovesickness: The Science of Sex, Gender Difference, and Pair Bonding* (Baltimore: Johns Hopkins University, 1980): p. 5.

22. C. Barnett, P. Lederma, R. Crobstein, and M. Klaus, "Neonatal Separation: The Maternal Side of Interactional Deprivation," *Pediatrics* 45 (1970): p. 198.

23. Michael Rutter, "Maternal Deprivation, 1972–1978: New Findings, New Concepts, New Approaches," *Child Development* (1979): p. 291.

24. Cited in Anthony Walsh, *Human Nature and Love: Biological, Intrapsychic and Social-Behavioral Perspectives* (Lanham, Md.: University Press of America, 1981), p. 150.

25. Ashley Montagu, *Touching: The Human Significance of the Skin* (New York: Harper & Row, 1978), p. 63.

26. Peter Klopfer, "Mother Love: What Turns It On?" *American Scientist* 59 (1971): pp. 404–407.

27. Niles Nelson, "Trebly Sensuous Woman," *Psychology Today* (July 1971): p. 68.

28. Ashley Montagu, *Growing Young* (New York: McGraw-Hill, 1981), p. 106.

29. M. Hofer, "Early Social Relationships: A Psychobiologist's View," *Child Development* 58 (1987): pp. 633–647.

30. C. Hoeffer and M. Hardy, "Later Development of Breast Fed and Artificially Fed Infants," *Journal of the American Medical Association* 96 (1929): pp. 615–619.

31. Staff writer, "Human Milk Aids in Health, Fosters Love," *Science Digest* (Winter 1979): p. 99.

32. A. Weisenfeld, C. Malatesta, P. Whitman, C. Granrose, and R. Uili, "Psychophysiological Response to Breast- and Bottle-Feeding Mothers to Their Infant's Signals," *Psychophysiology*, 22 (1985): pp. 79–86.

33. G. Morsbach and C. Bunting, "Maternal Recognition of Their Neonate's Cries," *Developmental Medicine and Child Neurology* 21 (1979): pp. 178–185.

34. G. Peterson and L. Mehl, "Some Determinants of Maternal Attachment," *American Journal of Psychiatry* 135 (1978): pp. 1168–1173.

35. Ibid., p. 1170.

36. Ibid., p. 1171.

3

Love and the Triune Brain

Love resides in the brain; it is the organ of love.—Paul Chauchard

The human brain is an immensely complicated and awe-inspiring organ. Every cell in the body, every movement, thought, memory, emotion, and feeling is governed by it. Sir Charles Sherrington, a giant of the neurosciences, rhapsodized about the "enchanted loom" within which "millions of flashing shuttles weave a dissolving pattern, always a meaningful pattern, though never an abiding one." Although the neural sciences are increasing their knowledge of the brain at an exponential pace, it is still very much an infant science. What is yet to be discovered about that spherical body that Plato called our "divinest part" far exceeds what we presently know. A book such as this can hardly be said to do justice to the complexity of the brain; perhaps no book ever can. Treading where angels (as well as less arrogant mortals) fear to tread, this chapter attempts to link an ageless emotion to what an infant science presently knows about its subject matter. Our divinest part and our divinest emotion: what other coupling of subject matter could be more intellectually exciting?

Paul MacLean, chief of the Laboratory of Brain Evolution and Behavior at the National Institute of Mental Health, has advanced the notion of the triune (three-in-one) brain. His hypothesis is that the brain has three distinguishable anatomical and functional components, which reflect the evolutionary history of the species. Although these areas are anatomically and functionally distinct and capable of independent functioning, they are fully integrated and carry on a lively exchange with one another. These brain areas are the *reptilian*, *limbic*, and *neomammalian* systems.

The functions controlled by the three respective areas are remarkably similar to the functions controlled by Freud's id, superego, and ego—basic biological drives, emotions, and rationality, respectively. While this analogy may be overly simplistic, for Freud's tripartite structure is merely a convenient way of accounting for and thinking about the human personality, it may help us to understand how three conceptually distinct mentalities function as a whole in our day-to-day lives. MacLean uses a literary metaphor to summarize his notion of the triune brain. He sees the reptilian brain as providing the basic plots and actions in our lives, the limbic brain as providing the emotional components accompanying our life plots and actions, and the neomammalian brain as guiding and expounding on these plots in ways unique to each author.[1]

THE REPTILIAN SYSTEM

The first of these structures is the brain stem, made up of the spinal cord, the medula oblongata, the pons, and the midbrain. MacLean calls this structure the reptilian brain to emhasize its primitiveness. The reptilian brain is found in all vertebrates from lizards to human beings. The reptilian system controls the basic survival functions of the body such as respiration and heartbeat. It is also the seat of the highly patterned instinctive forms of behavior such as territoriality, ritualism, nesting, and reproduction. (MacLean lists 23 patterns of behavior.) As I indicated, it can be viewed as the physical analog of the Freudian id—basic biological drives pressing for expression. The structures of the reptilian system come hard-wired and can only be channelled, albeit with utmost difficulty, and never eliminated. Such a primitive structure lacks the neural substrate to generate a mother/child primary bond or adult male/female pair bonds—the reptiles are quintessential "rugged individualists."

Although all vertebrates, including you and I, have a reptilian brain structure, only among the cold and heartless reptiles does it sit unopposed in the executor's chair. It sits thus unopposed because that's about all the brain reptiles have. But then, if you are a reptile cruising the rocks and swamps all day just munching and mating, or slithering through the undergrowth looking for something to swallow, you really don't need much more.

It may be a bit disconcerting to know that we have such a primitive structure lurking beneath our human grey matter. Learn to love it though, because we can't do without it. We can injure other brain structures and still survive, but if we injure the reptilian structure it's curtains for us. As newborn infants, we all responded to our new and frightening world almost exclusively from this primitive hard-wired structure. Our breathing, grasping, suckling, and the satisfaction of other survival needs depended on it. The automatic walk, the support reaction of the legs, and crawling movement, behaviors which many new mothers see tested in the pediatrician's office, are reflexive reptilian reactions. The reptilian system controls these motor responses at this stage of life because the neuronal tracts between the spinal column and the "higher" brain mechanisms require time to functionally connect and to become completely myelinated. The reptilian system *retains control* of the infant's responses for about two to four months, after which control is surrendered to the more human, neural subsystems.[2]

After the transfer of neural control, most of the reflexive behaviors are dropped from the infant's behavioral repertory, and he or she has to learn to crawl, support the body, and walk. This is one of the small prices humans pay for our relative freedom from the reptilian system's control of our behavior; included in this price is the uniqueness and adaptability of the human species. No other species experiences such a behavioral discontinuity. Other species simply build directly upon their hard-wired reflexes from day one to accomplish their species-specific tasks.

One such reflexive behavior considered to be important to the human bonding process is the smile. A newborn infant's smile is totally reflexive (nonelicited) and indiscriminate. It has been suggested that the infant reflexive smile has been selected into the human behavioral repertory in order to evoke caregiving behavior on the part of parents. We know that the newborn's smile is entirely unlearned because even blind infant's smile during the period of reptilian control. A blind infant ceases to smile after control of the smile response is transferred to other areas of the brain. Being unable to see and no longer governed by reflex, the blind baby has no basis for learning the so-called "social smile." The social smile, as distinct from the reflex smile, has to be learned by sighted imitations. The smiles of sighted infants become much more discriminating after the reflexive period is past, focusing now on parents and later on significant others. At this point the infant is providing the caregiver with a visible sign of the pleasure it is experiencing from the caregiver's love.[3]

The infant's smile is a strong reinforcer for the caregiver to continue to administer to its needs. In turn, the love and attention evoked by the smile reinforces smiling behavior. This love-smile-love-smile feedback loop provides the infant with its first real lesson in human relationships. "It's good to smile; it's good to affiliate; it's good to love." In short, "It's good to be nice because when I am I feel real good, and others are nice to me too." Such a lesson will provide the infant with a sound basis for affiliative behavior for the rest of its life. If the feedback loop is never developed or constantly interrupted, the infant receives no reinforcement for its smiles. Consequently, smiling behavior is infrequent. One only has to visit a home for abused and neglected children to see how infrequently they smile. It is no wonder that abused children have difficulty forming intimate relationships in later life. As the old saying goes, "Smile and the world smiles with you; cry and you cry alone."

Consistent with the claim that women are the more loving of the two sexes, newborn infants have been shown to exhibit significantly more frequent reflexive smiling. The trend started in the crib continues throughout infancy, childhood, adolescence, and adulthood. No doubt we can point to the frequently reported greater solicitude accorded female infants to account for their greater frequency of social smiling, but it does not explain why female infants exhibit more *reflexive* smiling. Remember, reflexive smiling is, by definition, unlearned and nonelicited; this smile simply appears without regard for the positive consequences of the infant's doing so. Additionally, females have more sensitive skin, and infants who have more sensitive skin, regardless of sex, smile more frequently. This is but another indication that females are "primed" from the earliest moments of life to both receive and to give love.[4]

The reptilian system is not modified by experience the way the other two brain structures are. However, responsive (loving) mothering can be vital to the infant's well-being during the transition period from reflexive to learned behavior. Lewis Lipsitt, professor of psychology and medicine at Brown University, has conducted a very interesting series of studies of sudden-infant-death syndrome (SIDS), or crib death.[5] SIDS is responsible for about 10,000 infant deaths per year in the United States; it is listed as the cause of death only when there is no other clearly specified cause. It has been noted that victims of SIDS tend to be lethargic and unresponsive infants. This could be the result of some congenital physiological problem, or it could be the result of a lack of stimulation in the infant's environment.

Lipsitt points out that many of the victims of SIDS have great difficulty in dealing with threats to their breathing capabilities when the brain is switching the coping mechanisms from reflexive to voluntary responses. When responses to respiratory difficulties are under the exclusive control of the reptilian system, the infant reflexively thrashes about and flails its arms to remove blockages to breathing, such as mucous or a food particle. With the shift of control to learned behavior, it is assumed that the neurological systems of SIDS victims have not sufficiently developed to produce the behavior necessary to eliminate any blockage previously eliminated reflexively, and death results.

What could love have to do with all this apart from the possibility that lack of stimulation could be responsible for the lethargy and unresponsiveness of the infant? Lipsitt feels that a mother (or other caretaker) who is responsive to infant discomfort can greatly assist the infant who is susceptible to SIDS during the brain's transition period. If the infant is rewarded by being picked up, cuddled, or placed at the breast when it cries and thrashes about (for whatever reason), the comforter is reinforcing the kinds of behavior that may save the infant's life. As we know, rewarding a behavior increases the probability that it will be repeated. The tactile stimulation received by the infant during comforting, as we have seen, increases the speed of neural maturation through increased myelination and thus a speedier "freedom" from reptilian-system control. Some mothers may cringe at the thought of reinforcing crying and thrashing about, *but such behavior is precisely what is necessary* should the infant be confronted with a respiratory crisis when he or she is alone in the crib.

You can be sure that mothers don't comfort their crying infants in order to reinforce crying or because they have read Dr. Lipsitt. They do it simply because they love their children. Thus love confers survival benefits even when the lover is totally oblivious to the specific benefits being conferred on the loved one. Love is like this: just love and the details will take care of themselves. Needless to say, this certainly doesn't mean that parents who have suffered the tragic loss of an infant to SIDS didn't dearly love their infant. There may well be yet undiscovered organic causes for the problem, and Lipsitt's program calls for assiduous attention to the infant that probably goes beyond the norm.

THE LIMBIC SYSTEM

Surrounding the reptilian system like a huge protective claw is the paleo-mammalian brain or limbic ("border") system. The limbic system is a kind of balancing system between its "lower" and "higher" cranial neighbors (the reptilian complex and the neocortex, respectively). It lends sensitivity and emotion to the reptilian system, without which we would be monsters, and permits an interplay of emotion and reason within the neocortex, without which we would be robots. It is the limbic system that reacts to stresses, both internal and external and directs the chemical (neuropeptide) reactions to them via the hypothalamus, which itself directs the pituitary gland, the body's master gland. The limbic system is also where we experience sensation and emotion—our pleasures and pains. It is this system which moves us to fasten tenaciously and unthinkingly to the symbols that define our social being—a flag, a cross, a particular race or group—and to violently uphold the principles of these symbols to the detriment of others who define themselves by a different set. But the limbic system is also the seat of the noblest feelings of humankind: of love, altruism, devotion.

The limbic system is more important than the rational neocortex in terms of simple nurturing behavior. The limbic system is able to function in the absence of the neocortex (the "thinking brain"). Scientists have prevented the development of the neocortex in animals and observed that the animals are able to breed, nest, and nurture their young. If sections of the limbic system are prevented from developing, however, maternal behavior is severely circumscribed and an inability to enjoy pleasure and play is observed. Although this suggests a great deal of genetic hard-wiring in the limbic system, it is open to modification through experience.

Within the limbic system are two regions of importance to the present discussion—the *amygdala* and the *septum pellucidium*. While I wish to avoid the charge of a too-narrow brain localizationism, we may say that the amygdala is generally the site of violence and aggression and that the septum pellucidium is generally considered to be the pleasure center. One view of violence holds that the amygdala and the septal-hippocampal circuit are in competition for control of the emotional-behavioral system of the organism. Neuropsychologist James Prescott has shown in laboratory experiments with animals that there is an either/or relationship between the two centers. If an animal is experiencing pleasure, the artificial stimulation of its violence center will result in the cessation of pleasure and produce instant rage. Likewise, the stimulation of the pleasure center will instantly calm a raging animal.[6] It is clear that pleasure and violence can eliminate one another, depending on which system is dominant.

While it has not been fully demonstrated, the amygdala may be naturally more dominant than the septum pellucidium. It is located closer to the reptilian complex, and since reptilian violence and aggression evolved before mammalian love and altruism, it is a reasonable speculation. Certainly, evolutionary theory informs us that for countless eons love did not exist. When our distant relatives slithered and crawled in the mud, all that was required for the perpetuation of the species was the mating of male and female genitals. The competition for mates (and for food and territory) rendered the amygdala a very necessary little brain mechanism. We can't slough it off now simply because the competition is less sanguinary. (Some exceptionally violent criminals have had the amygdala surgically removed, resulting in the elimination of their violent behavior.) If the amygdala is naturally more dominant, all that we have to do to assure its ascendency is nothing. If love and violence are neurologically mutually exclusive as Prescott asserts, it behooves us as a society and as a species *to give love all the help we can.*

We do have experimental evidence that suggests the dominance of the aggression response when neither love nor aggression has been modeled. This evidence comes from a series of studies conducted by psychologist Harry Harlow and his colleagues at the University of Wisconsin over the past three decades. Dr. Harlow raised a number of monkeys in isolation from parents and peers. Each monkey was placed in a separate cage, their only companions being two surrogate "mothers" fashioned out of wire mesh. One mesh mother was given a terry-cloth covering, the other was fitted with a bottle from which the infant monkey could feed.

These experiments produced two interesting and profoundly important findings. The first of these was the great need of the monkeys for tactile contact. Each monkey spent the overwhelming proportion of its time clinging to the cloth mother. Even when feeding from the bare-wire mother, they endeavored to maintain contact with the cloth mother. Harlow commented that his experiments showed that there is a tremendous need among primates for frequent and intimate contact between mother and child that goes far beyond nursing as a simple feeding mechanism. He went so far as to suggest that the primary function of nursing as an affectional variable was to assure this intimate mother/infant contact.[7] Subsequent research on the effects of mother/infant separation on endorphin levels, brain structure and function, and immune-system functioning, done in the 70s and 80s, muted much of the cynicism with which Harlow's early studies were initially received.

The second, and perhaps more important, finding was that monkeys deprived of real mothering did not behave as normally raised monkeys do when they were introduced to other monkeys following prolonged separation. When surrogate-raised monkeys were put with other monkeys, many responded with greater than expected aggression and others exhibited bizarre schizoid behavior, such as withdrawal, endless rocking, and catatonic posturing. These responses were obviously unlearned socially since this was their first contact with other monkeys. Furthermore, when female isolates were introduced to normally raised males for reproduction purposes, the females insisted on remaining chaste. Harlow and his colleagues had to devise "rape racks" in order to achieve their purpose. When the offspring of these rapacious unions were born, their mothers ignored, attacked, or killed them. Harlow described these lacklove mothers as "helpless, hopeless, heartless mothers devoid, or almost devoid, of any maternal feeling."[8]

Predictably, the offspring of these brutal mothers were found to be significantly more violent and aggressive than normally raised monkeys. Later on, we will see that such a relationship is also true of human children of brutal, unloving parents. Whether we are talking about young monkeys or young humans, the evidence is plain and compelling: Infants have a desperate need for maternal attachment as it is expressed in contact comfort. If they do not get it, bad things will happen to them, and these bad things will influence their view of the world for the rest of their lives.

All this suggests that the cruelty, coldness, and aggression of the reptilian complex will be dominant behaviors in the absence of experience that moves us in the opposite direction. Aggression is not so much learned as unlearned. It is a part of our primeval legacy, of our evolutionary baggage. It is love that has to be learned in our mothers' arms. In order to become a tender, caring, and loving person, one has to have been tenderly loved and cared for oneself. As Stephen Suomi, one of Harlow's proteges noted, it is important to realize that the aberrant behavior of their deprived monkeys was the direct result of abnormal dendritic wiring, which, in turn, was the direct result of love deprivation.[9]

The reader may balk at the idea of using experiments with monkeys to raise issues pertinent to the development of human beings, for are we not different from mere simians? Of course we are different, but in degree rather than in kind. To assert that there is a radical discontinuity between other primates and ourselves promotes a distorting anthropocentricity by dividing the world into the "natural" and the "human." Such a strict dividing line is not tenable. It has been estimated that we share between 98 and 99 per cent of our genes with our hairier cousins, thus being separated from them by only about 2 per cent of our genetic endowment. There are no reasons to doubt that roughly similar infant experiences would not have roughly similar consequences for human infants as for simian.

The 2 per cent or so of genetic material separating us from monkeys is what makes us cultural animals. Since we are cultural animals—meaning that our behaviors are more open to learned patterns than are the lower animals—we are even *more* likely to be influenced by experience than are monkeys. Our plastic brain internalizes experience, we remember it, we respond to further experience influenced by it, we stew over it—and we get even.

It is not enough to point out genetic similarities between humans and primates. We must also provide evidence that love deprivation does indeed have similar consequences for human infants. We will see when we discuss physical illness in the next chapter that motherless infants raised in institutions have died from lovelessness, even though their other needs were adequately met. Although no study of deprived human infants reports them as being subjected to the drastic levels of deprivation suffered by Harlow's monkeys, all similar studies report negative consequences accompanying deprivation. Consequences attributed to early maternal separation and institutionalization are antisocial and aggressive behavior, the inability to establish social relationships, social withdrawal, self-rocking, and excessive autoerotic activity. All these behaviors are identical to the behaviors displayed by Harlow's monkeys.[10]

In one heart-tugging study of institutionalized children, researchers found that infants were being subjected to almost the same degree of isolation that Harlow's monkeys experienced. They were kept in isolation cubicles almost continuously from birth. This was ignorance in action rather than deliberate cruelty. Hospital staff isolated the children as protection against infectious diseases. The children's contact with other humans was limited to having their bodily needs met by overworked attendants with little or no time to provide them with tactile comfort. When these children were compared with normally (family) raised infants, they showed serious impairments of their social-psychological development. Their reactions to other human being were fear and apathy rather than joy and interest. When distressed, they rarely approached others for comfort and reassurance. Instead, their reaction was most likely to be to huddle in a corner and rock back and forth.[11] The parallels between these human infants and Harlow's monkeys indicate that the lack of early love experiences have similar consequences across primate species. Neurologist Richard Restak sums up the importance of early tactile stimulation and sets up the subject matter of the next two chapters for us when he writes:

> Touch, it turns out, is as necessary to normal infant development as food and oxygen. Mother opens her arms to the infant, snuggles him, and a host of psychobiological processes are brought into harmony. Disrupt this process because the mother cannot or will not caress, touch or otherwise make skin-to-skin contact with the infant and psychobiological processes go askew . . . physiological imbalances, behavioral peculiarities, hostilities, suppressed anger and rage.[12]

In the days when neuroscience was little more than descriptive anatomy, the genius of Sigmund Freud suspected that the origin of love lay in the tactile pleasures infants received from their mothers. The infant, living as it does in a world of pure sensation, "loves" the bodily (erotic) pleasures of warmth, a full stomach, and a dry bottom, as well as the tactile manifestations of mother love because such pleasures are intrinsically rewarding. The child's love of intrinsically rewarding stimuli is an example of what psychologists call an "unconditioned response." When the child is able to identify the source of its pleasure as another human being, it extends its love to the source or sources, a "conditioned response." Needs and their satisfaction are indispensable components of all human relationships; those who satisfy our needs become valuable to us. This is as true of our love needs as it is of any other needs. In a very real sense, love can be viewed as a psychic by-product of physical imperatives. Observe how Freud, writing in 1926, anticipated Montagu's concept of utero- and exterogestation and the vital role of love during exterogestation when he wrote:

> The biological factor is the long period of time during which the young of the human species is in a condition of helplessness and dependence. Its intrauterine experience seems to be short compared to that of most animals, and it is sent into the world in a less finished state. . . . The dangers of

the outer world have a greater importance for it, so the value of the object
[by object, Freud is referring to mother] which can alone protect it against
them and take the place of its former intrauterine life is enormously enhanced.
This biological factor then establishes the earliest situation of danger and creates
the need to be loved which will accompany the child through the rest of its life[13]
[Emphasis added].

The evolution of the limbic system was a very important juncture in
making humans the kind of beings we are today. It was the evolution of
the limbic system that made for the evolution of the primary biological
mammalian bond, that of mother and infant. It is also the neural structure
responsible for adult male/female pair bonds. However, the limbic system
by itself is not responsible for human love relationships. Nonhuman primates do not integrate the two fundamental biological bonds to form kinship bonds. The human species does tightly integrate these bonds, and from
these bonds arise our basic sociocultural structures. The integration of these
two biological bonds was made possible by the evolution of the third part
of our triune brain—the neomammalian system.

THE NEOMAMMALIAN SYSTEM

The evolutionary switch from the genetically programmed behavior of the
reptilian system to the emotionally governed behavior of the mammalian
limbic system is only part of the story. Love in its adult state is not simply
the goings on in our limbic system. Mature love requires a shift from the
seething tropics of the limbic system to the cooler and more rational climate
of the neomammalian brain. The neomammalian brain (also called the
neocortex or cerebral cortex) is the third component of MacLean's triune
brain. It is the neocortex and its capabilities that define the human species.
It is the site of abstract reasoning and the internalizer of social prescriptions and moral strictures. It is this thinking ability that allows us to sacrifice the immediate discomfort of our loved ones for their future well-being.
All mammals will protect their young from pain and suffering, but only
human mammals will allow outsiders to inflict pain on their young, such
as the surgeon's knife or the teacher's admonitions, for their long-term good.
Thus, any maternal instinct that might exist is modified by the knowledge
and foresight stored in the neocortex of the human mother.

Our brain is able to override genetic instructions in instances in which
it becomes necessary, because the sheer weight of the number of "bits"
of information contained in the brain exceeds by a wide margin the information contained in the genes. It is estimated that we have approximate-

ly 100,000 genes governing the basic functions of our bodies. The various permutations of such a large number of genes are more than enough to produce billions of genetically unique individuals, but not enough to allow us to respond to the sheer complexity of the human world. The human animal requires many more information "bits" than is provided by its genetic endowment. These bits have to be numerous, flexible, and capable of interaction with many other bits. We call these marvelous bits designed for information gathering, processing, and responding neurons, those amazing little creatures we met in chapter 1. As was mentioned there, the number of neurons in each individual's brain is as high as 100 billion, and each one of them is capable of making thousands of connections with other neurons. If you can take one more number, and if you can trust my mathematics, this works out to about 1,000 trillion "bits" of information!

With such limitless capacity as this, it is difficult to think of limbic-system feelings such as love, pleasure, attachment, or maternalism not being informed by social knowledge and imagination. We have seen how these limbic feelings in monkeys, while innate, have to be actualized by experience. This is so much more true of humans, whose limbic system occupies a much smaller proportion of the cerebrum in relation to the neocortex than does the limbic system of monkeys. If mothering were simply a matter of gender and sex hormones uninformed by experience, we would not be able to observe that adoptive mothers, who have not undergone hormonal "priming," sometimes show themselves to be superior to biological mothers. Adoptive mothers (incidentally, it is almost always the female rather than the male who is the architect of the adoption decision) are a carefully selected group of individuals. In all likelihood, their experiences as infants were more loving and nurturant than any sample of other females chosen at random. They are incurring the considerable expense of time and money to care for and love another human being who is not biologically connected to them. Biological mothers who mother poorly, on the other hand, were in all probability treated during their infancy and childhood in a way more inimical to the growth of love than one would find in a randomly selected sample of mothers.

Even at the level of the neocortex there exists evidence for a greater potential for love in women. Thanks largely to the work of Nobel Prize-winning psychobiologist Roger Sperry, it is common knowledge today that we have two separate but interacting cerebral hemispheres.[14] These two sides of the brain are joined by a thick band of fibers called the corpus callosum ("hard body") which serves as a bridge for the nerve tracts running from one hemisphere to the other. The left side of the brain specializes in logical, linear skills such as mathematics and language, but is also fragmentary in its processing of information, somewhat like a computer. The right side of the brain functions more holistically; it specializes in visual-spatial arrangements and the processing of emotion.

Although these two sides are linked, working like two lumberjacks at either end of a saw, the severing of the corpus callosum bridge between them has, surprisingly, few adverse effects on personality or behavior. In fact, some severely epileptic patients have undergone a complete hemispherectomy (removal of one complete hemisphere) and are still able to function. Such drastic surgery is best done during early childhood when the brain is most plastic, because it does inhibit completely normal functioning. If performed early enough, the specialized functions of the excised hemisphere can be transferred to the intact hemisphere. However, the transferred functions do not operate as efficiently as they can within their "native" hemisphere any more than a single lumberjack can operate efficiently without his teammate.

The importance of this for our present discussion is that the female brain is less specialized or "lateralized" than the male brain. Man's evolutionary history as a hunter necessitated the selection of motor and visual-spatial skills needed for this task. Scientists today observe male superiority in those very visual-spatial skills that have been so important for more than 99 per cent of the history of the species. Females were more diverse in the tasks they had to perform in hunting and gathering societies, and so they were subjected to different evolutionary selection pressures. Woman's role as nurturer, caregiver, comforter, and peacekeeper exerted pressure for the selection of social skills such as language and greater emotional sensitivity, skills that are demonstrably superior in women today.

This does not mean that women cannot excel in occupations requiring visual-spatial skills (e.g., engineering), or that men cannot excel in occupations requiring social-nurturing skills (e.g., nursing). But it does not seem that occupational gender-sorting is solely a matter of arbitrary, sexist role-assignment after all. Psychiatrist Willard Gaylin's survey of the biological and genetic research in this area leads him to the conclusion that nature has infused women with biological drives toward nurturance and attachments, while men have been handed a biological orientation toward certain kinds of work and skill mastery.[15]

Having said all this about the left-right brain dichotomy, I should add that we must be cautious about making too much of it. Roger Sperry himself has called it "an idea with which it is very easy to run wild."[16] Male and female brains are much more alike than they are different. The functioning of the integrated brain is more important to human activity than the differential functioning of its separate hemispheres. The data on brain hemisphericity most definitely does not mean that males are "smarter" than females, as some who have "run wild" with it have asserted. Women have been injured by societies that have taken their greater capacity to love and assigned that as their sole function. We need both love and meaningful work to be fulfilled, yet for so long women were chained to home and hearth and denied satisfying work outside of the home. Gaylin decries this deprivation, but he also sees that the deprivation of a sense of the importance of love in males "is at least as egregious an injury."[17] I suggest that the male deprivation is much more egegrious an injury, both to the individual male and to society at large. As Freud often pointed out, blessed indeed is the man or woman who fulfills both the capacities for love and work.

The lesser degree of brain lateralization in females confers many advantages. For instance, female stroke victims regain more of their former functioning than men do because of the relatively easier transfer of brain processes from the damaged hemisphere to the healthy hemisphere. Sandra Witelson of the department of Psychiatry at McMaster University in Canada points out that it is this greater plasticity of the female brain that protects them from many developmental disorders associated with hemisphere dysfunctions.[18] We certainly do observe a much greater frequency of aphasia, dyslexia, autism, early-onset schizophrenia, psychopathy, and many other developmental disorders among men than among women.

Christine de Lacoste-Utamsing and Ralph Holloway of the Department of Neurology at the University of Texas have found what they believe to be an anatomical basis for greater interhemispheric transfer of information in the female brain. They found that the splenium, the posterior portion of the corpus callosum, is significantly larger in females that in males. While they are justly cautious in their interpretation of this finding, the implication is that the more fibers there are in the splenium, the greater the capacity for information transfer.[19] If the greater thickness of the splenium does mean a greater ability to transfer functions controlled by the stroke-affected hemisphere to the unaffected hemisphere, we can see why women do recover more readily from the ravages of a stroke than do male victims.

The findings of Lacoste-Utamsing and Holloway lead us to wonder if the corpus callosum is influenced in its development by experience. If neuronal branching and myelination are affected by experience, it is reasonable to suppose that the corpus callosum may be also. Victor Denenberg of the Department of Biobehavioral Science at the University of Connecticut believes that it is. His work has shown that just as early stimulation of the sensory systems enhances their growth and development, tactile and cognitive stimulation enhance the growth and development of the corpus callosum among animals. He has also argued that a more fully developed corpus callosum results in better integration of brain functions, and hence greater protection of either hemisphere is subsequently damaged.[20] Could it be that the greater frequency of female infant reflexive smiling, leading to a greater propensity for caregivers to stimulate them, is in some way responsible for the thickness of the female splenium? This is an intriguing question for which there is no answer at present.

What does this mean in terms of love? We have seen that the process of evolution has gradually provided the organism that was to become Homo sapiens with more and more complex brain mechanisms. When our distant ancestors were concerned only with feeding, fighting, fleeing, and reproduction (the four F's), the reptilian system served its purpose efficiently. As we evolved into mammals the selection for emotion, particularly love and nurturing, became important for species survival; hence, the limbic system developed. When we became complex culture-making creatures, we needed more complex brain mechanisms, and the neocortex slowly evolved. The rational neocortex enables us to temper the raw emotions of the limbic system with reason.

The prefrontal area of the neocortex appears to be the most recently evolved area of the brain. There is a pronounced difference in size between the areas of the skull housing the prefrontal cortex in Neanderthal man (who had a low brow) and in Cro-Magnon man (high brow), meaning that the prefrontal neocortex probably evolved in the relative brief period of a few thousand years. I emphasize that this line of thinking is speculative, and relies on an assumption of evolutionary continuity between Neanderthal and Cro-Magnon, as well as the assumption of a direct link between cranial morphology and brain development. Not all anthropologists think that such a linearity exists. Many believe that Neanderthal and Cro-Magnon were distinct subspecies and that the Neanderthal lineage became extinct. Still others believe that Neanderthal and Cro-Magnon, although once distinct subspecies, intermated and became a single lineage. If Neanderthal and Cro-Magnon were once distinct lineages, Cro-Magnon's possession of the prefrontal cortex may well be a factor in explaining why he survived to become modern man while the Neanderthalers disappeared.

According to Paul MacLean, the prefrontal area evolved in close relationship to the part of the limbic system involved in maternal care.[21] Through its connection with the limbic system it helps us to empathize, to gain insight into the felt life of others, and to understand it as if it were our own. It is the mechanism that leavens our rationality with feeling and that guides our emotions through thought. French neurophysiologist Paul Chauchard goes even further in his praise of the prefrontal brain:

The prefrontal is the brain of involvement. Reflection not only makes us decide what is suitable for us. It gives us the taste, the enthusiasm for what we choose. It does not give us merely a barren notional knowledge, but makes us assent with our whole hearts to what we know. And this is what would appear to be the full significance of the prefrontal. Its real name is the brain of the heart, the organ of love.[22]

As we have seen, parental behavior has a biological basis for women but is probably an entirely socially learned behavior in males; the evolution of the limbic system brought with it the development of the mother/infant and adult male/female bonds. The bond that is missing among nonhuman primates is that of fatherhood, a purely human *cultural* concept. If the human male was to contribute something more to the survival of the species other than stud service, the species had to become sufficiently intelligent to recognize and grasp the abstract concept of *relationship*. With the ability to grasp such a concept came the integration of the two biological bonds— mother/infant and male/female—with the cultural bond—fatherhood. The fusion of these basic bonds became a template for the evolution of ever more complex human relationships and bonds:—kinship, family, tribe, and on up to society itself. The pivotal figure in the extension of basic biological bonds to cultural bonds is woman, for she is the only figure common to both biological bonds.[23]

Such a pivotal figure might be expected to possess some special features within her neomammalian brain. Given the close relationship between the prefrontal cortex and the limbic system involved in parental care, it is reasonable to assume that the emotional messages arriving from the limbic system will retain more of their power after cortical integration in women than they will in men. In fact, it has been shown experimentally that women enjoy a greater capacity than men to integrate pleasurable experiences into the neocortex.[24] Other experiments tracing blood flow through the cortex during language tests have shown that while there is a tight fit between brain areas in the left frontal lobe involved in language and the motor areas (jaw, tongue, etc.) required for its expression in males, the fit is far more diverse in females. Neuropsychologist Cecille Naylor's experiments led her to exclaim that it is almost as though a female's brain is "ablaze" when she is processing language. Blood flow is not limited to the left hemisphere as it is in males, but is also observed in the right hemisphere. Naylor sees this as an "additional imaging function," and speculates that women bring a "richer, more expanded emotional component into play" than do men when processing language.[25]

As suggested by Naylor's research, this capability may well be a function of the female brain's lesser degree of laterality. Psychoneuroimmunologist Paul Pearsall believes so. He sees the tendency of males to be generally more self-oriented to be a function, at least in part, of their left-brain tendency. He also sees the "whole-brain" tendency of females as producing beings more "other" and "us" oriented. The female orientation to the world is viewed by Pearsall as being more in tune with the principles of healthy living.[26] The implication is that a woman's greater capacity for love within the limbic system, and its associated endocrinal processes, is augmented and reinforced within her rational brain and is thus more capable of wide diffusion.

We have seen that evolutionary survival imperatives have been instrumental in the development of increasingly more complex neural mechanisms. Each of these new mechanisms has played its role in muting the substrata of violence and aggression laid down during periods when such behavior was important to the survival of the organism. We have also seen how love is apparently indispensable to the process of becoming human in the fullest sense of the word. Early love deprivation seriously impairs an infant's ability to establish later affectual relationships of all kinds. The series of experiments by Harlow and his colleagues, surely some of the most meaningful ever conducted, have pointed out just how vitally necessary love is.[27] To be a loving person, one has to have been loved—it's as simple and as profound as this.

We ask ourselves if the insidious effects of early love deprivation can be overcome. The answer seems to be a very cautious and hopeful "yes." Based on subsequent "rehabilitative" work on Harlow's monkeys, biologist Melvin Konner offers a hopeful but hedging response. Konner is aware that the ability to form love relationships throughout the lifespan depends to a great extent on early affectional experience. But there are powerful, built-in, neuroendocrinal forces, says Konner, that make us crave closeness and love that will insure that most of us, whatever our early experience, will develop some form of affectionate behavior.[28] When entwined lovers whisper that they "need" each other, they are giving voice to hundreds of thousands of years of evolutionary selection for this need to give and receive love.

A 1972 study by Suomi and Harlow, involving the social rehabilitation of monkeys, showed a significant decline in abnormal behavior patterns of monkeys who had been isolated for six months when exposed to "therapists." These were normally raised monkeys who were three months younger than the isolates. The simian therapists showed great persistence and patience in clinging to the isolates, stroking them, and initiating play behavior. Not coincidentally, the best "therapists," the most interested and concerned, were female monkeys.

During three 60-day periods of therapy, in which the isolates were compared to the "therapists," there was a decline in the difference between "patient" and "therapist" in both abnormal behavior and socially desirable behavior. At the end of the 180-day period there were no significant differences between the two groups. The authors concluded their study by remarking that the isolation experience does not necessarily destroy all potential for adequate social development.[29] But "potential" is something which may or may not be realized. Unfortunately, subsequent studies have shown that this potential is never completely realized. It appears from these later studies that many of the abnormal behaviors reappear, albeit at somewhat lower levels, by the time the isolates reach sexual maturity (three years of age) and that rehabilitation is more complete the earlier it is attempted and the longer it goes on.[30] There's a lot of wisdom in the old adage: "Those who deserve love the least need it the most."

NOTES

1. Paul Maclean's original conception of the triune brain is contained in *A Triune Concept of the Brain and Behavior* (Toronto: University of Toronto Press, 1973). A more recent exposition is contained in "Brain Evolution: The Origins of Social and Cognitive Behaviors" in *A Child's Brain*, ed. M. Frank (New York: Haworth Books, 1984).

2. Rhawn Joseph, "The Neuropsychology of Development: Hemispheric Laterality, Limbic Language, and the Origin of Thought," *Journal of Clinical Psychology* (1972): p. 11.

3. N. Anastasiow, *Development and Disability* (Baltimore: Paul H. Brooks, 1986), p. 45.

4. D. Freedman, *Human Infancy: An Evolutionary Perspective* (Hillsdale, N.J.: Lawrence Erlbaum Associates, 1974), pp. 64–68.

5. Lewis Lipsit, "Critical Conditions in Infancy: A Psychological Perspective," *American Psychologist* 34 (1979): pp. 973–80.

6. James Prescott, "Body Pleasure and the Origins of Violence," *Bulletin of the Atomic Scientists* (1975): p. 11.

7. Harry Harlow, "The Nature of Love," *American Psychologist* 13 (1958): pp. 673–85, and "Social Deprivation in Monkeys," *Scientific American* 206 (1962): pp. 137–44 (with Margaret Harlow).

8. Harry Harlow, "Lust, Latency and Love: Simian Secrets of Successful Love," *The Journal of Sex Research* 11 (1975): 79–90.

9. Stephen Suomi, *A Touch of Sensitivity* (Boston: WGBH Educational Foundation, 1980), p. 10.

10. For a review of studies detailing consequences of human maternal separation, see S. Wolkind, "The Components of 'Affectionless Psychopathy' in Institutionalized Children," *Journal of Child Psychology and Psychiatry* 15 (1974): pp. 215–20.

11. S. Provence and R. Lipton, *Infants in Institutions* (New York: International Universities Press, 1962).

12. Richard Restak, *The Infant Minds* (Garden City, N.Y.: Doubleday, 1986), p. 141.

13. Sigmund Freud, "Inhibitions, Symptoms and Anxiety" in *The Works of Sigmund Freud*, Standard Edition (London: Hogarth, 1955), p. 7.

14. Roger Sperry, "Some Effects of Disconnecting the Cerebral Hemispheres," *Science* 217 (1982): pp. 1223–1226.

15. Willard Gaylin, *Rediscovering Love* (New York: Penguin, 1986).

16. Roger Sperry, "Some Effects of Disconnecting the Cerebral Hemispheres," p. 1223.

17. Willard Gaylin, *Rediscovering Love*, p. 193.

18. Sandra Witelson, "Sex and the Single Hemisphere: Specialization of the Right Hemisphere for Spatial Processing," *Science* 193 (1976): pp. 425–26.

19. Christine de Lacoste-Utamsing and Ralph Holloway, "Sexual Dimorphism in the Human Corpus Callosum," *Science* 216 (1982): pp. 1431–1432.

20. Victor Denenberg, "Hemispheric Laterality in Animals and the Effects of Early Experience," *Behavioral and Brain Sciences* 4 (1981): p. 1–49.

21. Paul MacLean, *A Triune Concept of the Brain and Behavior*, p. 58.

22. Paul Chauchard, *Our Need of Love* (New York: P. J. Kenedy & Sons, 1968), p. 30.

23. For a discussion of women as the pivotal point of the integration of the two basic human biological bonds, see P. Wilson, *Man, the Promising Primate* (New Haven: Yale University Press, 1980).

24. Mary Long, "Visions of a New Faith," *Science Digest* 89 (1981): pp. 36–42.

25. Cecille Naylor's research cited in Kathryn Phillips, "Why Can't a Man Be More Like a Woman . . . and Vice Versa?" *Omni* (October 1990): p. 46.

26. Paul Pearsall, *Superimmunity* (New York: Fawcett, 1987): p. 33.

27. Harry Harlow, "The Nature of Love."

28. Melvin Konnor, *The Tangled Wing: Biological Constraints on the Human Spirit* (New York: Holt, Rinehart and Winston, 1982): pp. 300–301.

29. Stephen Suomi and Harry Harlow, "Social Rehabilitation of Isolate-reared Monkeys," *Developmental Psychology* 6 (1972): pp. 487–96.

30. Mark Cummins and Stephen Suomi, "Long-Term Effects of Social Rehabilitation in Rhesus Monkeys," *Primates* 17 (1976): pp. 43–51.

Part Two

Kin Love

4

Love and Physical Illness

The main reason for healing is love.—Paracelsus

St. Augustine saw love as the one true human emotion. All other emotions he saw as derivatives of this single source: "Love eager to possess its object is Desire; possessing and enjoying it is Happiness; shrinking from what opposes it is Fear; being aware of effective opposition is Sorrow."[1] Freud might have added that its thwarting is aggression, its rejection is hate, and its protracted absence is pathology, illness, death, and destruction.

So men of God and men of science look upon love as something we humans need, and need very badly. But what an overworked word *need* is. A simple enumeration of the many things some behavioral scientist or another has considered to be a human need would fill many pages. The term has been tossed around so casually and carelessly that much of the meaning has been washed out of it. Let's agree that the term *need* implies an urgent necessity, the absence of which undermines the well-being, or even the survival, of the organism. A force so central to our human existence as love must surely qualify as a need in its most precise sense, for love alone among the many needs of seemingly abstract nature meets this demanding criterion.

The best demonstration of the functional importance of A to B is to view what becomes of B in the absence of A. Deprived of oxygen, the survival time for the human organism is measured in minutes and seconds. Deprived of food and water it is measured in weeks and days. While the lack of affectionate mother love has sent many a poor infant to an early grave, many other unloved souls have lived out their threescore years and ten. This observation does not diminish the status of love as a basic human need one iota. Few human beings are totally deprived of warmth and affection throughout their entire lives. Nevertheless, as Plato once commented: "He whom love touches not, walks in darkness." The results of such a pointless and lonely journey are numerous and tragic.

In apparent agreement with St. Augustine, Howard Whitman, in an article entitled "The Amazing New Science of Love," saw love as a kind of panacea for all that ails when he wrote:

> The psychiatrists, in their lurid battle against mental illness have finally concluded that the great taproot of mental illness is lovelessness. The child psychologists, wrangling over scheduled versus demand feeding, spanking versus non-spanking, have found none of it makes much difference so long as the child is loved. The sociologists have found love the answer to delinquency, the criminologists have found it the answer to crime, the political scientists have found it the answer to war.[2]

Is love really so powerful a need as to be responsible, at least in part, for all the problems wrought by its absence as Whitman suggests? The reader may be forgiven for feeling that Dr. Whitman (as well as myself) invests love with too much power as an explanation for the various pathological syndromes enumerated. A thorough examination of the dynamics of such syndromes demands that attention be paid to biological, psychological, and sociocultural variables and their interaction. Nevertheless, perusing the literature relating to these syndromes, I am struck with the consistency with which researchers of stature include the lack of warm and loving relationships in their lists of causal factors.

This does not mean that love deprivation is considered to be a necessary and sufficient cause of any one thing. It is best considered as a precipitating or predisposing variable that interprets and specifies the relationship between the existing syndrome and the more proximate cause. By this, I mean that if we observe, say, a relationship between frustration and violence, love deprivation helps us to interpret the mechanisms through which the relationship occurs and specifies those most at risk for responding violently to frustration.

The idea that disease may result from a disharmonious relationship between human beings and their environment is not a new idea; it is rather the resurgence of an old idea. It had been buried for over a century by the spectacular successes of the germ theory and the infectious model of disease. According to extreme proponents of the germ theory, illness is simply the result of some pathophysiological activity exacerbated by unhealthy physical habits such as smoking, poor hygiene, lack of exercise, and so forth, or the result of some external force, such as an invading virus. There is certainly nothing wrong with this model; we have all been beneficiaries of its remarkable fruits. The only problem with it is that it doesn't go far enough in recognizing the human factor in disease. Until quite recently, any assertion that disease could result from and/or be exacerbated by a lack of loving ties with other human beings would be met with icy silence among medical professionals. Today, health and general well-being is viewed more holistically. "Health," says the World Health Organization, "is a state of complete physical, mental, and social well-being and not merely the absence of disease or infirmity."[3]

We now know that stress, the kind of people we are, how we interpret and evaluate the world, and how we interact with others have consequences for our health. These things can alter brain chemistry, making us susceptible to such pathologies as deprivation dwarfism, debilitating depression, schizophrenia, and suicide. Stress can also suppress the functioning of the immune system, thus impairing our ability to fight off all manner of infections, and it can affect the level of fatty lipids in the blood, leaving us open to a number of cardiovascular ailments. In short, modern medicine is catching up with the genius of Freud, who wrote: "A strong ego is protection against disease, but in the last resort we must begin to love in order that we may not fall ill, and we must fall ill if, in consequence of frustration, we cannot love."[4]

ILLNESSES OF INFANCY AND CHILDHOOD

The annals of psychosomatic medicine contain numerous studies which point to the importance of love for the healthy functioning of human beings. The lack of love, in its various manifestations, is seen largely in terms of inducing stress. Stress is a psychophysiological syndrome that has damaging effects on the cardiovascular, gastrointestinal, respiratory, and endocrinal systems. This is not to say that love deprivation "causes" illness in a sense analogous to an invading virus. It is rather a major stressor, which has the effect of generating harmful biochemical changes in the body. Exposure to stress over an extended period may eventually lead to the exhaustion of the body's hormonal defensive capacity, thus weakening its capacity to deal with future stressors. As Hans Selye, the father of the modern stress concept once noted, it is the one who hates and confronts the world full of negativism who will get ulcers, hypertensions, and heart disease, not those who are hated. He went on to insist: " 'Love thy neighbor' is one of the sagest bits of medical advice ever given."

One of the earliest studies of the tragic consequences of early love deprivation was René Spitz's work in the 1940s with institutionalized infants.[5] Spitz was concerned with the high mortality rates of infants in foundling homes. Abnormally high numbers of infants were dying of no apparent organic causes in these institutions, despite high standards of hygiene and nutrition. In an effort to determine the cause, Spitz compared conditions in a foundling home with those existing in a nursery in a penal institution for delinquent girls. While the conditions (medical care, hygiene, nutrition) in the foundling home were superior to those in the penal institute, there was significantly less illness and death among infants in the penal institute.

Spitz also compared the two sets of infants, all of whom were less than one year old, on six indices of development: peception, body mastery, social relations, memory, relations to inanimate objects, and intelligence. These measures yield a general "developmental quotient" (DQ). Initially, Spitz found the infants from the foundling home to have superior average DQ's (124 versus 101). He attributed the relatively low scores of the penal infants to their "psychically defective" delinquent mothers. However, while the DQs of the nursery children improved normally over time, the DQs of the found-ling-home children declined the longer they were institutionalized. Upon retesting the children one year later, he found that the penal infants average DQ was 105, while the average DQ of the foundling children had plummeted to 72. The real tragedy of the story is that within two years after the start of the study 37 per cent of the foundling children were dead, while all of the penal children were still alive five years later.

Given all the apparent advantages of the foundling-home infants, why such tragic consequences? For Spitz, the answer was obvious. The penal children were cared for by their own mothers, "psychically defective" though they may have been. They were given exclusive care by their mothers—kissed, cuddled, stroked, talked to, fed, played with—in short, they were loved. The foundling-home children had no opportunity to develop this kind of relationship with caregivers. Despite the greater technical efficiency of the professional nursing staff of the foundling home, nurses simply did not have the time, even if they had the inclination, to develop this kind of bond with all the babies in their care.

If the lack of love can literally kill, a remarkable long-term study by Harold Skeels bears testimony to the curative property of love. Skeels ran-domly divided a number of institutionalized "mentally retarded" two-year-old children into two groups. One group of children was placed in the care of individual substitute mothers, who were themselves classified as mentally deficient and institutionalized. The other group remained behind in the orphanage. As was the case with the Spitz study, Skeels observed dramatic results. Over the years of testing the IQs of the two groups of children, it was found that those in the care of surrogate mothers showed an average increase of 28 points, while those still institutionalized showed an average decrease of 30 points.

Thirty years later, Skeels decided to trace his subjects to determine what became of them. He found that all those who were placed in the care of surrogate mothers were self-supporting members of the community. The average IQ of this group was 92. Such an IQ hardly qualified them for membership in MENSA, but it is within the normal range and a long way from mental retardation. His search for the unfortunate members of the control group left behind in the institution found that they were all either dead or still institutionalized.[6] Both of these studies accent the power of love to organize, nourish, extend, and preserve life.

PHYSICAL GROWTH AND DEVELOPMENT

The lack of love has adverse effects on physical as well as intellectual growth and development. An early study of neglected children at the Cleveland Jewish Orphans Home found that love deprivation (termed "socio-emotional deprivation" by the authors) played a crucial role among the factors responsible for retarded physical growth and generally poor physical health. Another early study conducted at the Massachusetts General Hospital concluded that no physical cause could be detected to account for the dwarfism among children subjected to extreme emotional deprivation. And a study conducted at the Menninger Clinic in Topeka, Kansas, found that osteoarthritic patients in the study all had histories of some kind of early neglect, rejection, and other adverse emotional deprivations.[7]

The most dramatic and well-studied syndrome of physical "failure to thrive" is psychosocial or deprivation dwarfism. Children suffering from psychosocial dwarfism are severely retarded in physical growth, usually falling below the third percentile in height for their age, meaning that about 97 per cent of their age peers are taller than they. Dwarfism can occur within loving families; that is, it can have a purely physiological cause that is totally independent of psychosocial factors. In such instances, dwarfism is secondary to hypopituitarism, meaning that the pituitary gland is underactive because of some inherent physiological pathology. Biochemical malfunction is certainly at the bottom of most illness states, but as one British scientist put it: "Love is biochemistry's chief assistant."[8]

In two classical papers in the same issue of the New England Journal of Medicine, Powell and his colleagues outlined a number of criteria for distinguishing hypopituitary dwarfism from psychosocial dwarfism, that is, for distinguishing between organic and emotional causes.[9] First, does the child have a history of strange behavior patterns that suggest emotional disturbance, such as social apathy and withdrawal? Is he accident prone, have delayed language and IQ development, and bizarre feeding habits such as polyphagia and polydipsia? Polyphagia and polydipsia are excessive and bizarre eating and drinking behavior, respectively. These behaviors include gorging, vomiting, hoarding, eating from garbage, and drinking stagnant water, dishwater, and toilet water.

The second criteria focuses on mothers. Do they exhibit pathological behaviors, such as anxiety, depression, abuse of children, and social and marital instability? Alcoholism and absence of the father are also fairly frequently observed in the homes of psychosocial dwarfs. These parental behaviors are certainly indicators of emotional deprivation. A study by a team of French pediatricians at the Hopital des Enfant-Malades in Paris concluded that a number of tests have shown that the crux of the psychosocial dwarfism problem to be the absence of loving mother-child relationships.[10]

Third, if abnormal endocrine function is observed in the dwarf children (it is in about half of the cases) and if it is rectified upon removal from the home without hormonal or psychiatric treatment, we have clear evidence of the pernicious effects of an abnormal home environment, one bereft of love. Conversely, we have evidence of the medicinal power of love in its ability to normalize endocrine functioning. Researchers Green, Campbell, and David indicate that psychosocial dwarfs typically show dramatically accelerated rates of emotional and physical growth when they are removed from a loveless environment and placed in a less stressful and emotionally positive environment.

Lastly, malnutrition should be ruled out as a major contributory cause. Malnutrition is certainly a major causal variable in retarded growth, so this must be ruled out in psychosocial dwarfism. Few psychosocial dwarfs are underweight for their height. The abruptness and magnitude of growth spurts upon admission to the hospital, and the equally abrupt cessation of growth upon discharge if returned to the home of origin, have convinced researchers that psychosocial deprivation, and not malnutrition, is the crucial variable. Taken together, these four criteria confirm a diagnosis of psychosocial dwarfism in cases where hypopituitary dwarfism has been ruled out.

The precise endocrinal mechanisms leading to psychosocial dwarfism are less clear than is its origin in love deprivation. Clearly the fear, anxiety, and depression wrought by parental hostility, maltreatment, and rejection somehow inhibit the secretion of pituitary hormones, including the growth hormone, in the same way that an observable organic pathology does. Some medical researchers have hypothesized that an emotionally deprived environment results in abnormal sleep patterns.[11] Specifically, such an environment leads to a sleep pattern that alternates between insomnia and stupor. The regulated release of growth hormones (somatotrophin), which increase sharply during the early hours of sleep, requires normal sleep patterns. The outward manifestations of love—tactile stimulation and cuddling—lead to muscular relaxation and a sense of security (the brain's endorphins at work). Muscular relaxation and a warm feeling that "all is right with the world" is a prerequisite for healthy sleep. Muscular rigidity and anxiety, as we all know, is inimical to a good night's sleep. In early childhood, the lack of a good night's sleep can evidently lead to less than adequate amounts of growth hormones and ultimately to the agonies of being exceptionally short in a world that values tallness.

Summing up their review of the literature on psychosocial dwarfism, Wayne Green and his colleagues speculate that the processes that translate love deprivation into psychosocial dwarfism proceed something like this. The child perceives it is not loved. This perception is relayed to the hypothalamus, where the deprivation is emotionally experienced. The emotional experience of not being loved leads to sleeping difficulties, which upsets the normal cortisone/endorphin balance. Due to this imbalance, hypothalamic releasing factors are inhibited when sleep does occur. Although Green and his coworkers acknowledge that the precise mechanisms are far from clear, they conclude: "The presence of a strong emotionally positive relationship may enhance physical growth more than has previously been suspected." [12] Another prominent researcher in this area writes similarly: "Deprivation dwarfism is a concrete example—an 'experiment of nature,' so to speak—that demonstrates the delicacy, complexity and crucial importance of infant-parent interaction." [13]

CARDIOVASCULAR DISEASE

Heart disease is still the number-one killer of adults in the United States. Hypertension, or high blood pressure, is a major precursor of many of the other heart diseases, such as coronary artery disease, myocardial infarction, chronic renal failure, strokes, and so on. Essential, ideopathic, and primary hypertension are the various terms applied to hypertension when an observable pathophysiological cause cannot be identified. Approximately 80 per cent of hypertensive cases fall into this category. [14]

The role of love in the exploration of heart disease should satisfy the romantics among us, since poets have long written about "broken hearts" resulting from the loss of loved ones. Some hard-nosed scientists are also beginning to see the importance of the fracture or disruption of human relationships on the heart. In fact, James Lynch, scientific director of the Psychosomatic Clinic at the School of Medicine at the University of Maryland, entitled a 1977 book *The Broken Heart: The Medical Consequences of Loneliness*. In this book, Lynch states that: "Growing numbers of physicians now recognize that the health of the human heart depends not only on such factors as genetics, diet, and exercise, but also to a large extent on the social and emotional health of the individual." [15]

Underlying much of the research into ideopathic hypertension is Hans

Selye's theory of stress. Simply put, Selye's theory states that various psychosocial experiences with an emotional content have the effect of generating neuroendocrinal reactions that adversely affect the cardiovascular system.[16] To illustrate the physiology of the stress process: suppose that an immigrant's country of origin is the butt of some negative remarks as he sits with his coworkers at lunch. His cerebral cortex will perceive the remarks as insulting and derogatory. His perceptions will be communicated to the limbic system, arousing negative feelings such as anger and embarrassment. These limbic-system feelings influence the hypothalamus to communicate with the autonomic nervous system, resulting in the secretion of the somatic activating hormones epinepherine and norepinepherine from the adrenal glands. These are the so-called "fight or flight" hormones that prepare our bodies to more efficiently confront or to flee from a challenge. If the result of experiencing stressful stimuli is fight or flight, the stress hormones are rapidly metabolized by the lipoprotein lipase enzyme after they have accomplished their task.

In modern society where stressors are perhaps more frequent, if not as immediately threatening as those facing our ancestors, the response is likely to be far less energetic. Our insulted alien is not too likely to punch his country's detractors in the nose or to flee the lunchroom. He is much more likely to "sit and seethe" than to fight or flee. Such a response is socially acceptable, but it does not activate enzymes to restore hormonal balance. If he has experiences such as this fairly often, his biological legacy will be an unhealthy accumulation of unconsumed fatty lipids in his blood stream. One of the outcomes of this accumulation is elevated blood pressure.

One of the most useful instruments in evaluating the amount of stress that an individual experiences is the Holmes-Rahe Life Change Scale. This instrument is an attempt to quantify the degree of stress an individual experiences in a year in response to major life changes. Each life change is assigned a numerical score according to how stressful the change is determined to be. According to this scale, the death of a spouse is assigned the maximum score of 100. The next three highest scores are all assigned to other disruptions of interpersonal relationships (divorce, marital separation, and death of a close family member). A large number of subsequent studies have found that the higher a person's life change score—and hence his or her stressful experiences—the higher the probability of the occurrence of many types of diseases, particularly cardiovascular diseases.[17]

My own research in this area has been on the effects of the twin processes of immigration and assimilation on blood-pressure levels.[18] There are surely few more profound and comprehensive life changes that an individual can undergo than moving to alien shores. Immigration changes almost everything, especially if one's sources of love and security are left behind in the native country. Hippocrates noted many centuries ago that whenever people migrated into new social settings, "a terrible perturbation always followed." A whole library of studies has documented the fact that immigrants have significantly higher rates of many types of chronic diseases and psychiatric problems than host nationals, regardless of the country of origin or country of settlement. Careful analyses have shown that generally these high rates are not attributable to preexisting symptoms but rather to the stresses and strains of the immigration experience.[19]

In a study conducted by myself and Patricia Walsh, it was found that social support was second only to age in explaining variation in blood-pressure levels among a sample of 137 immigrants from 17 different countries. Social support is a powerful adaptive mechanism in primate evolution. Social support was conceived of in our study as a network of valued others who provide the immigrant with emotional sustenance that acts as a buttress to the stresses of adjusting to a new culture. Those immigrants who were secure in the knowledge that they had valued others upon whom they could lean when necessary, and who appreciated, respected, and cared for them had significantly lower blood-pressure levels than those immigrants who lacked such a network. The relationship between social support and blood-pressure levels held true after adjusting for the effects of other variables known to influence blood-pressure levels such as age, sex, diet, exercise, and smoking habits, as well as income and educational levels and occupational status.[20]

An earlier study conducted by Sam Sisca, Patricia Walsh, and myself among faculty, staff, and students at the University of Toledo found that love deprivation was significantly and positively related to elevated blood-pressure levels (the greater the love deprivation the higher the blood pressure). Love deprivation was measured by two questionnaire scales that tapped each person's subjective perceptions of the degree to which he or she felt loved or unloved. The relationship between love deprivation and blood-pressure levels was particularly strong among older subjects, but less so among younger subjects. Since the accumulation of fatty lipids in the blood requires the passage of time to show up as elevated blood pressure, the fact that older respondents manifested more clearly the effects of love deprivation than did younger respondents should not surprise us. The significant relationship between love deprivation and blood pressure levels was independent of age and weight. In other words, after the ravages of age and excess weight on the cardiovascular system had been accounted for, love deprivation exerted its own independent toll on the system.[21]

The therapeutic action of social support must be balanced against the capacity of those needing the support to form or integrate himself or herself into a network of supportive others. Some people can move with ease and assurance into new social networks, others with difficulty, and some hardly at all. Our review of Harlow's work showed the importance of early bonding on the ability to establish subsequent bonds. The amount and quality of support experienced at any given time, then, would appear to be to a large extent contingent on the quality of the individual's early bonding.

A study conducted by Joseph Flaherty and Judith Richmond lends credence to this supposition. They studied 211 first-year medical students at the University of Illinois Medical School and found a significant correlation between the quality of their subjects' early relationships with their fathers and mothers (especially with their mothers) and the quality of their current support systems. The better the quality of their early relationship with their parents, the better and more widely diffused were their adult relationships.[22]

What about the possible effects of love in the recovery process for those already afflicted by cardiovascular problems? After reviewing a wide range of literature attesting that poor interpersonal relations can produce dangerous or even lethal cardiac changes, James Lynch states that the evidence is strong that the reverse is also true. "If the lack of human love or the memory of earlier traumas can disturb the heart, then just as clearly the presence of human love may serve as a powerful therapeutic force, helping the heart to restore itself."[23]

It has been shown under laboratory conditions that tactile stimulation prevents hardening of the arteries among dogs. Drescher and Gantt subjected a number of dogs to repeated painful electric shocks. They found that petting animals after they had received the shocks reduced the dogs' increased heart rates that normally accompany electric shocks. Contact comfort mitigated the harmful effects of stress for the experimental animals by dampening the body's fight-or-flight response to threatening stimuli through tactile assurances of love and security. The dampening of the stress response meant lower levels of fatty lipids in the bloodstream. Control animals who received the same shocks but who were not "loved up" afterwards did have hardening of their arteries from the accumulation of stress-induced lipids.[24]

Touching, stroking, and holding have similarly been shown to be beneficial in reducing heart rate in human beings in a number of studies. A recent study by Vincent Drescher and his colleagues at Johns Hopkins School of Medicine showed a significant reduction in heart rate following an aversive stimulus after being touched on the wrist. Subjects in this experiment were subjected to painful ice-water stimulation under two conditions. In one situation the experimenters held the wrist of the subjects while their hands were immersed in the ice water, and in the other the subjects' hands were not held. Average heartbeat rates were significantly lower in the first experimental situation. More importantly for our purposes is the explanation offered by the researchers for their finding: "Our speculation is that touching represents a potent primitive mechanism for establishing an emotional attachment between mother and infant which persists into adulthood."[25]

Perhaps the most dramatic study of the effect of human relationships on the heart was carried out recently by William Knaus and his colleagues at the George Washington University School of Medicine. The study involved 5,030 intensive care unit (ICU) patients (many of whom were cardiac patients) in a variety of hospitals across the United States during a five-year period. The researchers set out to find out what variable was the single most important one in terms of its impact on the survival of ICU patients. They examined many variables, such as the prestige of the hospital, technological sophistication, levels of professional expertise of physicians and nurses, level of research funding, and patient/caregiver ratio. To their expressed surprise, none of these variables turned out to be the crucial one. The crucial variable was the quality of the relationships existing between caregivers and patients. The hospitals in which nurses were allowed to interact with patients at an emotional level—talking, reassuring, and holding patients—were the hospitals with the best ICU survival rates.[26]

This study shows that all the buzzing and clicking of expensive monitoring equipment and the extensive knowledge of armies of MDs cannot match the more wondrous life-giving power of human love. It is a great pity that the type of human care exposed in this study—what nurses call primary-level nursing—is falling afoul of cost-containment practices in modern hospitals. Hospital administrators understand and can justify the purchase of wondrous technological equipment, but they do not seem to be able to understand or justify the financial cost of the practice of loving, primary-care nursing.

LOVE AND IMMUNOLOGY

Imagine you are peacefully fishing by a stream, only dimly aware of the throbbing in your thumb where you stuck yourself with a dirty fishhook 30 minutes ago. Unknown to you, a virus has entered your bloodstream via your wound. As it moves swiftly through the veins and arteries carrying blood throughout your body, a life and death drama is taking place. If the virus is allowed to live and multiply, you will soon be as dead as the fish in your basket. Doing its best to see that no such fate befalls you is a vast army of chemical creatures who collectively comprise your immunological system.

The body's immunological system is a fascinating one with a complexity approaching that of the brain itself. Unlike other body systems such as the central nervous, cardiovascular, and digestive systems, the immunological system exists as distinct subsystems scattered throughout the body. We often use the analogy of machines, pumps, and pipes to describe the physically connected cardiovascular system. The immunological system is more analogous to a society of separate but interrelated families. It is a society of well-knit subsystems that is constantly on a war footing. Its many enemies (antigens) include invading bacteria, viruses, pollens, and genetically unrelated human fluids and tissue. Unfortunately, like a Central American army, it sometimes revolts and attacks its own host body. When it runs amok it produces a number of *autoimmune diseases* such as rheumatic fever, some kinds of anemias, rheumatoid arthritis, allergies, multiple sclerosis, and deadly cancers.

Since chemical foreign substances can invade the body at many different sites, nature wisely dispersed the immune system throughout the body. The lymphocytes, the masterminds of the immune system, come in two varieties: T-lymphocytes, which are under the influence of the thymus, and B-lymphocytes, formed in the lymph nodes scattered throughout the body. Other components of the immune system such as natural killer cells, granulocytes, and complement proteins are manufactured in the bone marrow and the liver. These chemical defenders destroy invaders by several different mechanisms. For instance, lymphocytes work in concert with antibodies to combat viral infections; the lymphocytes cause cells containing viruses to disintegrate, and the free-floating viruses are then destroyed by circulating antibodies.

Most relevant for our discussion is the discovery that *receptors* for a variety of chemical messengers—sex hormones, endorphins, and cathecholamines—have been discovered on the surface of lymphocytes.[27] This discovery may have profound implications for a mind-body connection more intimate than heretofore considered. It strongly suggests that since there are receptors for neuroendocrines, neurotransmitters, and neuropeptides on lymphocytes, these brain chemicals must influence their activity in terms of where to go and what to do.

Perhaps even more surprising is the discovery that *macrophages* themselves release neuropeptides. Macrophages ("big eaters") are giant, circulating white blood cells. Under the microscope, macrophages look like a nightmare from some science-fiction movie. They are slimy, slithery, scavenging blobs, but they are the "shock troops" of the immune system. They reach out and gobble up cells damaged by foreign invaders and release protein fragments from the invaders that are then recognized and attacked by T-cells. The ability of macrophages to release neuropeptides leads some to speculate that macrophages may be free-floating nerve cells able to engage in two-way communication with the brain either directly or via hormones.

The discovery of chemical links to the brain may be the key to explaining how lymphocytes "remember" encounters with invading organisms so that they can mount a stronger and more speedy attack in future encounters. The brain encodes chemical memories of our conscious day-to-day life experiences so that we can more efficiently deal with similar experiences in the future. The intriguing discovery of receptors for neurotransmitters on lymphocytes makes for the possibility that both memory processes (the conscious and the immunological "unconscious" processes) are intimately linked. Since the brain can apparently "talk" with the immune system, it is hardly far-fetched to assume that one's emotional state can influence one's immunological system for better or for worse.

A new breed of adventurous scientists calling themselves *psychoneuroimmunologists* have begun to investigate the possibility that "real" organic diseases can be linked to how we feel and think about ourselves and our relationships. These scientists have published a large number of papers showing that loneliness, loss, bereavement, and other life stresses are associated with sometimes dramatic *decreases* in immune-system functioning, leaving us susceptible to a wide range of diseases. Their growing ability to delineate the precise mechanisms linking our experiences and how we relate emotionally to them have given a new respectability to holistic medicine. They have gone beyond the "psychobabble" of earlier holistic theorists by opening the "black box" to discover the hows and whys of the mind-body, or perhaps more correctly, the brain-body, relationship.

One of the pioneering studies in psychoneuroimmunology conducted by R. W. Bartop and his colleagues found significantly lower levels of T-lymphocytes circulating in the systems of 26 bereaved spouses in comparison to 26 control subjects. Another study found that natural killer-cell activity was significantly different among women, depending on how depressed and lonely they were. Natural killer-cells are another kind of lymphocyte that have the ability to recognize and attack harmful and malignant cells without having previously encountered them. The same researchers also found an increase in the ratio of T-suppressor to T-helper cells as loneliness and depression became more severe.[28] T-helper cells are the field commanders of the immune system. They do not themselves attack the invaders, but they are experts in identifying their chemical structure. Upon recognizing a foreign substance, they rush to recruit and activate the killer T-cells and guide their activity. T-suppressor cells, on the other hand, down-regulate the production of antibodies and are associated with an increase in *autoantibodies* that attack the host body.

Yet another study among the lonely and loveless by Kiecolt-Glasser and her associates found that "high loneliness" subjects showed significantly lower levels of natural killer-cell activity and significantly elevated levels of cortisol than "low loneliness" subjects. Cortisol is a stress-related hormone that has the effect of suppressing the immune system.[29] These and many other studies tend to show that a lack of connectedness with other people leaves victims both more prone to stress-related diseases and less able to effectively combat autoimmune diseases, as well as invading pathogenetic substances.

From the Harlow monkey studies and other related animal and human studies, we know that one of the cruelest and most deleterious events that young primates can suffer is separation from their mothers. We have also seen how this experience leaves its imprint on the very *structure and function of the brain*, and how it often leads to behavioral aberrations. It is not surprising to discover that psychoneuroimmunologists have also explored the effects of maternal-love deprivation on the immune system. One such piece of research studied lymphocyte activity in mothers and infant monkeys during and after a 14-day separation. The researchers found a significant decrease in lymphocyte activity among the infant monkeys relative to pre-separation baseline levels. Lymphocyte activity returned to baseline levels following mother/infant reunion. The infants' mothers showed a similar decrease in lymphocyte activity during separation and a similar return to baseline levels upon reunion.[30]

Other recent studies have shown that immune-system-suppressing cortisol is significantly elevated among infant monkeys separated from their mothers. If infants are placed in adjacent cages to the mother, allowing visual and auditory, but no tactile access, cortisol levels are elevated, but not by as much as they are when the monkeys are totally isolated. Totally isolated monkeys, after a period of severe agitation, slip into deep depression and adopt freezing postures.[31] It is plain from the psychoneuroimmunology literature that the lack of love leaves us open to disease just as its presence protects and preserves health. As psychoneuroimmunologist Paul Pearsall put it, "To love and be loved is perhaps the single most important result of being healthy. When we fail to love, our supersystem [the immune system] is jeopardized."[32]

MULTIPLE SCLEROSIS

Multiple sclerosis (MS) is a progressive disease of the central nervous system. Symptoms are characterized by exacerbations and remissions in some cases, while in others they are chronic and progressive. While multiple sclerosis is not usually fatal, it can be seriously disabling both physically and psychologically.

The precise cause of MS is not known. A slow-acting virus and/or autoimmunity are currently the most favored explanations. In MS the body's own immune system attacks, at many locations, the myelin sheath around the axons, possibly because of the presence of a virus, leaving multiple scars (scleroses). The destruction of the myelin sheath causes interruptions and distortions of nerve impulses. The symptoms of the disease vary greatly according to the site of the sclerotic lesions. Lesions in the spinal cord produce such symptoms as loss of sensation in the limbs, weakness, loss of fine motor coordination, partial paralysis, and bowel and bladder dysfunction. Lesions in the cerebellum lead to vision, speech, and gag-reflex problems. Usually occurring later in the progression of the disease are lesions of the cerebrum. Lesions here affect the patient's thinking and memory patterns.

In chapter 3 we saw that females were less at risk than males for a large number of developmental disorders because of the finer integration of the two hemispheres of the female brain. Females are also better protected immunologically than males. The female hormone, estrogen, has the effect of enhancing the activity of T-cells while the male hormone, testosterone, has a depressing effect on T-cell activity. Males suffering from some kinds of cancers are often therapeutically castrated or given estrogen to counteract the effects of testosterone. The reason for this is that testosterone is an anabolic steroid that promotes tissue growth, including, however, the growth of cancerous tissue. Estrogen, on the other hand, is catabolic. It helps to break down proteins and helps promote the storage of fat. The enhanced immunological protection of the female is nature's way of recognizing that females are more valuable to the species than males. Unfortunately, women pay a price for their more efficient immune systems in the form of greater susceptibility to autoimmune diseases compared to males. Multiple sclerosis is one of the autoimmune diseases that disproportionately affects women, at a rate of about 2 to 1.

Stress is not known to be a major causal variable in multiple sclerosis, as is the case with cardiovascular diseases; however, there is a good deal of evidence to suggest that stressful events may hasten the onset of the disease among those predisposed and/or exacerbate symptoms among diagnosed patients. Many theories have been advanced regarding the causes of MS by virologists and other scientists. Among the studies reporting emotionally stressful experiences prior to the onset of MS, one found that 35 out of 40 (87.5 percent) had such experiences, and another found exactly the same percentage experiencing stress prior to onset (28 of 32 patients).[33] Yet another study found a significant difference between 100 MS patients and 100 control subjects in the number of emotionally stressful events for the two-year period prior to onset of the disease.[34] Thus, while emotional stress may or may not be a predisposing cause, these studies are highly suggestive of the notion that such stress (almost always of an interpersonal nature) can hasten and exacerbate the symptoms of the disease.

When I discussed cardiovascular disease, we saw how the "fight or flight" stress response has been selected into our evolutionary physiological repertoire because it confers survival benefits by preparing the body for vigorous action. It was also pointed out that, in our less immediately life-threatening and more sedentary environments, the fight or flight response more often than not works to our cardiovascular system's disadvantage. With multiple sclerosis we may be witnessing another example of an evolutionary benefit turning traitor on us. It has been pointed out that the experience of stress prompts the adrenal glands to pump out cortisol, which suppresses the immune system.

Why would suppression of the immune system be selected by evolution as beneficial? Imagine a hominid ancestor being severely wounded while hunting (or being hunted) or in a skirmish with other hominids. An over-zealous, "pumped-up" immune system might well attack healthy tissue, as it sometimes does today while attacking damaged tissue and foreign matter. Cortisol, acting like a battlewise general, would in effect be restraining the enthusiasm of the immune system by instructing it to wait for the opportune time to attack. This delaying tactic would do no harm, because it takes a while for infection to set in. With the real enemy correctly identified and differentiated from the healthy tissue, cortisol levels gradually fall as stress is less immediately experienced and the immune system is released to do battle.

Modern stresses are less immediately life-threatening and severe, but possibly more protracted. What was a beneficial response to the stressors of our prehistoric ancestors over their brief lifespan may be harmful to modern humans over our much longer lifespan. The typical age of onset for multiple sclerosis (20 to 40 years of age, with a peak onset at 33) generally exceeds the prehistoric hominid lifespan. What I am speculating is that a series of stressful responses over a long period of time among people somehow predisposed to multiple sclerosis may weaken their immune systems due to frequent cortisol-induced suppressions. This "weakening" may be in the form of rendering the immune system incapable of discrim-inating between healthy myelin tissue and a foreign body, such as a slow-acting virus.

There is no preventative or cure for MS; the best thing we can do for MS patients is to help them to cope with this debilitating disease. Researchers Matson and Brooks found a positive self-image to be the best predictor of adjustment to MS.[35] The self-image, or self-esteem, is that measure each of us has in our "mind's eye" about our worth and dignity as human beings. If that measure of our worth is strong we are better able to cope with the obstacles life puts in our way. If we are confronted with such a heavy cross that our self-image is insulted and damaged, we tend to lose confidence in ourselves, to become fearful, and to withdraw. The embarrassing symptoms of MS can result in a damaged and insulted self-image, which may lead to social isolation of the patient. But the effects on self-esteem wrought by the symptoms of MS can be counteracted by warm interpersonal relationships with caring others.

William Glasser has asserted that all human beings have two basic psychological needs: the need to love and be loved, and the need to feel worthwhile.[36] While these needs appear to be separate, they are intimately connected. A person who loves and is loved will feel worthwhile, and a person who feels worthwhile is usually one who loves and is loved. Of course, to give and to receive love, and hence to feel worthwhile, we have to be involved with others. Being involved with others in a positive way has been shown to reduce depression levels among MS patients, and even remission of symptoms has been indicated by patients who report improved interpersonal relationships.[37]

Because one of my dearest friends has MS and because my wife is the MS resource specialist at the Boise VA hospital, I have an active interest in MS research. Patricia Walsh and I recently completed a research project to test the hypothesis that self-esteem is positively related to loving human relationships among MS patients. Our sample consisted of 135 patients residing in southwestern Idaho. Among the significant correlations that came out of the study, we found that self-esteem was positively related to the amount of love patients perceived themselves as receiving, the amount of contact the patient had with his or her family, and membership in a MS support group. On the other hand, self-esteem was negatively related to the degree of social isolation. We also looked at the effects of degree of infirmity, attitude toward the disease, number of years since diagnosis, and a number of other variables, on self-esteem. None of these variables came anywhere near love in terms of their effect on self-esteem levels.[38]

We also found a significant relationship between the amount of love a patient was receiving and the severity of MS symptoms. We cannot say definitely that a lack of love and support, and the stress implied by such a lack, has a direct causal effect on severity of symptomology. It is just as likely that the severity of symptoms affected the level of love and support experienced because of patient withdrawal. But it is suggestive to note that among the divorced members of our sample, 86 per cent were divorced after the onset of MS and that this group reported receiving less love and support than those divorced prior to onset of symptoms or the still married. Nevertheless, our study showed rather conclusively that those MS patients who are surrounded by caring others gather unto themselves the inner strength, as provided by high self-esteem, to cope with this pernicious disease.

We can conclude from the numerous studies presented in this chapter that the role of love in the prevention of "real" organic illness, as well as its ability to help those who are afflicted, is becoming more and more recognized by modern science. Any physician or nurse will tell you that in their care of the sick it is the individual who is well-loved, happy, and contented with life—all other things being equal—who has the best chance of a speedy recovery. Expressions of love and affection are the greatest medicines we can give one another. Man or woman, young or old, whatever our race, creed, or ethnicity, we need to know that we are loved and are important to somebody.

Four hundred years before the birth of Jesus, Hippocrates emphasized the importance of the "laying on of hands." How very modern was his recognition that touch conveys concern and reassurances to patients and turns an anatomical technician into a physician: "for where there is love of man, there is also love of the art. For some patients, though conscious that their condition is perilous, recover their health simply through their contentment with the goodness of the physician."

NOTES

1. St. Augustine quoted in J. Barnaby, *Amor Dei, A Study of the Religion of St. Augustine* (London, Hodder and Stoughton, 1938), p. 95.

2. Howard Whitman, "The Amazing New Science of Love," *Journal of Lifetime Living* (August 1955): p. 76.

3. World Health Organization's definition of health quoted in M. Terris, "Approaches to the Epidemiology of Health, "*American Journal of Public Health* 65 (1973): p. 1037.

4. Sigmund Freud, "On Narcissism," in *Collected Papers of Sigmund Freud*, vol. 4 (New York: International Psychoanalytic Press, 1924), p. 42.

5. René Spitz, "Hospitalism," in *The Psychoanalytic Study of the Child* (International Universities Press, 1945).

6. Harold Skeels, "Adult Status of Children with Contrasting Early Life Experiences," *Monographs of the Society for Research in Child Development* (1966).

7. Studies of "socio-emotional deprivation" cited in Ashley Montagu, "A Scientist Looks at Love," *Phi Beta Kappan* 51 (1970): pp. 463–467.

8. Michael Young, *The Rise of the Meritocracy* (Middlesex, England: Penguin, 1975), p. 30.

9. G. Powell, J. Brasel, and R. Blizzard, "Emotional Deprivation and Growth Retardation Simulating Ideopathic Hypopituitarism. I. Clinical Evaluation of the Syndrome," *New England Journal of Medicine* 276 (1967a): pp. 1271–1278. G. Pow-

ell, S. Raiti, and R. Blizzard, "Emotional Deprivation and Growth Retardation Simulating Ideopathic Hypopituitarism. II. Endocrinologic Evaluation of the Syndrome," *New England Journal of Medicine* 276 (1967b): pp. 1279–1283.

10. M. Bouras, H. Bourneuf, and G. Raimbault, "La relation mere-enfant dans le nanism dit d'origine psycho-social," *Archives Francaises de Pediatric* 39 (1982): pp. 263–265.

11. R. Patton and L. Gardner, "Deprivation Dwarfism (Psycho-Social Deprivation): Disordered Family Environment as a Cause of So-Called Ideopathic Hypopituitarism," in *Endocrine and Genetic Diseases of Childhood and Adolescence*, ed. L. Gardner (Philadelphia: W. B. Saunders, 1975).

12. W. Green, M. Campbell, and R. David, "Psychosocial Dwarfism: A Critical Review of the Evidence," *Journal of the American Academy of Child Psychiatry* (1984): p. 46.

13. L. Gardner, "Deprivation Dwarfism," in *The Nature and Nurture of Behavior: Developmental Psychobiology* (readings from *Scientific American*), ed. W. Greenough (San Francisco: W. H. Freeman, 1973), p. 107.

14. W. Phipps, B. Long, and N. Woods, *Medical Surgical Nursing* (St. Louis: C. V. Mosby, 1983), p. 1177.

15. James Lynch, *The Broken Heart: The Medical Consequences of Loneliness* (New York: Basic Books, 1977), p. 13.

16. Hans Selye, "The Evolution of the Stress Concept," *American Journal of Cardiology* 26 (1970): pp. 289–299.

17. T. Holmes and R. Rahe "The Social Readjustment Rating Scale," *Journal of Psychosomatic Research* 11 (1967): pp. 213–218.

18. Anthony Walsh and Patricia Walsh, "Social Support, Assimilation, and Biological Effective Blood Pressure Levels," *International Migration Review* 21 (1987): pp. 577–591. Anthony Walsh, "The Prophylactic Effect of Religion on Blood Pressure Levels among a Sample of Immigrants," *Social Science and Medicine* 148 (1980): pp. 59–63. Sam Sisca, Anthony Walsh, and Patricia Walsh, "Love Deprivation and Blood Pressure Levels among a College Population: A Preliminary Investigation," *Psychology* 22 (1985): pp. 63–70.

19. See D. Hull, "Migration, Adaptation, and Illness: A Review," *Social Science and Medicine* 13a (1979): pp. 25–36, for a review.

20. Anthony and Patricia Walsh, "Social Support."

21. Sam Sisca, Anthony Walsh, and Patricia Walsh, "Love Deprivation."

22. Joseph Flaherty and Judith Richmond, "Effects of Childhood Relationships on the Adult's Capacity to Form Social Supports," *American Journal of Psychiatry* 143 (1986): pp. 851–855.

23. James Lynch, *The Broken Heart*, p. 113.

24. V. Dreschner and W. Gantt, "Tactile Stimulation of Several Body Areas (Effect of Person)," *Pavlovian Journal of Biological Sciences* 14 (1979): p. 2.

25. V. Dreschner, W. Whitehead, E. Morrill-Corbin, and F. Cataldo, "Physiological and Subjective Reactions to Being Touched," *Psychophysiology* 22 (1985): p. 99.

26. William Knaus study cited in D. Holtzman, "Intensive Care Nurses: A Vital Sign, "*Insight* 1 (1986): p. 56.

27. R. Ornstein and D. Sobel, "The Healing Brain," *Psychology Today* (March 1987): pp. 48–52. R. Adler and N. Cohen, "CNS-Immune System Interactions: Conditioning Phenomena," *The Behavioral and Brain Sciences* 8 (1985): p. 380.

28. R. Bartop, L. Lazarus, E. Luckhurst, L. Kiloh, and R. Penny, "Depressed Lymphocyte Function after Bereavement," *Lancet* 1 (1977): pp. 834–836.

29. J. Kiecolt-Glasser, D. Ricker, J. George, C. Messick, C. Speicher, W. Garner, and R. Glasser, "Urinary Cortisol Levels, Cellular Immunocompetency, and Loneliness in Psychiatric Inpatients," *Psychosomatic Medicine* 46 (1984): pp. 15–23.

30. E. Tecoma and L. Huey, "Minireview: Psychic Distress and the Immune Response," *Life Sciences* 36 (1985): pp. 1799–1812.

31. F. Bayart, K. Hayashi, K. Faull, J. Barchas, and S. Levine, "Influence of Maternal Proximity on Behavioral and Physiological Responses to Separation in Infant Rhesus Monkeys (Macaca mulatta)," *Behavioral Neuroscience* 104 (1990): pp. 98–107.

32. Paul Pearsall, *Superimmunity* (New York: Fawcett, 1987), p. 287.

33. G. Philippoulos, E. Wittkower, and E. Cousineau, "The Etiological Significance of Emotional Factors in Onset and Exacerbations of Multiple Sclerosis," *Psychosomatic Medicine* 20 (1958): pp. 458–474.

34. V. Mei-tel, M. Meyerowitz, and G. Engel, "The Role of Psychological Process in a Somatic Disorder: Multiple Sclerosis," *Psychosomatic Medicine* 32 (1970): pp. 67–85.

35. R. Matson, R. and N. Brooks, "Adjusting to Multiple Sclerosis: An Exploratory Study," *Social Science and Medicine* 11 (1977): pp. 245–250.

36. William Glasser, *Reality Therapy: A New Approach to Psychiatry* (New York: Harper & Row, 1975), p. 11.

37. G. McIvor, M. Riklan, and M. Reznikoff, "Depression in Multiple Sclerosis Patients as a Function of Length and Severity of Illness, Age, Remissions, and Perceived Social Support," *Journal of Clinical Psychology* 40 (1984): pp. 1028–1033. S. Warren, S. Greenhill, and K. Warren. "Emotional Stress and the Development of Multiple Sclerosis: Case Control Evidence of a Relationship," *Journal of Chronic Disease* 35 (1982): pp. 821–831.

38. Anthony Walsh and Patricia Walsh, "Love, Self-Esteem, and Multiple Sclerosis," *Social Science and Medicine* 29 (1989): pp. 793–798.

5

Mental Health and Illness

He whom love touches not walks in darkness.—Plato

A distinguished British physician once wrote: "By far the most significant discovery of mental science is the power of love to protect and restore the mind."[1] Similarly, American psychoanalyst Reuben Fine has asserted that, at bottom, the psychoanalytic explanation of mental illness is a simple equation: love equals mental health, lovelessness equals mental illness.[2] Across the wide spectrum of mental-health professions we hear the same thing. Whether they call themselves psychoanalysts, client-centered therapists, reality therapists, transactional analysts, rational-emotive therapists, or even behaviorists, we hear the same equation being preached: we must love and be loved if we are to be mentally wholesome beings.[3] Without love, life is a lonely, barren treadmill, devoid of all joy and creativity. One can either leave the treadmill by discovering the power of love, or one can withdraw into mental illness, crime, substance abuse, or completely, into the oblivion of suicide.

SCHIZOPHRENIA

Schizophrenia may be the most widespread of the psychotic disorders. Schizophrenia is a very broad term covering a wide variety of disorders with varying degrees of malignancy. Schizophrenics are identified emotionally and behaviorally by the degree to which they exhibit the so-called "four A's: *autism* (living in a subjective fantasy world), *ambivalence* (having simultaneous conflicting feelings), inappropriate *affect* (feelings and emotions incongruent with the situation), and *associations* that are loose (incongruent connections between sets of experiences and ideas).

There are four "classical" subtypes of schizophrenia defined by the kinds of symptoms exhibited. The first subtype, *hebephrenia*, most closely conforms to popular notions of insanity. The hebephrenic exhibits incoherent and bi-

zarre behavior, and is subject to sudden fits of laughing, crying, and bab-
bling. The second type, *catatonia*, often involves the patient maintaining
immobility in weird positions for long periods of time in a so-called catatonic stupor. Occasionally he or she will go to the opposite extreme of catatonic excitement, becoming dangerous at such times to self and to others.

The *paranoid schizophrenic* is possessed of an elaborate set of delusions
involving persecution or grandeur. Such individuals are extremely tense and
suspicious at all times, but do not usually behave in ways that too closely
resemble stereotypes of "madness." The final subtype is the *simple
schizophrenic*. Rather than exhibiting dramatic symptoms of the affliction,
the simple schizophrenic is identified more by his or her aimless, shallow,
transient, and alienated lifestyle.

There is considerable overlap in the symptoms of the four subtypes,
with a hebephrenic sometimes acting like a catatonic, and a simple schizophrenic occasionally acting like a paranoid, and so on. Some clinicians and
researchers have suggested that a simpler classification system, one emphasizing the route to schizophrenia rather than its behavioral symptoms, might
be more useful. The terms *process* and *reactive* schizophrenia are gaining
prominence as alternatives to the classical subtypes. Process schizophrenia
is a diagnostic term applied to individuals who slowly deteriorate into full-
blown schizophrenia over a long period of time. Such individuals show early
in childhood a marked inability to function normally, to make friends, to
handle schoolwork, and to behave acceptably. Reactive schizophrenics do
not show early histories of social and psychological maladjustment. Their
decent into schizophrenia is sudden, marked by an acutely stressful experience. As might be expected, the prognosis for improvement of functioning is much better for reactive schizophrenics than for process schizophrenia.

Up until quite recently, some otherwise clever behavioral scientists made
reputations by denying the existence of a definable set of symptoms we could
collectively call schizophrenia. Mental illness was called a "myth," which disguised moral conflicts between those labeled mentally ill and those with the
social power to impose the label.[4] We are rarely exposed to such denials
these days, because we can now actually "see" schizophrenia using computer-
imaging techniques in the same way that a physician sees a broken bone on
an X-ray. The tool enabling us to do this is a scanning technique known
as positron emission transaxial tomography (PETT). The PETT-scan is similar
to the more familiar CAT-scan. The difference is that CAT-scans reveal
information about brain *structure* only, while PETT-scans reveal information
about brain *functioning*, as well as structure. Biochemical "maps" of neurometabolism are achieved by the PETT-scan when the patient is injected
with radioactive glucose isotopes. The radioactive glucose is taken up by the
brain, and radiation is emitted in those parts that are most active. The radia-

tion is collected by detectors surrounding the brain and displayed on a screen. The computer images projected by a schizophrenic's brain are radically different from those projected by a mentally normal person's brain.[5] PETT-scans also allow psychiatrists to view the ventricles (communicating cavities) of the brain. Typically, schizophrenics have ventricles that are about twice the normal size.

We now know that schizophrenia is associated with definite physical malfunctions of the brain and that it is not simply a mentalistic or a "social power differential" phenomenon as some doctors once claimed. Perhaps we should cease to make any distinctions at all between somatic and psychological illness. After all, it's not the heart that decides that the loss of a loved one is too much to bear, nor is it the ulcerated stomach that perceives an experience as stressful any more than a disembodied mind decides to withdraw into the abyss of schizophrenia. It is the brain that makes those decisions, the brain that knows, that feels, and that responds.

Schizophrenia afflicts both sexes, but it afflicts males more seriously. Pierre Flor-Henry, one of the leading researchers in brain hemisphericity, tells us that not only is schizophrenia more deadly and more chronic in the male than in the female, but that among people under the age of 35 there is an overwhelming excess of male schizophrenics. Flor-Henry views schizophrenia as a syndrome related to dysfunction of the dominant left hemisphere of the brain, particularly of the left limbic system regions. The left hemisphere is more vulnerable to dysfunction than the right because it is at the same time larger and less well-irrigated.[6]

In chapter 3 we said that males are less secure in the verbal left-hemisphere than females and more secure in the visual-spatial right hemisphere, although the left is the dominant hemisphere in both sexes. Major stressful events are experienced differently by males and females because of this sex-based brain difference. Evidence from brain researchers in many countries indicates that negative feelings tend to be expressed in the right hemisphere, and that positive feelings tend to be expressed in the left hemisphere. The stress response in females often leads to a decrease in norepinepherine (the "action" hormone) secretion and a decrease in right-hemisphere activity. Such a neuroresponse leaves females more prone to depression, as the left-hemisphere takes over and dwells on the stressful event. The opposite effect is usually seen in males; that is, an increase in norepinepherine and an increase in right-hemisphere motor functioning. With the left-hemisphere partially disengaged and the right-hemisphere given free reign, aggressive and bizarre behavior can result.

Among men, vulnerability to schizophrenia decreases with age but it actually increases for women. Nature is more protective of females while they are in their child-bearing and child-rearing ages. After all, one healthy

male can potentially father hundreds of offspring in the time it takes a female to be a mother of one. The species cannot tolerate the loss of many
females, but the male is far more expendable, in reproductive terms. While
the female is in her child-bearing years, she is protected by the female hormone, estrogen. Estrogen protects females not only from heart disease but
also from falling victim to left-hemisphere dysfunctions. When she is past
her child-bearing years, her estrogen levels drop and she begins to catch up
to male rates of diseases from which she was formerly protected. In other
words, sexual dimorphism is greatest during child-bearing years, after which
there is a blurring of hormonal differences between the sexes.

If you want an inkling of what the schizophrenic experience is like,
think of the scariest and most vivid dreams you've ever had. When we
dream our neurons are making haphazard connections. They are not responding to external stimuli; since we are sleeping there are none. The brain
has an inherent need for structure, so it does the best it can by drawing
on our past experiences to achieve some sort of structure and harmony
from these chance neuronal firings. Both schizophrenic and dream states
are evoked from a private reality which may be scary and incoherent. The
difference between the two states—and what a difference it is—is that when
we dream we wake up, know that we were dreaming, and begin responding
to stimuli from the external world.

The visual and auditory hallucinations experienced by schizophrenics
can be viewed as the brain's attempt to fashion some sort of order from
neurochemical chaos. The chaos is either the result of excessive secretion
of neurotransmitters (or hypersensitivity of their receptors) or a deficit in
enzymatic material responsible for removal of these neurotransmitters. One
study found twice as many receptors for the excitatory neurotransmitter
dopamine in the limbic systems of deceased schizophrenics as in the limbic
systems of deceased nonschizophrenics.[7] The work of Gary Lynch, mentioned in chapter 1, suggests that these extra receptors may have resulted
from a large number of high-frequency firings of neurons in response to
experiences with high emotional content.[8]

Neuroleptic (nerve modulator) drugs, such as *chlorpromazine*, act to block
dopamine receptors at the synapse and thus relieve the buzzing activity in the
schizophrenic's brain and help the sufferer to function more normally. These
drugs, however, don't affect behavioral symptoms of schizophrenia such as
flattened affect, social withdrawal, motivation, or anhedonia (inability to experience pleasure; cocaine addicts appear to have the same supersensitivity to
dopamine, and they suffer like schizophrenics from chronic anhedonia when
not using the drug.) It is the success of the neuroleptic drugs and the similar
symptomology experienced by cocaine addicts that convince modern researchers
that schizophrenia is at bottom a disease involving neurochemical imbalances.

The brain manufactures its own chemicals to remove excessive dopamine, as well as many other neurotransmitters. These specialized chemicals are proteinaceous molecules produced by our cells called *enzymes*. Enzymes produce or accelerate reactions to convert chemical molecules into other kinds of molecules. One study found that schizophrenics had significantly *lower* levels of an enzyme called *monoamine oxidase* (MAO) in their blood than a control group of nonschizophrenics.[9] MAO is an enzyme that removes a variety of neurotransmitters by oxidation after they have performed their task. A deficit in MAO would leave excess neurotransmitters at the synapses transmitting "information" which is, in reality, not there. That is, it's not there as far as the observer is concerned, but it is very much part of the schizophrenic's reality.

There is now quite a bit of convincing evidence indicating a strong *genetic* component to schizophrenia. The influence of genes in schizophrenia is primarily determined by studies using monozygotic (identical) twins as subjects. Since identical twins are produced from the same fertilized egg, they share an identical genetic endowment. A large number of studies have shown that if one member of a pair of identical twins is schizophrenic, the other member has a much higher probability of becoming schizophrenic than if the pair were dizygotic twins (fraternal twins developed from separate ova), who share only 50 per cent of their genes. After reviewing a number of such studies, one researcher concluded that the average concordance rate (the rate that both members of a pair have an identical trait) for schizophrenia is about 55 per cent for monozygotic twins and about 12.5 per cent for dizygotic twins.[10]

Although genetic studies have shown conclusively that there is a definite biological predisposition to schizophrenia, a concordance rate of 55 per cent means that 45 per cent of genetically identical individuals are discordant for schizophrenia. In other words, there is a lot of room for environmental factors to play a role in the onset of schizophrenia. We should realize that genes are biochemical units of *potential* that are differentially realized in different environments. One of the world's leading researchers on the genetics of schizophrenia, Seymour Kety, has stated that we cannot ignore environmental factors in seeking to explain its causal origin. Biologically oriented researchers, Kety insists, must understand that environmental factors can precipitate, intensify, or ameliorate the symptoms of schizophrenia. To ignore such factors will confound the biological picture and lead researchers astray, just as surely as pure environmentalists were led astray by their refusal to consider biological factors.[11]

Many of those involved in the treatment of schizophrenics view love deprivation as the major predisposing environmental variable. We know that experience can alter synaptic strength, and that stimuli deprivation can result in diminished quantities of essential neurotransmitters. Some scientists investigating MAO activity speculate that events occurring in early life could influence future MAO activity in ways not fully understood at present. It is worth recalling at this point that Harlow's love-deprived monkey exhibited schizophrenic-like behavior such as catatonic posturing and rocking, as well as social withdrawal and other bizarre behaviors. We saw how the deprivation experience also visibly altered normal dendritic patterns in the brain. Since the experience altered brain structure, it is quite possible that it also changed the pattern of MAO activity. There is no doubt that the secretion patterns of other neurochemicals are adversely affected by separation of mother and infant, especially the *catecholamines*. Dopamine, norepinepherine, acetylcholine, and serotonin are among the class of neurotransmitters called catecholamines. Since MAO is a regulator of these chemicals, changes in MAO-secretion patterns may be responsible at this level for the observed patterns of catecholamine activity.

Psychotherapist Arnold Buss offers us a typical, environmentally based view that schizophrenia may have its origin in love deprivation. Humans are social beings, says Buss, so we must all learn to view the world without suspicion and to trust and care for others. The origin of care and trust lies in parental love. If we did not receive this love, if instead we experienced parental coldness and rejection, we will be predisposed toward passivity, isolation, and suspicion. Depending on how severely deprived of love we were, this passivity, suspicion, and isolation may balloon into schizophrenic proportions.[12]

The picture painted by Buss fits the common developmental pattern found in study after study of the onset of schizophrenia. It cannot be too hard to see that it is difficult to experience the world as exciting and pleasurable if misery has been one's lot early in life. One who has grown up in a barren, colorless, and loveless environment is bound to exhibit to some extent the "flattened" affect of the schizophrenic; it is not at all surprising that neuroscientists find this flatness of affect reflected in brain physiology and chemistry.

Few researchers deny a correlation between growing up in the kind of environment I have just described and schizophrenia. But correlation does not prove causation. A correlation is simply a mathematical relationship between variables that may or may not be indicative of some underlying causal relationship. To the extent that schizophrenia is a genetic disease, one or both parents share some of the pathological genes with their offspring. These genes may be responsible for the way the parent or parents interact with their offspring, making the correlation between developmental environment and schizophrenia, in effect, spurious. Furthermore, having a child who is exhibiting the early stages of process schizophrenia, even in a normal family, is not conducive to a loving relationship. Even very loving parents may eventually be turned off by a child's lack of response to their efforts to love it. *This may suggest that the observed negative home environments of many schizophrenics may be an effect rather than a cause of schizophrenia.*

We may respond to this observation by again turning to Harlow's monkeys for suggestions as to how early environmental experiences could produce, or cause, the symptoms of schizophrenia. It has long been established that *anhedonia* is a characteristic of schizophrenia. Studies by Robert Heath at Tulane University have indicated that this inability to experience pleasure is physiologically linked to disturbances in the septal region, the pleasure center of the limbic system. Heath conducted depth-electrode studies on some of Harry Harlow's love-deprived monkeys at the request of James Prescott. Prescott was anxious to have his cerebellum-limbic system theory (discussed in chapter 1) tested in the laboratory. Heath discovered that all the deprived monkeys were found to have severe septal disturbances. Heath concluded: "This was the first evidence that aberrant electro-physiological activity occurs in deep cerebellar nuclei, as well as in other deep brain structures—most pronounced in the limbic system—in association with severely disturbed behavior resulting from maternal-social deprivation."[13] Heath's studies provided compelling evidence for Prescott's theory.

Commenting on Heath's conclusions, neurologist Richard Restak says: "The infant who is deprived of movement and physical closeness will fail to develop the brain pathways that mediate pleasure. In essence, such people may be suffering at the neuronal level from stunted growth of their pleasure system."[14] Since Harlow did not select the monkeys he subjected to deprivation by genetic screening, essentially he "controlled" for the influence of genes, leaving their cold and loveless early experiences as the only variable influencing the observed outcome. Furthermore, since all deprived monkeys in all studies of this kind exhibit schizophrenic-like behavior, we cannot conclude that the deprivation experience served only to catalyze a genetic predisposition.

Whenever we extrapolate from animal studies to humans, we must be aware of the point made earlier that similar experiences affect human development more strongly than nonhuman development. The attitudes, ideas, and behavioral patterns of others, experienced by the child, are consciously and subconsciously incorporated into his or her own personality. Once the human child introjects its early experiences into its personality, there is a great tendency to become more and more sensitive to the introjected version of reality. Once this version of reality is strongly ingrained in the child's personality, he or she then responds to the world from this personal reality as opposed to the reality shared by others. This disjunction between one's private reality and the reality experienced by others is, of course, the essence of schizophrenia.

Psychiatrist Michael Liebowitz, whose work focuses on the chemistry of love, sees the pleasure and displeasure centers of the brain being activated differentially according to how "well-trodden" the neuronal circuits to these centers are. If the infant or child introjects negative experiences, these will be reflected in his or her neuronal circuitry. Later experiences that may be only mildly negative for most of us will, for the adult who was love-deprived as a child, produce a cascade of biochemical switches along the well-worn synaptic routes to awaken infant or childhood memories or feelings. These memories will then color his or her responses to the present experience. In his delightful book, *The Chemistry of Love*, Liebowitz writes:

> If someone grows up in a cruel, neglectful, uncaring, or cold atmosphere [read "love deprived"], the chances are that as an adult he or she is going to have a store of painful memories. What this means is there will be a series of well-established links between memory and displeasure centers. As adults these people will be more prone to depression, sadness, or pessimism. Any time an unhappy childhood memory is evoked, the displeasure circuits will be activated.[15]

Schizophrenia may very well be the result of the effects of early negative childhood experiences on the mechanisms of neurotransmitter metabolism for individuals with a schizophrenic predisposition. The reverse may also be true, suggesting the strong possibility that love can "over-ride" any biological predisposition to schizophrenia, just as its absence can precipitate it. Of course, similar experiences have different effects on different infants. Love deprivation may have little effect on some infants and truly devastating effects on others. Among those infants most severely affected, the consequences can differ radically. Some may become schizophrenic, some psychopathic, and others may be propelled toward any one or a combination of other pathologies, depending on many other factors including genetic factors.

One such physiological factor linking genetics to experience may be differences in the reactivity of the *autonomic nervous system (ANS)* among different people. We have seen how the ANS, among its other functions, regulates short-term bodily changes in response to external stimuli by pumping out chemicals preparing us for fight or flight. These ANS responses— fear, anxiety, heart thumping, "butterflies," cold sweats, and so on—are unpleasant and uncomfortable. The unpleasantness of ANS responses is nature's way of making sure that we take threats to our well-being seriously and that we take steps to eliminate whatever it is that threatens us. When we successfully eliminate threats to our well-being, our ANS is restored to its formerly balanced state and we feel greatly relieved.

Danish researcher Sarnoff Mednick has conducted long-term research with children at genetic risk for schizophrenia. Comparing children who did and who did not suffer a psychotic breakdown among these at-risk individuals, he found two major differences. The first difference was that those who succumbed to the disease had abnormally reactive ANSs. An abnormally reactive ANS means both that it is activated relatively easily, and that when it does react it reacts wildly. The second difference was that these unfortunate individuals were found to have suffered considerably more maternal separation and adverse environmental conditions than those who did not succumb.[16]

Are these two variables causally linked, or are they simply variables common to the schizophrenic syndrome but causally independent of each other? Mednick theorizes that genetic factors largely determine the reactivity of the ANS response, but that harsh and loveless environments build on this disposition to produce schizophrenia. He reasons that children growing up in harsh environments frequently have to find safe havens from threat and fear, conditions that activate the ANS. Lacking any real alternatives, safe havens for young children may be nothing more than entering into a fantasy world of irrelevant thoughts and feelings. We have all done this at one time or another. When confronted with something fearful, worrisome, or anxiety-provoking we often advise ourselves to think of something else "to take our minds off it." This is often sage advice, but what if we were genetically predisposed to schizophrenia, and what if as children we continued to invent ever more bizarre thoughts to escape the reality of a continually threatening environment and the ANS upheaval it engenders?

The functioning of the ANS is thought to interact with a harsh environment to produce the onset of schizophrenia not only in terms of its hyperactivity but also in terms of its recovery rate. Suppose an at-risk child is confronted with a threat from the environment and the child's ANS begins to react wildly. Further suppose that previous experience has taught the child that the physiological consequences of the threat are less severe if he or she mentally withdraws from the threat in the way described above. If this mental disassociation results in a fast recovery of the child's ANS, he or she will be reinforced in this kind of avoidance behavior, and it will tend to be elicited more readily when confronted with similar threats in the future. If the autonomic recovery rate is slow rather than fast, the bizarre avoidance behavior is not so strongly reinforced and may not become an enduring part of the child's avoidance repertory; hence, schizophrenia may be avoided.

In sum, Mednick's theory of schizophrenia rests on four variable conditions: (1) a genetic predisposition, (2) an overly responsive ANS, (3) a cruel and neglectful environment from which the child withdraws into a private fantasy world, and (4) an ANS that speedily recovers when the avoidance response is activated. The theory nicely integrates physiological and environmental variables, and has the rare quality of being based on data gathered over a long period of time. It does not specifically take into account findings that report excessive dopamine and/or low levels of MAO in the brains of schizophrenics. But given the link between the peptides mediating autonomic responses, emotions, and thought processes, it is not unreasonable to suppose that the process described by Mednick could upset the delicate balance of the neurochemical system as posited by researchers cited earlier in this section, and especially the research of Kandell and Lynch I discussed in chapter 1.

I do not claim to have disentangled the messy web of potential causes of schizophrenia here. Hard facts in this area are sparse; hence the opportunities for speculation are rich. What I hope I have succeeded in doing is to have pointed out how love deprivation may interact with the other known social and biological correlates of schizophrenia.

DEPRESSION AND SUICIDE

Many are the immediate conditions that lead people to take their own lives. Whatever the immediate condition may be, it can be viewed as the last straw added to the bale of Liebowitz's "painful memories." The most immediate or proximate cause of suicide is severe depression. Shakespeare's Hamlet perhaps described depression most succinctly when he said: "How weary, stale, flat, and unprofitable seem to me all the uses of the world." When we are depressed the pleasure centers in our brain are closed down; we can't sleep or eat, we don't want sex, and some of us don't want to live.

Akiskal and McKinney have proposed what they call a "multilevel interaction" theory of depression. Psychosocial experiences such as a lack of relatedness, rejection, and lovelessness lead to reduced brain *catecholamines*. Decreased catecholamines lead to behavioral disturbances such as insomnia, loss of appetite, and the slowing or agitation of psychomotor functioning. Chemically speaking, low levels of the various catecholamines are responsible for the anhedonia, feelings of hopelessness, and the seeming inability to control what goes on in one's life. If not enough of these vital neurotransmitters are available, the neurons will be unable to respond normally to impulses from the environment that should evoke cheerfulness, and the person will be more prone to depression. Depression is evoked most severely and most often by the loss of loved ones, whether through death, separation, or breakups, and appears to be more or less a constant among the lonely and emotionally unattached.[17]

Patients with unipolar depression (depression resulting from chemical imbalances within the brain) are sometimes treated with drugs that block the activity of monoamine oxidase (MAO). The so-called MAO inhibitors prevent MAO from breaking down the catecholamines, so they remain available for activating synapses. MAO inhibitors relieve depression in about 70 per cent of its victims, and take about one month to do so.

In one of the first pieces of scientific sociology, the nineteenth-century French sociologist Émile Durkheim showed that suicide varied inversely with the strength of the ties one enjoyed with other people. Suicide is higher in urban areas, where there is greater anonymity, than in rural areas; it is also higher among the unmarried and the divorced than among the married, higher in marriages that are childless than among marriages that produce children, and higher among the lonely than among the socially active. Thus, we can see that love ties one to life itself. If one is sensitized to pathological reactions by love deprivation during the early years of life, subsequent rejections, breakups, and the vagaries of life in modern society are less well coped with in a nonpathological manner.

It should be noted that appearing to love too intensely and exclusively can be as conducive to suicide as not loving at all. "Altruistic" suicide is Durkheim's term for this type of suicide.[18] Religious and political martyrdom are examples of altruistic suicide committed by individuals who have totally surrendered themselves to a "cause." Such people tend to be rigid ideologues incapable of seeing the value of other people or other causes. The terrorist who drives a truckload of dynamite into a barracks full of U.S. Marines has no compassion or love for eithe his victims or for himself. He has subjugated all other human emotions to the single emotion of hate—and he does this in the name of love for cause or country. Is it any wonder that George Bernard Shaw termed patriotism "a particularly pernicious form of psychopathic idiocy"? There is nothing wrong with loving our own people or land or country, but when such "love" turns us against other parts of humanity and we begin mouthing clichés such as "My country right or wrong," we have become loveless morons.

In a less general sense, it is also possible to be "hooked" so strongly on some other person that the addicted person will attempt suicide at the loss, or threat of loss of the loved one. Such is a style of loving termed "manic" love by sociologist John Lee. (See chapter 9.) The manic lover is extremely possessive and jealous, clinging to the lover like a leech and sinking into deep depression at any hint of nonresponse from him or her. This is the kind of love that Abraham Maslow calls "D-[deficit] love."

Such a person seems to love so intensely because he or she, ironically, is loved so little. D-lovers have been so deprived of loving experiences that they crave love in the worst way. The partner is valued for his or her ability to satisfy an intense hunger, resulting in a selfish and growth-inhibiting feeling some call love but which is not really love. Those who so singularly invest their "love" are at greater risk for suicide in the event of a breakup than those whose love is more freely given in an adult manner.

We are all, of course, deeply grieved at the loss of a loved one. But if we are part of a wide circle of loving human beings, we can share our tribulations with them. "A trouble shared is a trouble halved," as an old saying goes. Social support at a time of loss is crucial, regardless of whether we are talking about a loss of a loved one by death or a fracture in a relationship. Those unfortunate souls lacking wide social support are hit with a cross that they may find impossible to bear alone. It was the lack of a wide circle of loved ones that led the aggrieved to invest so much of the self in the loved one in the first place. With the departure of the love object, life is all the more lonely and brutal during the interlude. For such people, it is not "better to have loved and lost than never to have loved at all."

A number of studies support the view that love functions as a shield against suicide. This is particularly true for young people between the ages of 15 to 24. Suicide is the third leading cause of death (after accidents and homicide) among this group of young people. Adolescence is a trying period, regardless of early childhood experiences. Psychologists Rosenthal and Rosenthal found among a clinical sample of behaviorally disturbed children that abused and neglected children were significantly more likely to attempt suicide than nonabused and nonneglected children.[19] J. Arthur Beyer and I compared 39 juvenile delinquents who had attempted suicide with delinquents who had not. We found that those who attempted suicide had been significantly more love-deprived than those who had not.[20] Similarly, a study conducted by Deykin and her colleagues found that abused and neglected boys were 3.8 times more likely to attempt suicide than a control group of nonabused boys; the corresponding ratio for girls was 6.1.[21]

This last finding agrees with national figures indicating that while about twice as many females attempt suicide, about twice as many males succeed. This makes sense in terms of our discussion in the section on schizophrenia of the differential neuroresponse to stress. Females are more likely to become depressed than males, but their suicide attempts tend to be less violent, and hence less successful. Females favor more passive methods, such as overdosing on pills, which can be countered by medical intervention. Males, on the other hand, favor more violent and drastic measures such as hanging and shooting, methods that are very unlikely to be effectively countered by medical treatment.

Nevertheless, regardless of the pathways to suicide or the methods employed to implement it, the fact remains that if parents demonstrate by their abuse and neglect that they do not consider their children loveable and worthwhile, this evaluation will be internalized by the abused child and become his or her own evaluation. Suicide is often considered a cry for help—"love me, value me, respect me, treat me right."

Sorokin and Hansen sum up the relationship between love and suicide thus: "We know that the main cause of suicide is psycho-social isolation of the individual, his state of being lonely in the human universe, of not loving or caring for anybody and not being loved by anybody . . . . [however] Each time one's love and attachment to fellow men multiply and grow strong, one's chances of suicide decrease. This means that love is indeed the intensest vital force, the central core of life itself."[22] To which I add, amen!

THE NEUROSES

Neurosis is a generic term for a large number of sociopsychological disorders characterized by anxiety and self-defeating attempts to deal with that anxiety through memory distortion, repression, and a number of other defense mechanisms. Like many other forms of mental illness, neurosis manifests itself in different degrees of severity. Typically, a neurosis does not require hospitalization, but in its severest forms it can be quite destructive. The overwhelming number of neurotics, however, are able to control or hide their symptoms enough, at the right times, to continue functioning in society—even though they continue to experience great anxiety and tension.

Broadly conceptualized, neurosis is a form of mental withdrawal from the fullness of life. It is also a failure of the personality to develop fully. Many neurotic people are adjusted to their world; in fact, they may be overly adjusted, in the sense that they are overly conformist, constantly worrying over the propriety of their behavior and whether or not they are liked. They are wracked by guilt, anxiety, phobias, and compulsions that they don't understand. Minor suspicions, small financial setbacks, or even something like an untidy office can turn into nightmares of inadequacy for neurotics. They are afraid to get too close to others lest they reveal themselves, and they frequently bolster their low sense of self-esteem in conspicuous consumption. They want love—nay, crave it—but they are victims of ambivalent impulses. They desire to be loved and esteemed for themselves, but they cannot easily love in return; hence, we see the frequent sublimation of the impulse toward love into neurotic activity.

There is essentially no disagreement within psychology and psychiatry that manifestations of neurosis result from past memories or feelings intruding into the individual's present perceptions. The residual emotion, etched as it is into neuronal circuitry, is so strong as to "take over" perceptions of present situations and render them more threatening than they objectively are. We know that past experiences can alter patterns of synaptic activity and neurotransmitter secretion, and that the frequency and intensity of similar experiences "habituates" and strengthens these neurological processes. At the neurophysiological level, then, the anxiety experienced by the neurotic results from atypical activity (relative to the activity of nonneurotics) in the neurotransmitter-receptor systems. In other words, an experience that many people may view as rather innocuous seems to result in the pumping of excess excitatory neurotransmitters and generating exaggerated physiological and behavioral responses.

The neurotransmitter *gamma-aminobutyric acid (GABA)* plays an inhibitory rather than excitatory role in the brain. GABA receptors induce calm by inhibiting or modulating neurons that might be stimulating neurotic overreaction. Drugs such as Valium and Librium assist the calming action of GABA receptors, thus reducing anxiety. We are more interested in the experiences that may have habituated the neurotransmitter-receptor systems to overreact in the first place rather than in the chemical processes. Love, nature's "Valium," means the endorphins are at work to make us feel secure, and a sense of security is a bulwark against anxiety. Those who have a legacy of a loveless childhood are likely to feel most insecure, and hence to react neurotically to mildly threatening situations.

I think it fair to say that most mental-health professionals see the origin of neurosis in some form of emotional deprivation. Neurosis is viewed as a condition generated by the inability to have basic human needs for affection, emotional security, and self-esteem gratified. Neurotic behavior is viewed as either a compulsive effort to satisfy these needs, or an equally compulsive effort to deny their existence. The neurotic is a person who generally comes from an emotionally cold or controlling family background, although not necessarily a physically abusive one. Emotional coldness is most often expressed by parents rebuffing the child's needs for closeness and its attempts to express love or controlling the child so that he or she is unable to develop fully or made to feel "bad'" if he or she rebels against the controlling parent. The constant thwarting of these needs for love and autonomy leads children to feel that there is something wrong with them, that they are not worthy of being loved or trusted to be themselves. Self-derogatory feelings experienced time and time again crystallize into permanent feelings of worthlessness and inadequacy.

A particularly pernicious form of neurosis is *hysteria*. Subsumed under this diagnostic label are *disassociative reaction* and *conversion reaction*.

Disassociative reaction is the multiple-personality syndrome made familiar by the book and movie *The Three Faces of Eve*. Slipping in and out of apparently different personality constellations may be seen as a way of avoiding unpleasant situations with which the person is not psychologically equipped to deal.

Conversion reaction produces psychosomatic symptoms: severe headaches, loss of body sensation, hyper- or hyposensitivity to various foods and substances, motor paralysis, respiratory difficulties, and various degrees of deafness and blindness. More interesting than the symptoms, for our purposes, is the statement of British psychologist John Bowlby: "Regardless of the individual's inborn tendencies, he will not develop hysteria unless he is subjected during childhood to situations causing him to crave affection."[23] Note that while Bowlby is not suggesting that love deprivation is a sufficient cause of neurosis, he is emphatic that it is a necessary cause.

Empirical (as opposed to clinical) evidence linking love deprivation to the neuroses is sparse, primarily because of methodological hazards. There is certainly plenty of evidence to show that unattached individuals—the unmarried, the childless, the lonely—have much higher rates of neurosis than attached individuals. But are they neurotic because they are unattached or unattached because they are neurotic? It is certainly possible that being unattached for much of one's life could eventually lead to neurotic behavior. It is more likely, though, that the causal relationship runs the other way. Neurotic persons do not exactly endear themselves to others. Their lack of early affectionate experience has not equipped them to be skilled in forming interpersonal relationships.

The neurotic's difficulty in forming attachments has been studied by Scot Henderson, director of the National Health Medical Research Council at the Australian National University. Henderson argues that neurotics crave attachments more desperately than other individuals, but the very desperation of their need leads others to avoid them. Neurotics often use what Henderson calls "care-eliciting behavior" in an attempt to draw others closer to them. Care-eliciting behavior is functionally equivalent to behavior observed in neglected infants and children. Like such children, neurotics may cry, cling, use verbal appeals for pity, or use other "please-love-me" signals that cause distress both to themselves and to others. Sometimes it works; often it does not. Henderson affirms that what he calls *anophelia* (lacking in care, love, succor, support) is the major cause of the neuroses, and care-eliciting behavior is a way of attempting to rectify the deficit.[24]

Care-eliciting behavior is a way, albeit a negative way, of making emotional contact with others, and is an apt description of Maslow's deficit love, which I have already described. Individuals, neurotic or not, must make contact with other individuals; it is an imperative deep within the human biological legacy. Those who have little experience in loving and being loved too often express this imperative in inappropriate and annoying ways, but they must express it nonetheless. Maslow likens the search for love among the seriously deprived to the instinctive ways animals seek to rectify deficiencies in certain minerals and vitamins vital to their health. If these dietary deficiencies can't be rectified, sickness results. Likewise, "If this healing necessity [love] is not available, severe pathology results . . . . The sickness 'love hunger' can be cured in certain cases by making up the pathological deficiency. Love hunger is a deficiency disease exactly as is salt hunger or the avitaminoses."[25]

We should not berate or bemoan individuals for trying to fulfill their needs in naive and unsophisticated methods any more than we should scold starving dogs for rummaging for food in the garbage. We can demonstrate and cultivate our own love by helping them to satisfy their craving in more mature ways. To offer love, succor, and support to those who need it most is the love, succor, and support that most affirms ourselves as loving human beings.

ALCOHOL AND DRUG ABUSE

Alcohol and drug abuse extracts a terrible price from the addict and from his or her family and society. Alcohol, at once the most popular and most deadly of our chemical comforters, is a depressant drug that acts as a disinhibitor of behavior. The more alcohol we ingest, the more the higher brain center surrenders to the raw emotionality of the primitive brain center. Under the influence of alcohol, a man or woman is not simply acting to express repressed emotions; rather, he or she is acting with drugged emotions. Dazed emotions lead people to do such nasty things as molest young children, assault spouses, drive cars into trucks, and sometimes to kill one another. It has been estimated that 92 per cent of all arrests for violent crimes and 55 per cent of all arrests are associated with drunkenness.[26]

As with the other destructive syndromes we have examined, alcoholism has a genetic component. *Acetaldehyde (AcH)* is the first metabolite of alcohol, and it produces unpleasant reactions, such as nausea and headaches. Those individuals who rapidly convert alcohol into AcH have a built-in guardian against drinking too much. In fact, disulfiram (Antabuse) is used in the treatment of alcoholics because it functions to maintain high levels of AcH in the body by retarding further metabolic reactions. It appears that those who become physically addicted to alcohol tend to have metabolic systems that both produce more than the usual amount of AcH and convert it too quickly into a morphinelike substance called tetrahydropap-averoline (THP). Most of us retain AcH in sufficient quantities to experi-ence the punishing effects of alcohol, but alcoholics experience the euphoric effects of THP more than the aversive effects of AcH. This line of inquiry perhaps explains why the vast majority of those who drink do not become alcoholics.[27]

This physiological explanation of alcoholism is not the whole story of the etiology of problem drinking. Many people who do metabolize AcH normally drink themselves into stupors with depressing regularity. Alcohol is an artificial method of making ourselves more confident, successful, and powerful. Note the images of power, wealth, success, masculinity, and sensuality implicit in alcohol advertising and the names we give to some of our most popular alcoholic concoctions—Manhattans, Margaritas, pile-drivers, pink ladies, and boilermakers.

Alcohol is also taken to reduce anxiety and tension. It works rather like Valium in that it has potentiating effects on GABA synapses. Those who resort to alcohol to dull the pains of life, rather than as a simple and pleasurable diversion, are obviously missing something vital in their lives. The difference between the problem chronic drinker and the occa-sional imbiber, according to the President's Task Force on Drunkenness, is that the chronic drinker "has never attained more than a minimum of integration in society . . . he is isolated, uprooted, unattached, disorganized, demoralized, and homeless."[28] We cannot say to what extent these charac-teristics are consequences rather than causes of alcoholism. Nevertheless, the Task Force's conclusions again point to the importance of reciprocal love relationships for healthy human functioning.

Although alcohol is a drug, we can separate alcohol abuse from drug abuse in this analysis because alcohol is a legal method of drugging our-selves whereas heroin, LSD, cocaine, and methamphetamines are not. There are far too many varieties of illegal drugs to allow us to address them here. The factor they all have in common, however, is that they alter moods from the undesirable to the desirable—as viewed from the perspective of the drug-taker. Depending on the drug taken, the individual's moods, feel-ings, and behavior are stimulated or mellowed, intensified or reduced, speeded up or slowed down according to how they affect brain chemistry.

Why do people take these self-destructive and illegal substances? Would a happy, contented, loved, and loving person risk such a life for a few fleet-ing moments of chemical euphoria? I think not, although I suppose some people who match this description do manage to get themselves hooked be-cause they once decided to experiment under the misguided notion that they could "handle it." Most of the many addicts I have dealt with, however, conform with the characterization offered by Chein, Gerhard, Lee, and

Rosenfeld: "In almost all addict families, there was a disturbed relationship between parents, as evidenced by separation, divorce, open hostility, or lack of warmth."[29]

Many addicts began their drug taking for the same reasons that alcoholics started drinking: to be sociable, to conform, and be "with it." They also continue to take drugs for the same reasons that an alcoholic continues to drink: to escape tension, stress, and chronic boredom. They become dependent on them because they find little pleasure, comfort, solace, or meaning in their lives. They come to think of their chemical comforters as friends that temporarily relieve them of the pains of life. Those who find more pain than pleasure in their lives need all the artificial pleasure they can get. They become emotionally attached to their drugs in the same way others become attached to other people. Lacking in experiences that prepare them for loving relationships with people, addicts find their warmth and pleasure pharmacologically. Lacking attachments, heroin substitutes for the brain's own endorphins; lacking romantic attraction, cocaine and other stimulants stand in for the brain's own phenylethylamine (a brain chemical associated with romantic attraction discussed in chapter 8).

We tend to be pessimistic about the prognosis for addicts: "Once a junkie, always a junkie." Most drugs, alcohol or otherwise, are indeed powerful substances that do not easily surrender their hold on their victims. But addiction is partly a function of the power of the drug and partly a function of the psychosocial resources of the individual in its grasp. For instance, a very large percentage of U.S. troops in Vietnam used heroin to help them to cope with the horrors and turmoil of that war. Upon returning from Vietnam, all troops were given tests to detect the presence of heroin in their bodies. It has been reported that 90 per cent of those troops who tested positive for heroin were able to kick their habits without undue difficulty or discomfort. Once these troops were back in the United States among family and friends and away from the pressures of war and once they were again afforded opportunities for constructive activity, the need for heroin quickly dissipated.[30] Attachment, involvement, and commitment are the attributes most noticeably missing in the lives of people who continue to use and be used by drugs.

NOTES

1. G. Vickers, "Mental Health and Spiritual Values," *Lancet* (March 1955): p. 524.

2. Reuben Fine, *The Meaning of Love in Human Experience* (New York: John Wiley, 1985), p. 336.

3. For an analysis of love as the underpinning of a wide variety of mental health therapies, see Anthony Walsh, *Understanding, Assessing, and Counseling the Criminal Justice Client* (Pacific Grove, Calif.: Brooks/Cole, 1988), chapters 7 and 8.

4. See Thomas Szasz, *Psychiatric Slavery* (Garden City, N.Y.: Doubleday, 1977).

5. Jack Fincher, *The Human Brain: Mystery of Matter and Mind* (Washington, D.C.: U.S. News Books, 1982), pp. 140–143.

6. Pierre Flor-Henry, "Gender, Hemispheric Specialization and Psychopathology," *Social Science and Medicine* 12b (1978): pp. 155–162.

7. P. Seeman and T. Lee, "Chemical Clues to Schizophrenia," *Science News* (November 1981): p. 112.

8. Ibid., note 9, chapter 1.

9. R. Wyatt, D. Murphy, R. Belmaker, C. Donnelly, S. Cohen, and W. Pollin, "Reduced Monoamine Oxydase Activity in Platelets: A Possible Genetic Marker for Vulnerability to Schizophrenia," *Science* 179 (1983): pp. 916–918.

10. S. Snyder, *Biological Aspects of Mental Disorder* (New York: Oxford University Press, 1980), p. 59.

11. Seymour Kety cited in M. Duke and S. Nowicki, *Abnormal Psychology: Perspectives on Being Different* (Monterey, Calif.: Brooks/Cole, 1979), p. 183.

12. A. Buss, *Psychopathology* (New York: John Wiley, 1966), p. 352.

13. Robert Heath's work cited in Richard Restak, *The Brain: The Last Frontier* (New York: Warner, 1979), p. 150.

14. Ibid., p. 151.

15. Michael Liebowitz, *The Chemistry of Love* (New York: Berkley Books, 1983), p. 45.

16. Mednick's research cited in R. Trotter, "Schizophrenia: A Cruel Chain of Events," in *Psychology 79/80: Annual Editions*, ed. C. Borg (Guilford, Conn.: Dushkin Publishers, 1979).

17. H. Akiskal and W. McKinney, "Overview of Recent Research in Depression," *Archives of General Psychiatry* 32 (1975): pp. 285–305.

18. Émile Durkheim, *Suicide* (Glencoe, Ill: Free Press, 1951).

19. R. Rosenthal and S. Rosenthal, "Suicidal Behavior by Preschool Children," *American Journal of Psychiatry* 141 (1984): pp. 520–524.

20. Anthony Walsh and J. Arthur Beyer, unpublished data.

21. E. Deykin, J. Alpert, and J. McNamara. "A Pilot Study of the Effect of Exposure to Child Abuse or Neglect on Adolescent Suicidal Behavior," *American Journal of Psychiatry* 142 (1985): pp. 1299–1303.

22. P. Sorokin and R. Hanson, "The Power of Creative Love," in *The Meaning of Love*, ed. A. Montagu (Westport, Conn.: Greenwood, 1953), p. 126.

23. John Bowlby, *Child Care and the Growth of Love* (Hamonsworth, England: Penguin, 1977), p. 42.

24. Scot Henderson, "The Significance of Social Relationships in the Etiology of Neurosis," in *The Place of Attachment in Human Behavior*, ed. C. Parkes and J. Stevenson-Hinde (New York: Basic Books, 1982).

25. Abraham Maslow, "Deficiency Motivation and Growth Motivation," in *Personality Dynamics and Effective Behavior*, ed. J. Coleman (Chicago: Scott Foresman, 1960), p. 482.

26. L. Taylor, *Born to Crime* (Westport, Conn.: Greenwood Press, 1984), pp. 107–108.

27. For material on the physiology of alcoholism, see P. Applewhite, *Molecular Gods: How Molecules Determine Our Behavior* (Englewood Cliffs, N.J.: Prentice-Hall, 1981) and A. Rosenfeld, "Tippling Enzymes," *Science* 81, 2 (1981): pp. 24–25.

28. President's Commission on Law Enforcement and Administration of Justice, *Task Force Report On Drunkenness* (Washington, D.C.: U.S. Government Printing Office, 1967), pp. 11–13.

29. I. Chein, G. Gerhard, R. Lee, and E. Rosenfeld, *The Road to H: Narcotics, Delinquency and Social Policy* (New York: Basic Books, 1964): p. 273.

30. Stanton Peel, "Addiction: The Analgesic Experience," *Human Nature* 1 (1978): pp. 61–66.

6

Lovelessness and Lawlessness

Criminal, delinquent, neurotic, psychopathic, asocial behavior can, in the majority of cases, be traced to a childhood history of inadequate love.

—Ashley Montagu

THE CRIMINAL

Jimmy Kain is a small man of 5'5" and weighs in at around 130 pounds. At 26 years of age, he had accumulated one of the worst criminal records I had ever seen: burglary, robbery, rape, aggravated assault—name it, Jimmy has probably done it. As he sat opposite me in his jail cell, it was obvious from his many scars and his pug nose that this little tearaway had been in his fair share of street battles. I was there to interview him after his arrest for the brutal rape and attempted murder of a 45-year-old barmaid.

I was aware of the story behind Jimmy's arrest before going to see him. He had entered an unlocked bar one night after closing time to find a lone barmaid attending to some final cleaning chores. Brandishing a knife, Jimmy forced the barmaid into the kitchen, ordered her to strip, and then proceeded to rape her. After he completed his dirty business, he became enraged because the terrified woman had not been sexually responsive. Jimmy reacted to this affront to his "manhood" by placing the woman's head over a sink and attempting to decapitate her. Fortunately, Jimmy's knife was as dull as his conscience. Further incensed, Jimmy threw the knife down, picked up a bottle of liquor, and smashed it over her head. As the barmaid lay moaning on the ground, he poured more liquor over her while telling her "I'm going to burn you up, bitch." Before he was able to complete his threat, he was disturbed by the bar owner and ran off.

One of the first things Jimmy said to me was to ask what I would do if he attacked me. Since I outweighed him by a good 50 pounds and since I kept in fairly good shape in those days, I felt confident in replying that I would "take care" of him. He then laughed and replied that he didn't care about pain, and even liked it. He proudly displayed his numerous scars to me, scars, he added, that he had received from "guys bigger'n you." After all this chest expanding, we put that macho stuff behind us and Jimmy began to talk about his crime. He seemed to enjoy retelling the story, even embellishing it with more sick details than the barmaid herself recalled. A nasty piece of work was little Jimmy Kain: an emotionless, guiltless, walking id.

Documents from court psychiatrists and psychologists in my possession revealed that Jimmy had had the most abominable home life imaginable. His alcoholic father would regularly beat his mother while Jimmy sat and watched. Jimmy would also be beaten with fist, foot, and belt just as regularly. According to Jimmy, he eventually came to like these beatings as he got older: "I'd cuss, and my dad would whip me, and that felt good. I would laugh and tell him to do it again; I liked the pain. I'd feel good inside and feel important when he whupped me." In his later years, Jimmy and his father would get into numerous knockdown, drag-out fights with each other, but they would operate as a team in drunken barroom brawls against others. Jimmy's only interests in life were sex, booze, and violence, preferably all in one package.

THE CRIMINAL PSYCHOPATH

Examining psychiatrists and psychologists had no trouble in arriving at a diagnosis for Jimmy: he was an out-and-out psychopath. But it's a lot easier to label people on the basis of their behavior than to explain how they got that way. Just as many behavioral scientists used to deny the objective existence of schizophrenia; many still deny the existence of the psychopath. They do not deny that behavior that we choose to call "psychopathic" exists, but they do not believe that we can identify psychopaths independently of their behavior. Crime is best explained, say the sociologists, by reference to social conditions such as class, race, unemployment, poverty, discrimination, and so on. Not all sociologists subscribe to this narrow view, but the climate of tolerance within the discipline leads many sociologists and social workers to stoutly defend criminals from allegations that they might somehow be different from the rest of us. Everything and everyone— except, of course, the criminal—is responsible for crime.

There is an increasing awareness among criminologists that they must come to terms with individual differences and with the biological foundations of criminal behavior. European criminologists long ago recognized this by employing biologists and other natural scientists in their criminological departments. The American criminologist C. Ray Jeffery has made the case for an interdisciplinary approach to criminology that includes insights from sociology, psychology, biology, and biochemistry.[1] I agree with Jeffery that any theory not taking such an eclectic approach is less than adequate.

The one factor that weaves in and out, affecting and being affected by the processes studied by the four disciplines mentioned is love. Ashley Montagu has written: "Show me a murderer, a hardened criminal, a juvenile delinquent, a psychopath, or a 'cold fish' and in almost every case I will show you a tragedy that has resulted from not being properly loved during childhood."[2] Psychiatrist William Glasser estimates that 85 per cent of incarcerated criminals are there because they have not had their basic needs for love and feelings of self-worth met, and I agree.[3] Of course, many crimes are committed by those not having such a background. There are cultural, subcultural, and social-class pressures that lead to crime. In America's ghettoes, membership in a gang is often a rational response to survival imperatives that is quite independent of one's love experiences. As a former police officer and probation officer, I have dealt with many offenders whose offenses could best be explained sociologically, that is, without reference to uniquely personal experiences.

But our concern here is with criminality rather than with crime. Crime is any socially defined behavior forbidden by the penal codes. These penal codes list so many diverse forbidden acts as to make any comprehensive causal explanation for their violation impossible. Asking a criminologist "What causes crime?" makes as little sense as asking a physician "What causes disease?" Both the specific disease syndrome and the specific crime and its context must be articulated before any attempt can be made to address such questions. Trying to explain euthanasia and civil disobedience by appealing to the same principles used to explain murder and riot just doesn't wash. Just about every adult in America has committed some crime at one time or another for which he or she could have been jailed, just as we've all been sick. The difference between crime and criminality is something like the difference between occasional sickness and chronic, debilitating illness. Criminality is a chronic condition among individuals who are constitutionally predisposed toward crime. Such people seek out and manufacture opportunities to commit crime as a way of life, waking up every morning thinking, "Who can I rip off today?"

My interest in love began when I was perusing files on the family backgrounds of criminals during my days as a probation officer. I noticed that the very worst delinquents and criminals, the Jimmy Kains who kill, rob, rape, and mutilate without remorse, and often with pleasure, had the most abominable family backgrounds. Many grew up in fatherless homes, were illegitimate, and were physically and/or emotionally abused and neglected by promiscuous, substance-abusing "caretakers." Being consistently abused and rebuffed, these children spent much of their time in the streets and fell afoul of the law very early in life. Since they never developed ties of love and affection with any "significant other," they never acquired the ability to sympathize, empathize, or love. We call the worst of these emotionally flat criminals psychiatric names such as *psychopath*, or its synonyms, *sociopath* and *antisocial personality*.

Birth-cohort studies in a number of nations have shown that about 6 to 8 per cent of criminals account for approximately 66 to 67 per cent of all crimes. (A birth-cohort study studies all individuals of a certain type born in a given place within a given time-frame.) Marvin Wolfgang's study of a birth cohort of 10,000 males born in Philadelphia in 1945 found that 35 per cent of the arrestees (2.2 per cent of the full cohort) accounted for 52 per cent of all arrests and 66 per cent of all arrests for violent offenses![4] Another study of a larger cohort born in 1958 in the same city arrived at almost identical findings.[5] Interestingly enough, the percentage of serious chronic offenders found consistently in these cohort studies is almost exactly the percentage of criminals diagnosed as psychopaths (7 to 10 per cent) in American prisons in various studies done since 1918.[6] There are a lot of folks out there fishing in the crime pond, but a very small number of Jimmy Kains catch nearly all the fish. It's like a Satanic version of the biblical adage: "Many are called, but few are chosen."

What is it that distinguishes the psychopath from the one-time or occasional criminal? There is wide aggreement among students of the psychopath that lovelessness and guiltlessness most distinguish him (the psychopath is almost always male) from other human beings. While he is not really normal, he is not insane either. Many even seem to enjoy quite robust mental health. It is this "mask of sanity," to use a phrase coined by Harvey Cleckley, that makes the psychopath so dangerous.[7] While psychopaths appear to be mentally healthy, their behavior is far more destructive than that of the obviously mentally ill schizophrenic. Psychopaths leave heartbreak and destruction behind them everywhere they go, because many can hide their evilness behind a cultivated veneer of charm and trustworthiness. Cleckley sees the psychopath as an incomplete man, as a "subtly constructed reflex machine."[8] Psychopaths stand on that wavy, muddied line that criminologists call the "mad/bad" line. They know exactly what they are doing, and from their completely selfish perspective they believe it to be quite right and care not a hoot who they hurt.

Two fairly recent examples, John Wayne Gacy and Theodore Bundy, typify the loveless and guiltless criminal psychopath. Gacy was a well-respected member of the community, a successfully self-employed contractor, and an indefatigable volunteer in community affairs. (He was even a reserve police officer for a period.) This man nevertheless found time to sexually assault, torture, and murder at least 33 teenage boys and young men, and bury them in his basement. His veneer of respectability kept the police off his back for a long time despite many complaints from some of his more fortunate victims, those who lived. Never once did Gacy express remorse or guilt for his crimes, and he indicated that he felt not the least put off by sleeping in the same house night after night with his victim's corpses rotting beneath him.

Ted Bundy also wore a lily-white mask of respectability. He was a clean-cut law student, active in the affairs of the Young Republicans. He put his charm and his smile to use as a volunteer at a crisis hotline center, and was evidently quite good at it. When not putting his talents to work as a student or volunteer, he may have been responsible for the murders of at least 100 women and girls. Also like Gacy, Bundy never expressed remorse for his brutal crimes or pity for any of his victims until the last few days before his execution. These overdue expressions of remorse rang as hollow as his conscience, and they were doubtless a last-ditch effort to manipulate authorities into once again delaying his execution. He was a psychopath to the end.

There is disagreement among researchers as to whether psychopathy is a continuous or a discrete trait, that is, whether is is something that exists to varying degrees or is something that one either is or is not. I take the former position because the traits that define psychopathy—scope of conscience, impulsiveness, propensity for violence, capacity to love, and so on—are themselves continuous dimensions. At one end of the scale we have the Gacys and Bundys of the world, whose psychopathy is violently destructive and evidently total. At the other end we might have a person such as the great composer Richard Wagner. Wagner, who was called a "monster" by one of his biographers, had many psychopathic traits, but he was never accused of any crimes. Socially nondestructive psychopaths have even been called "a blessing to society" because of their genius, which almost by definition requires a certain degree of nonconformity and self-serving arrogance. But we are not concerned here with such people.

PHYSIOLOGY AND PSYCHOPATHY

Physiologically, psychopathy is related to atypical autonomic nervous system (ANS) functioning and exaggerated right-hemisphere brain functioning. We have seen that the sympathetic branch of the ANS functions to prepare the body for vigorous action when confronted with threat. When we discussed Sarnoff Mednick's theory of schizophrenia, we learned that individuals differ considerably in the strength of their ANS's response to stress. The greater the individual's autonomic response to fear-evoking stimuli, the less likely that person will be to put himself or herself into situations that will precipitate the unpleasantness of strong autonomic arousal. A person whose ANS is hyperreactive has a strong aversion to any sort of punishment or social displeasure and is highly conditionable to social expectations. It is this hyperreactivity, according to Mednick's theory, that leads to the autoconditioning of the schizophrenic response.

On the other hand, people who have hyporeactive (underreactive) ANSs do not fear punishment or social disapproval very much, and they are not very conditionable. Psychopaths are such people. Whether we study them in natural settings or under laboratory conditions, whether we study them in the United States, England, Canada, or Timbuktu, psychopaths consistently have been found to have unresponsive ANSs relative to nonpsychopathic criminals.[9] They seem unable to anticipate punishment, or if they do, to discount it. One study tested urinary catecholamine levels of psychopaths in jail just prior to sentencing. Catecholamine levels were compared to previously collected base-line levels and to urinary catecholamine levels of nonpsychopaths awaiting the same fate. Awaiting sentencing would seem to be a most stressful experience, and this experience should be reflected in the level of stress-related catecholamines in the urine. Indeed it was for nonpsychopaths, but psychopaths showed no elevation of base-line catecholamine levels as they were about to experience their punishment.[10] Psychopaths have also been found to differ significantly from nonpsychopaths on other indicators of autonomic arousal, such as electrodermal, cardiac, and vasomotor activity when exposed to threatening stimuli in laboratory settings.

Pierre Flor-Henry sees psychopathy as he sees schizophrenia—as a function of exaggerated right-hemisphere brain activity. Some extremely bright psychopaths notwithstanding, Flor-Henry says that they are generally characterized by diminished verbal capacity (and the diminished understanding and empathy it emplies) coupled with enhanced visual-spatial ability. The implication of this is that individuals deficient in their ability to talk themselves out of getting into trouble, but who have exaggerated visual-spatial skills, are likely to "act out" anger and frustration aggressively and impulsively.

A recent study of mine conducted among 256 juvenile delinquents lends support to the notion that poor verbal ability is related to a tendency to react violently to frustration. The lower the delinquents' verbal IQ, the more frequently and seriously they were involved in violent crimes (murder, rape, assault). Conversely, the higher the verbal IQ, the greater the frequency and seriousness of property crimes, crimes that take a certain amount of preplanning. The latter result should not be taken to mean that high IQ is related to the prevalence of property crime. It only means that within a sample of juveniles *already* involved with crime, the more intelligent among them tend to commit property crimes. Taking the sample as a whole, just over 60 per cent of the juveniles had IQs below normal, and only 8 per cent had IQ scores above normal.[11]

More important than IQ level per se is the discrepancy between verbal and performance IQ. The various Wechsler IQ scales have two primary components—verbal and performance. An individual's full-scale IQ is the arithmetic average of these two subscales. PETT scans of neurometabolism have shown that verbal IQ is localized in the left hemisphere of the brain, and performance IQ is localized in the right hemisphere.[12] Over 30 years ago, David Wechsler, the originator of these scales, noted that a *significant discrepancy* between the two IQ subscales is the most outstanding feature of the psychopath's test profile.[13]

Linking this with left-hemisphere dysfunction/right-hemisphere exaggeration, Flor-Henry's studies have shown dysfunction of the dominant left hemisphere of the brain is reflected in lower verbal IQ scores. Similarly, dysfunction in the right hemisphere results in diminished visual-spatial skills, and these diminished skills are reflected in low IQ scores. The literature on psychopathy, almost without exception, reports that criminal psychopaths show significantly higher performance IQ in relationship to their verbal IQ (P > V). A significant performance/verbal discrepancy is considered to be 12 points or more.[14] Jimmy Kain was found to have a much-below-average verbal IQ of 77 and a slightly-above-average performance IQ of 106, for a P > V discrepancy of 29 points.

It should be noted that while high P > V discrepant individuals are overrepresented among criminals and delinquents, individuals with the opposite profile, verbal IQ significantly greater than performance IQ (V > P), are underrepresented. In a "normative" (nondelinquent) sample of 2,200 juveniles, it was found that 16 per cent had a P > V profile.[15]

If P/V discrepancy scores, or the direction of the discrepancy, were unrelated to criminality, we would expect to find only chance departures from these percentages among criminals and delinquents. But this is not what we find. For instance, a study by June Andrew found the respective percentages to be 10.8, 55.6, and 33.8.[16] Another study conducted by myself and colleagues Thomas Petee and J. Arthur Beyer found the percentages to be 11.3, 51.6, and 37.1.[17] What this indicates is that individuals whose verbal skills are significantly greater than their performance skills are greatly underrepresented among criminals, and individuals whose performance skills are significantly greater than their verbal skills are overrepresented among criminals.

Interestingly, females in the normative sample were just as likely as males to show significant P > V discrepancies, and no more likely to show V > P. We know that females are much less likely to commit violent crimes than males, and there is no indication in the literature that P > V discrepancy is related to violence among females. This suggests that the relationship between IQ subtest scores, hemisphericity, autonomic-nervous-system functioning, and psychopathy is a very complex one, perhaps mediated by sex hormones.

For instance, "exaggerated males," that is, males with an extra Y chromosome (the XYY pattern) almost always show a significant P > V discrepancy. XYY males are usually taller than average, have lower overall IQ levels, and are somewhat more prone to violence than normal XY males. One review of 35 studies of the XYY males in prisons found that, on average, they were represented in prison populations over 20 times more frequently than would be expected from the incidence of XYY births (about 1 in every 1,000 male births) in the general population.

Just as exaggerated males have a significant P > V profile, "exaggerated females" (XXX and XO chromosomal patterns) invariably show a significant V > P profile. Turner's syndrome (XO) females have only one sex chromosome and hence are deprived of the fetal androgens that are apparently so important to visual-spatial and numeric abilities. In some cases they are so deficient in spatial perception (although they usually have normal or superior verbal IQs) that they are said to suffer from a syndrome known as "space-form blindness." These females are of diminutive stature and tend to be extremely shy and passive, and show very little interest in sex. They do show a great interest in and fondness for children and animals. In short, the exaggerated male tends to be big, nasty, brutal, visually and spatially astute, and nonverbal, while the exaggerated female tends to be petite, verbal, highly nurturant, and coy.

There is a possible sex-hormone explanation for why exaggerated right-hemisphere dysfunction only appears to translate into violent psychopathy for males. To begin with, it has been found in many MOA assays that males have on average about 20 per cent less MOA than females.[18] This datum by itself may account for a great deal of the difference between the sexes in schizophrenia, psychopathy, crime rates, and sensation-seeking behavior in general. Among male-only samples, psychopaths have been shown to have significantly lower levels of MAO activity than nonpsychopaths.[19]

How does this translate into an increased propensity to engage in criminal and violent behavior? We know that MAO is an enzyme that removes neurotransmitters through oxidation after they have performed their excitatory task. We have also seen that in males stress has the effect of increasing norepinepherine secretion and increasing right-hemisphere activity. Low levels of MAO would have the effect of allowing for prolonged activity of increased norepinepherine secretion during periods of stress, and hence an increased probability of violence.

Even in nonpsychopathic males, the male sex hormone testosterone has the effect of increasing the intensity of stress, resulting in greater secretion of norepinepherine. It is possible that a high level of testosterone, sometimes found to characterize violent or angry individuals, is itself responsible for low MAO activity. This conjecture is supported by findings indicating that MAO concentrations increase with age. Increasing age is also accompanied by a decrease in testosterone levels in males and in a decrease in the propensity toward violence and other antisocial behaviors. Declining testosterone levels perhaps allow for increased MAO activity and correspondingly better-behaved individuals. Social and psychological factors, such as an increase in responsibilities, moral maturity, and "burn-out" are also doubtless involved in decreased criminality among the aging.

Regardless of any exaggerated right-hemisphere dysfunction among females, the differential activity of norepinepherine should help to preclude a violent reaction to stress. Recall that women are more likely to exhibit violent reactions to stress during the paramenstrum period if they suffer from extreme PMS. Perhaps stress induces the male pattern of norepinepherine secretion and all that it implies during this period. Supportive of this view is the fact that women over 30 are responsible for nearly half of all crimes committed by women, but males over 30 are responsible for less than one-fourth of male crimes.[20] While women at all ages commit far less crimes than men at all ages, these figures reflect the changes in the balance of the sex hormones in men and women with advancing age. Testosterone/estrogen levels tend toward equilibrium in both sexes as we age. Men actually have higher levels of the major estrogen, estradiol, than postmenopausal women (although, of course, the male brain is less sensitive to it, and therefore less affected by it).

We have thus far attempted to link what we know about brain hemisphericity, $P > V$ discrepancy, MAO, and sex hormones to psychopathy. It remains to connect these variables to autonomic nervous system (ANS) functioning. In linking IQ scores to ANS functioning, I should point out that the performance test is primarily a test of short-term memory, and it is more productive of anxiety than is the verbal test. Anxiety plays havoc with short-term memory. That's why victim descriptions of criminal perpetrators are notoriously unreliable, especially if the victim has a hyperreactive ANS. On the other hand, individuals with hyporeactive ANSs suffer less disruption in those areas of the brain (the hippocampal circuits) that are thought to play a role in short-term memory retention.[21] In other words, individuals who don't become anxious and nervous (such as psychopaths) in short-term memory testing situations will score better on such tests than they will on verbal tests, which involve long-term memory.

To complicate the picture a little, there is a great deal of evidence indicating that psychopaths are hyperarousable when the central nervous system is considered. They are more easily aroused to anger and rage than nonpsychopaths, an observation which on the surface runs counter to the view that they possess relatively unresponsive autonomic nervous systems. A. R. Mawson and Carol Mawson of Loyola University have proposed a theory that seems to reconcile contradictory findings relating to autonomic responsiveness. They hypothesize that extreme oscillations of the autonomic nervous system, rather than hypo- or hyperresponsiveness as either/or conditions, characterize the psychopath.[22] Some kinds of noxious stimuli will barely faze him, while other kinds will send him into a violent rage. Stimuli to which he is relatively unresponsive include the fear of punishment and pain. Stimuli to which he is hypersensitive include being slighted, not getting his own way, being "crossed," or having his "manhood" threatened, the stimulus that sparked Jimmy Kain's outrage.

The theory put forth by the Mawsons is a complicated one involving the interplay of arousal and inhibiting neurotransmitters on the sympathetic and parasympathetic branches, respectively, of the ANS. We won't pursue the details of this theory. However, the Mawsons conclude their paper by making a point most germane for our purposes. They state: "It should be emphasized that neither the present theory nor the low arousal theory explains what is, perhaps, the major characteristic of the psychopath: namely, his lack of affect and inability to form close, personal relationships."[23] Despite the Mawsons's conclusion, there are clues out there that will enable us to link the psychopath's lovelessness to what is known about the psychopath's physiology. Let us explore those clues.

PSYCHOPATHY AND LOVE DEPRIVATION

In terms of environmental or experiential correlatives of psychopathy, Robert Hare, perhaps the world's leading researcher on psychopathy, tells us that disturbances in the family, parental loss, rejection, neglect, and abuse are almost always associated with psychopathy.[24] Criminologist C. R. Jeffery notes that psychopaths come from brutally neglectful homes, in which love and security are alien feelings.[25] We might reasonably expect that such protracted ill-treatment would adversely affect the structure and functioning of the emotional centers of the brain. In fact, EEG studies have consistently found atypical limbic-system functioning in violent psychopathic individuals. Could it be possible that, just as the neural circuits to the schizophrenic's pleasure centers are weak and undeveloped, the psychopath's neural circuits to the centers of violence and aggression are too well-formed by their violent and loveless experiences? There is no definitive answer to this question at present, but it is a plausible speculation. Ashley Montagu confidently predicts that if we take any violent individual and inquire into his background we will find that he had a love-starved childhood.[26]

The evidence concerning the childhood experiences of psychopaths must be linked with the physiological correlates of psychopathy if we are to gain a more complete picture. Few studies have attempted to link the two. This is perhaps not surprising since the ANS used to be considered a biological given (hence the term *autonomic*), which was impervious to experience. While the published studies demonstrate clearly a hereditary mechanism underlying autonomic responsiveness, research has shown that the autonomic nervous system can be conditioned to a remarkable degree.[27] In fact, the physiological line of thought reasons that socialization and the development of conscience (the internalized control of behavior) are largely a function of autonomic conditioning in early chidihood.

British criminologist Michael Wadsworth has suggested that the stress associated with a loveless and violent family background could result in a diminution of autonomic responsiveness. He reasons that children who are subjected to constant emotional stress are likely to develop some kind of internal mechanism that will be reflected in later ANS functioning. Wadsworth's own research supports his speculation. He found pulse rates (an indicator of autonomic activity) to be significantly lower among emotionally deprived boys. He also found that pulse rates could be used to predict later delinquent activity.[28] My own research in this area has supported the notion that love deprivation is related to the hyporesponsiveness of the ANS.[29]

Danish psychiatrist Wouter Buikhuisen makes a speculation similar to Wadsworth's. After writing at some length about the process by which a negative relationship develops between parents and child, he states: "After some time he feels rejected and no longer loved by his parents. The continuous stress he is experiencing makes it necessary to look for defense mechanisms. To avoid being hurt, he develops a kind of flat emotionality, a so-called indifference with its physiological pendant: low reactivity of the autonomic nervous system."[30]

Perhaps you have noted that the line of thinking presented by Wadsworth and Buikhuisen is somewhat similar to Sarnoff Mednick's theory of schizophrenia. The difference is that rather than withdrawing into a fantasy world and being reinforced in doing so by the fast recovery of a *hyperactive* ANS the child who becomes a psychopath develops a *hyporeactive* autonomic response. This suggests a mechanism mediated by the ANS by which severely deprived children may become either schizophrenic or psychopathic, depending perhaps on differing constitutional factors predisposing the individual's ANS to either hyper- or hyporeactivity. Similar experiences yielding radically different outcomes bring to mind the old German proverb: "The heat that melts the butter hardens the egg." The schizophrenic melts, the psychopath hardens.

Psychologist Richard Solomon suggests that physiological adjustment to constant emotional arousal (whether positive or negative) is necessary to prevent overtaxation and possible breakdown of physiological response mechanisms. He has shown that repeated aversive stimuli presented to laboratory dogs have a steadily decreasing effect on autonomic responses. Over a period of time, the administration of a negative stimulus has little or no effect on an animal's autonomic responses. The psychopath's ANS, like those of Solomon's laboratory dogs, may be unreactive to punishment or threat of punishment for the same reasons: the constant exposure to a cruel, brutal, and loveless environment.[31]

Richard Solomon's work led him to develop a theory of acquired motivation that he calls the "opponent-process." Following a long line of similar thinkers, Solomon states that pleasure and pain are inextricably bound together and that the "opponent" of one experience can acquire the properties of the other: pain can become pleasure and pleasure can become pain. He offers considerable evidence that repeated aversive events lose a lot of their unpleasantness and may become potential sources of pleasure. One example Solomon uses is that of military parachutists. Before the first jump even the bravest men show considerable anxiety. During the jump the feeling most frequently reported is sheer terror. After the jump the feeling is relief. After many jumps the parachutists actually look forward with considerable eagerness to the next one. Instead of feeling terror during the jump, they now report a thrilling feeling; the exhilaration that lasts for two or three hours after the jump has replaced the feeling of relief. What has happened is that a new source of positive reinforcement (exhilaration) now exists after habituation to a previously negative stimulus (fear). Otherwise stated, after repeated exposure, negative feelings lose some of their power to direct behavior while the positive feelings gain power, primarily because they last considerably longer.

Similarly, almost every law-enforcement officer becomes an "adrenaline junkie" after some time on the job, living for the code 3 call, the high-speed chase, the "robbery in progress." These are frightening experiences at first, but the exhilarating high felt during and after the call is most rewarding after repeated exposures. The successful culmination of such a call results in a high that lasts for the rest of the shift and beyond. Participation in painful sports such as boxing, karate, wrestling, and long-distance running also certainly contains elements of this opponent process.

Since the defining characteristics of the psychopath include stimulus seeking and the ability to discount pain and punishment, Solomon's opponent-process theory may have great applicability in explaining psychopathic behavior. I remind you again of Jimmy Kain. There is little doubt that he had an intense need to expose himself to danger and pain. Rather than being negative experiences for him, he sought them out as intensely rewarding experiences. Although Jimmy's ANS functioning was not directly tested, indirect testing via the P $>$ V discrepancy test seemed to indicate a most unresponsive ANS. Further indirect evidence of Jimmy's unresponsive ANS was his history of enuresis (bed-wetting), lasting long beyond the normal age a child stops, and his long history of setting fires (indicative of the stimulus hunger associated with slow ANS reactivity). Jimmy also had a history of cruelty to animals. This triad of childhood behaviors —enuresis, fire-setting, and cruelty to animals—have long been considered by psychiatrists as the single best predictor of future violence.[32]

The process of ANS adjustment to parental rejection might provide us with clues about how early childhood stresses tie in with the noted left-hemisphere dysfunction and exaggerated right-hemisphere functioning of psychopaths. With regard to brain laterality and environmental experience, there is a fair amount of evidence that early experiences of being handled and stroked positively influence hemispheric integration, at least in animals.[33] Parental rejection, by definition, means less interaction and communication between parents and child, leading to deficits in left-hemisphere development, which is reflected in the child's poor verbal abilities. Conversely, efforts to avoid punishment may favor the development of the visual-spatial skills of the right hemisphere. If abused children are to avoid as much punishment as possible, they have to become sensitive to environmental cues that punishment is imminent. They may develop exceptional visual-spatial skills and the ability to associate these cues with the parents' verbal cues. The constant association of verbal and visual cues as threatening may explain the abused child's tendency to respond to all sorts of verbal stimuli in a violent way as he or she grows older.

If this speculation has any merit, it would apply more to boys than to girls because of the greater hemispheric specialization of males. Females are better protected from exaggerated right-hemispheric functioning by less strict brain lateralization, perhaps due to the larger splenium of the corpus callosum that females have (as noted in chapter 3). Since, in addition to possessing significantly smaller spleniums, males are also generally less secure in the left hemisphere than females, it may be that a similar lack of communication experience will affect males more adversely. Boys do seem to suffer the trials of an abusive environment less well than girls, and it is often observed that it requires a greater degree of negative experience to push girls into criminality than it does boys. Perhaps this is because boys are more "modifiable," or because girls have more positive ways of dealing with stress, such as a more open display of emotion.

Some interesting observations relating to the greater propensity of women to openly express their emotions have been made by Fry and Langeth in their book *Crying: The Mystery of Tears*. It appears that crying offers not only psychological relief but also has positive somatic consequences. An analysis of tears reveals that they contain by-products of stress-related chemicals. By crying we rid ourselves of these damaging chemicals and more quickly restore our bodies to chemical balance. Crying also tends to decrease testosterone levels in both males and females when levels of this hormone are high.[34] The implication of this is that crying may have the consequence not only of helping to prevent stress-related diseases such as ulcers, hypertension, and other cardiovascular problems but also of reducing aggressive responses to stress.

It should be made quite clear at this point that visual-spatial skills are not dysfunctional per se. Creative scientists, artists, and mathematicians are noted for their right-brain brilliance. Creativity, imagination, and synthetic holistic thinking are right-brain functions. The "Eureka!" of creative discovery seems to be accomplished via synchronicity of the two hemispheres. What is dysfunctional is overdevelopment of the right hemisphere *relative* to the development of the left and when visual-spatial skills are used in the service of violence and aggression. In the extreme case of right-hemisphere exaggeration in the schizophrenic and the psychopath, right-hemisphere functioning may even be below population norms, but their left-hemisphere functioning is even more so.

Consistent with the preceding, it has been shown that criminal psychopaths with normal or above-normal verbal IQs tend not to be any more violent than nonpsychopathic criminals. On the other hand, psychopaths with low verbal IQs are extremely dangerous. Psychologists Heilbrun and Heilbrun's research in this area lead them to the overall conclusion that poor impulse control is mostly a function of low verbal IQ. This lack of impulse control in low-IQ psychopaths constitutes a mental deficit that compromises their ability to achieve goals without resorting to violence.[35]

An even deadlier combination predictive of violence is psychopathy, low verbal IQ, and severe love deprivation, a profile that fits Jimmy Kain. A study conducted by Beyer, Petee, and myself found that delinquents who conformed to this particular profile were 4.28 times more likely to have committed a violent crime than other delinquents, including less verbally deficient psychopaths. No other variable in this study predicted violence, psychopathy, or low verbal IQ more strongly than love deprivation. That is to say, the more deprived of love a juvenile was found to be, the lower was his verbal IQ, and he was more likely to be a psychopath, and to have a record that included arrests for violent offenses.[36]

SERIAL KILLERS

We could go on for many more pages reciting studies that have linked childhood love deprivation to violent crime. Rather than do this, it might be more interesting to take a brief look at the early experiences of some of the most notorious and violent criminals of the last few decades. Summing up Merilyn Moore's profile of serial killers contained in a manual used by about 2,000 law-enforcement agencies in the U.S., Dillingham writes: "The serial killer is likely someone who grew up in a single-parent home, was abused as a child, often sexually, and had family members who were addicted to drugs or alcohol."[37] The experiences outlined by Dillingham, along with a number of others, made up the measure of love deprivation used in the studies conducted by myself and my colleagues.

What if, rather than having exceptionally low overall intelligence, Jimmy Kain had exceptionally high overall intelligence? We cannot say what might have accrued under such a circumstance, but there is a possibility that he might have been able to rise above his early experience and become a productive, if not loving, member of society. On the other hand, he might have become a more dangerous creature. When high-IQ psychopaths (such as John Wayne Gacy and Ted Bundy) become serial killers, their greater intelligence enables them to be more efficient and "successful" at preying on their victims and eluding capture.

The quintessential example of psychopathy coupled with an intelligence that bordered on genius is that of Adolf Hitler, one of the most infamous killers in history. In his book *The Psychopathic God*, historian Robert Waite has much to say about Hitler's loveless childhood.[38] His central emotional experiences in childhood were anxiety, tension, and cruelty. Hitler often witnessed his father beating his mother in drunken rages, and was frequently the victim of such abuse himself. He was a hyperactive stimulus seeker, who at age 15 beat his own mother. Waite saw the child Adolf being overwhelmed by terror, fear, rage, and mistrust of his fellow human beings. Of such experiences are murderers made. Any calculation of the consequences of Hitler's terrible childhood must include not only the millions he had slaughtered but also the millions of lives it took to remove such a monster and the machine he built from the face of the earth.

Although Hitler was not technically a serial killer because he did not personally commit murders, he has a lot in common with several well-known serial killers. Carl Panzram once had the reputation of being "America's most violent prison inmate." Panzram's father deserted the family when Carl was a young child. He was frequently cuffed and beaten as a child and grew to hate his mother. As an adult, Panzram roamed the country as a rapist and serial killer. Jack Abbott, who wrote the once acclaimed *In the Belly of the Beast*, was the child of an abusive alcoholic father and a prostitute. Jack's parents were divorced when he was four years old, and he was thereafter shuttled from foster home to foster home. In at least one of these homes he was sexually abused. He killed 3 people and by 1990 had spent about 34 of his 46 years behind bars. Albert DeSalvo, the "Boston Strangler," came from a home in which his alcoholic father brutally tortured Albert and his mother, and in which there were forced incestuous relations. Charles Manson was born illegitimately to a 15-year-old girl, who was imprisoned shortly after giving birth. Manson was also farmed out to surrogate parents. The list goes on with monotonous regularity documenting the insidious effects of love deprivation.

After reviewing the life histories of these men, as well as many others, Colin Wilson was led to conclude in *A Criminal History of Mankind*: "And so insecure social bonds prevent a capacity for love and affection from being channelled into stable relationships, and the resentment lies dormant, like a volcano, waiting to be detonated into violence by stress."[39] Violence is the frustration of love. Sooner or later we all pay for the loveless abuse of children. Children are the heirs to our tomorrows; as long as we allow them to suffer today there is little cause for optimism for the future.

NOTES

1. C. Ray Jeffery, "Punishment and Deterrence: A Psychobiological Statement," in *Biology and Crime*, ed. C. Jeffery (Beverly Hills, Calif.: Sage, 1979).

2. Ashley Montagu, "A Scientist Looks at Love," *Phi Beta Kappan* (1970): p. 46.

3. William Glasser, *The Identity Society* (New York: Harper & Row, 1976): p. 187.

4. Marvin Wolfgang, Robert Figlio, and Thorsten Sellin, *Delinquency in a Birth Cohort* (Chicago: University of Chicago Press, 1972).

5. Paul Tracy, Marvin Wolfgang, and Robert Figlio, *Delinquency in Two Birth Cohorts* (Chicago: University of Chicago Press, 1985).

6. L. Bennett, T. Rosenbaum, and W. McCullough, *Counseling in Correctional Environments* (New York: Human Sciences Press, 1978): p. 76.

7. Harvey Cleckley, *The Mask of Sanity*, 4th ed. (St. Louis: Mosby, 1964).

8. Ibid., p. 406.

9. Sarnoff Mednick and K. Finello, "Biological Factors and Crime: Implica-

tions for Forensic Psychiatry," *International Journal of Law and Psychiatry* (1983): p. 3.

10. Daisy Shalling, "Psychopathy-related Personality Variables and the Psychophysiology of Socialization," in *Psychopathic Behavior*, ed. R. Hare and D. Shalling (New York: Wiley, 1978).

11. Anthony Walsh, "Cognitive Functioning and Delinquency: Property versus Violent Crime," *International Journal of Offender Therapy and Comparative Criminology* 31 (1987): pp. 285–89.

12. T. Chase, P. Fedio, N. Foster, R. Brooks, G. Di Chiro, and L. Mansi, "Wechsler Adult Intelligence Scale Performance: Cortical Localization by Fluorodeoxyglucose F 18 Positron Emission Tomography," *Archives of Neurology* 41 (1984): pp. 244–47.

13. David Wechsler, *The Measurement and Appraisal of Adult Intelligence* (Baltimore: Williams and Wilkins, 1958), p. 176.

14. Pierre Flor-Henry, "Gender, Hemispheric Specialization and Psychopathology," *Social Science and Medicine* 12b (1978): pp. 155–62.

15. A. Kaufman, "Verbal-Performance IQ Discrepancies on the WISC-R," *Journal of Consulting and Clinical Psychology* 5 (1976): pp. 739–44.

16. June Andrew, "Delinquency: Intellectual Imbalance?" *Criminal Justice and Behavior* 4 (1977): pp. 99–104.

17. Anthony Walsh, J. Arthur Beyer, and Thomas Petee, "Intellectual Imbalance: Comparing High Verbal and High Performance IQ Delinquents," *Criminal Justice and Behavior* 14 (1987): pp. 370–79.

18. M. Zuckerman, M. Buchsbaum, and D. Murphy, "Sensation Seeking and Its Biological Correlates," *Psychological Bulletin* 88 (1980): pp. 187–214.

19. L. Lidberg, I. Modin, L. Oreland, R. Tuck, and A. Gillner, "Platelet Monoamine Oxydase Activity and Psychopathy," *Psychiatry Research* 16 (1985): pp. 339–43.

20. L. Taylor, *Born to Crime* (Westport, Conn.: Greenwood, 1984): p. 89. Grace Balazs found that only 4 per cent of reported crimes are committed by people over 65. "The Elderly Offender: Literature Review and Field Interviews," paper presented at the Second Annual Idaho Conference for Students in the Social Sciences and Public Affairs, 1990.

21. T. Keiser, "Schizotype and the Wechsler Digit Span Test," *Journal of Clinical Psychology* 31 (1976): pp. 303–06.

22. A. Mawson and Carol Mawson, "Psychopathy and Arousal: A New Interpretation of the Psychophysiological Literature," *Biological Psychiatry* 12 (1977): pp. 47–74.

23. Ibid., p. 65.

24. Robert Hare, *Psychopathy: Theory and Research* (New York: Wiley, 1970), p. 95.

25. Ibid., note 1, p. 109.

26. Ashley Montagu, *Touching: The Human Significance of the Skin* (New York: Harper & Row, 1978), p. 178.

27. L. DiCara, "Learning in the Autonomic Nervous System," *Scientific American* 222 (1970): pp. 30–39.

28. Michael Wadsworth, "Delinquency, Pulse Rates and Early Emotional Deprivation," *British Journal of Criminology* 16 (1976): pp. 245–56.

29. Anthony Walsh, J. Arthur Beyer, and Thomas Petee, "Violent Delinquency: An Examination of Psychopathic Typologies," *Journal of Genetic Psychology* 148 (1987): pp. 386–92.

30. Wouter Buikhuisen, "Aggressive Behavior and Cognitive Disorders," *International Journal of Law and Psychiatry* (1982): p. 214.

31. Richard Solomon, "The Opponent-Process Theory of Acquired Motivation," *American Psychologist* 35 (1980): pp. 691–712.

32. D. Wax and V. Haddox, "Enuresis, Fire Setting and Cruelty to Animals in Male Adolescent Delinquents: A Triad Predictive of Violent Behavior," *Journal of Psychiatry and Law* 2 (1972): pp. 45–71.

33. Victor Denenberg, "Hemispheric Laterality in Animals and the Effects of Early Experience," *Behavioral and Brain Sciences* 4 (1981): pp. 1–49.

34. W. Fry and M. Langeth, *Crying: The Mystery of Tears* (New York: Winston Press, 1985).

35. A. Heilbrun and M. Heilbrun, "Psychopathy and Dangerousness: A Comparison, Integration and Extension of Two Psychopathic Typologies," *British Journal of Clinical Psychology* 24 (1985): pp. 181–95.

36. Ibid., note 29.

37. S. Dillingham, "Manual on Catching Ones Who Kill and Kill," *Insight* (February 1988): p. 24.

38. Robert Waite, *The Psychopathic God: Adolf Hitler* (New York: Basic Books, 1977). Although few would argue with my characterization of Hitler as evil, some may balk at my characterization of him as a genius. However, sociologist Michael Blain writes that Hitler was extremely "calculating in his approach to propaganda . . . and extremely successful in revving up his military machine to do battle." Blain's article makes abundantly clear that Hitler was an "evil genius," and an applied psychologist of the first order. Michael Blain, "Fighting Words: What We Can Learn from Hitler's Hyperbole," *Symbolic Interaction* 11 (1988): pp. 257–76.

39. Colin Wilson, *A Criminal History of Mankind* (London: Panther, 1984), p. 623.

7

Love and Society

In love the separate does remain, but as something united, and
no longer as something separate.   —Hegel

THE IMPORTANCE OF LOVE,
VIEWED CROSS-CULTURALLY

Most of the evidence examined so far, relating to the importance of love
to the individual, comes from Western industrialized societies. Do the characteristics associated with love and love deprivation hold true regardless
of the cultural context? Put another way, do cross-cultural studies corrob-
orate the findings of Western studies and thereby increase our confidence
that the development of love and attachment has universal implications?

Anthropologist Ronald Rohner set out to answer this question by
examining over a period of 15 years the effects of love and love deprivation
in 101 different cultures. His results are contained in a book entitled *They
Love Me, They Love Me Not: A Worldwide Study of the Effects of Parental
Acceptance and Rejection.* He concludes this delightful piece of comparative
anthropology by asserting that the need for love exists in all cultural settings
and that it is a universal need shared by all members of the human species.
Whether we are Bantus or Britons, Ainus or Americans, the need for love
is rooted in our common genetic makeup and evolution. If we don't receive
it, says Rohner, "pernicious things happen to us," and these malignant effects
"have implications permeating throughout both personality and the entire
social system."[1]

A tragic illustration of Rohner's assertion is provided by Colin Turnbull's study of the Ik tribe of Uganda. The Ik had been hunters and gath-
erers before being driven off their lands in the late 1930s by the Ugandan
government and forced to become farmers in a drought-stricken locale. The
Ik proved to be poor farmers, and only government relief prevented mass
starvation. But the relief was paltry, and hunger was the constant companion

of every Ik. Turnbull's account of the Iks' adaptation to their new, enforced lifestyle is a savage documentation of what happened to a people who came to feel that generosity, compassion, and love were inimical to personal survival. Young children were starved and turned out of the family hut at the tender age of three. The strong bullied the weak and stole food from the mouths of ailing kinfolk and parents. The suffering of others were occasions for amusement, and the dead were disposed of by rolling them unceremoniously over a cliff into a gorge. The Ik became a "community" of extreme "rugged individualists," scratching and clawing for personal survival; every other individual was considered no more than a competitor for scarce foodstuffs.[2]

Despite the hideousness of the Ik culture, enough of them survived to cause Turnbull to wonder if love is all that necessary. If it is, then it should be discernible among the Ik. But since, according to Turnbull, it isn't, we have ipso facto evidence that love is not necessary for survival.[3] The Ik study certainly shows that love is not absolutely necessary for short-term brute survival, strength and callousness being more functional under such circumstances. But certainly Rohner's "malignant effects . . . on the personality and on the entire social system" are starkly in evidence here.

The Ik experience does not gainsay the importance of love; it emphasizes it. There is no doubt that the pursuit of a full stomach takes precedence over emotional attachments in the hierarchy of sheer survival. But many Iks perished, more from brutality and neglect than from starvation. In fact, subsequent anthropological inquiry found that the entire tribe finally disintegrated into small bands of marauding bandits. There was total destruction of a centuries-old culture within three short decades. Assuredly, the forced relocation of the tribe, with its psychological blow to a distinct and successful way of life, plus the poor land and attendant hunger, precipitated the decline, after which the loss of human love made it inevitable.

Other cultural practices contribute to the level of decency and humanity within cultures. James Prescott tested his thesis, discussed in chapter 1, regarding the either/or nature of the pleasure and violence brain centers, using cross-cultural data. He hypothesized that low levels of body pleasure, defined as physical affection between parents and children and as adult sexual pleasure, would be associated with high levels of physical violence. In 36 of the 49 societies he examined he found the expected relationship. Twenty-two of the societies with high levels of physical affection for infants had low levels of adult violence, and 14 societies characterized by low physical affection for infants had high levels of adult physical violence. Of the 13 societies that could not be classified by level of violence on the basis of infant affectional practices, all but one could be classified by the presence or absence of sexual pleasure experiences during adolescence.[4]

The romantic Cheyenne we met in the Introduction is one culture that could not be classified on the basis of infant affectional practices. To read E. Adamson Hoebel's account of the tribe, there surely have been few cultures more solicitous of their infants and children than the Cheyenne. But Hoebel tells us that the Cheyenne were an intensely militaristic, bloodthirsty, and cruel people who practiced torture on their enemies with relish.[5] We saw that the Cheyenne were an extremely sexually repressed culture. According to Prescott's theory and data, the Cheyennes' violent propensities were attributable to the repression of pleasurable sexual activity outside the bonds of marriage.[6]

The message provided by Prescott's data is that physically affectionate societies are unlikely to be physically violent ones. The anthropological evidence is consistent with his neurophysiological thesis that the more often the pleasure centers of the brain are "turned on," the more one is likely to become a "pleasure-prone" individual whose violence centers in the brain are not easily activated; hence, pleasure drives out pain. If we are to enjoy life in a relatively peaceful society, we must emphasize personal relationships and encourage pleasure.

However, we encounter difficulties slipping from the imperative to the indicative mode. One of Prescott's prescriptions for a more peaceful and loving society is the same as that offered by Plato some 2,500 years ago: a more relaxed and open attitude toward sexuality, both premarital and extramarital. Prescott decries the West's puritanical attitudes toward sexuality, stating that the values we place on monogamy, chastity, and virginity lead to the frustration of pleasure and thus leave room for the ready emergence of violence.[7]

I am just enough of a hedonist to have agreed with him in those halcyon days prior to the appearance of the AIDS virus. Today, Prescott's might be a prescription for destruction. Somehow we have to go beyond the individual and his or her behavior to explore the behavioral context in any attempt to define the "good society," or the "loving society."

LOVE IN A SOCIOPOLITICAL CONTEXT

Love, in all its forms, requires a lover and a love object. It is born and sustained by the interactions of human beings, as is society itself. All of the things we have been discussing—maternal behavior, child abuse, aggression, feelings of self-worth, romantic love, and so forth—take place in a social context. The anthropological evidence shows strongly that there are well-founded reasons to believe that social living, and hence the life of our species, would have ceased were it not for the evolutionary selection of love. Freud saw love, along with work, as the twin parents of culture.[8] Work we must if we are to eat, clothe, and accommodate ourselves. Love we must if we are to cooperate in these endeavors and raise the next generation to continue what we have carried on from our ancestors.

There has been a tendency to view the Freudian eros in narrowly sexual terms. While this may be a valid interpretation of Freud's earlier writing, he later broadened the concept to include a universal form of love that includes self-love, parental love, civic love, and love (more or less) for all humanity. Love in its broadest meaning is therefore an indiscriminate concept that denotes a total love in all its manifestations. Eros should not be considered to be some spiritual force unamenable to investigation, nor should the term *sexual* apply solely to the urge to copulate.[9] Our self-love has to reach out and affirm the existence and worth of others with whom we share our society and our planet. All social and cultural life involves dependency and interdependency, no matter how much one's culture might value and and nurture personal independence. No person is an island; each of us relates positively to ourselves only insofar as we are related and connected positively to the rest of humanity.

Societies vary; some social forms are conducive to love and some are inimical to love. Just because humans have lived under all manner of sociopolitical systems, it does not mean that all are equally conducive to physical, psychological, and spiritual well-being. If a society fosters insecurity, anxiety, and hostility because of excessive competitiveness for scarce resources, as with the Ik—or even for ample resources, as is increasingly happening in America—there will be little love within it. The Harvard pediatrician Dr. T. Berry Brazelton says that a very great proportion of America's children are suffering psychological and physical deprivation, and that as "a pediatrician with 40 years' experience with 25,000 children, mostly middle class, I have begun to regard the growing neglect and poverty of the young as the biggest threat to the nation's future. I also see evidence that we could start preventing this terrible waste, with remedies available right now—*but we seem to have lost the will to even think about it.*"[10]

However, conversely, if there is little competition and conflict, there will be little creativity and progress, and the society will stagnate. Competitiveness, it is clear, has to be balanced with cooperation and concern in a loving society.

What is a "good" society? This question is a lot more difficult than asking what makes a good mother or a good husband. There is no way to prevent one's ideology from intruding into any attempt to answer this question. Certainly there will be much disagreement among those audacious enough to tackle it. Psychoanalyst Reuben Fine is such an adventurous soul. He divides societies into what he calls love cultures and hate cultures: "Love cultures are those in which the predominant feelings of people toward one another are positive and affectionate; hate cultures are the reverse." [11] Despite the circularity of this definition, it serves our purpose for the present.

Examples of love cultures given by Fine are the Tasaday, the Mangaia, the Ifaluk, the Hutterites, and the Arapesh. Fine agrees with Prescott that one of the defining characteristics of love cultures is the wide latitude allowed for sexual expression. He fails to point out, however, that these societies tend to be extremely small. (The Tasaday, for instance, consist of a small group of about 25 people.) They are also relatively isolated from other societies. Isolation means that there has been little or no need for such cultures to develop the technology of war or to experience out-group hatred, and their small size and simple lifestyles preclude excessive in-group competitiveness. Their cultures, being so vastly different from ours, provide us with little meaningful guidance as to how a large and complex society can become more loving.

Fine's cultures of hate include the Aztec, the Jivaro, the Tauade, the Dobu, Nazi Germany, and the entirety of Western civilization! Common threads running through hate cultures are patriarchy, devaluation of women, sexual repression, and some absolutist form of religious or political ideology. Hate cultures are, on the whole, considerably larger and more complex than love cultures, and have a well-developed and well-financed system of warfare. Since some of these hate cultures are more similar in size and complexity to modern Western cultures, they have more lessons to impart to us than do love cultures. The lessons they hold for us are negative rather than positive—what to avoid rather than what to adopt. With this in mind we can begin to explore what makes a good society within the context of modern society.

An excellent working definition of a good society, which spares us the circularity of Fine's, is offered by Erich Fromm:

> Whether or not an individual is healthy is primarily not an individual matter, but depends on the structure of his society. A healthy society furthers man's capacity to love his fellow men, to work creatively, to develop his reason and objectivity, to have a sense of self which is based on the experience of his own productive powers. An unhealthy society is one which creates mutual hostility, distrust, which transforms man into an instrument of use and exploitation of others, which deprives him of a sense of self, except inasmuch as he submits to others he becomes an automation. [12]

Few would argue with Fromm in general, but feathers would certainly fly in any discussion of particulars. How does a society create a capacity for love in its members, and how does it assure them creative work? The distasteful truth is that it cannot. Only those who view the abstraction called society as an all-powerful, prime mover and who view human beings as animated by nothing but social forces believe that society can live up to such a vision. Even the "best" societies throughout history have failed to create universal adherence to the Golden Rule or to compensate for the alienation among those who have had to perform stultifying but necessary work. Conversely, the "worst" societies have produced their share of loving saints and creative geniuses.

DEMOCRACY

The kind of society we live in generally makes a difference to the "average" level of love and compassion within it. I am convinced that democracy is the sociopolitical system most in tune with Fromm's definition of a good society. *Democracy* is one of those words that changes its meaning, depending upon who is using it. Few governments in the world, regardless of how oppressive they may be, fail to declare that they are guided by the voice of the people. My use of the term is in the Anglo-American, constitutional sense—that is, freedom of press, religion, and association, the rule of law and equality before it, the right to dissent and to petition, and the presence of two or more viable opposition political parties.

What is it about democracy that allows for a greater general level of loving relationships within society? I believe it is the sense of freedom; of having some say in the way things are done; of being left alone to develop one's creative capacities; in living under laws which prevent extremes of exploitation of others on the basis of privilege, race, or class; and of living in a system that encourages and rewards education. The strength—and perhaps the self-fulfilling prophesy—of most actual democracies is the society's universally accepted assumption, generally, of the rationality, worth, and dignity of the individual. In a perfect democracy, individuals can be entrusted to conduct themselves properly and are assumed to be wise enough to know what that means. Therefore, there should, ideally, be a minimum of state compulsion.

You will not like democracy if you are philosophically predisposed to the logic that concludes that the citizen finds his or her self-actualization in the subjugation of individual will to the state; you will not like it if you yearn for the dictatorship of the proletariat; you will not like it if you believe in racial, national, or sexual superiority; nor will you like it if, with Mussolini, you believe that the guiding principle of good citizenship is "Believe! Obey! Fight." These beliefs are part and parcel of the ideological absolutism of Fine's hate cultures.

It is no accident that the philosophical father of modern democracy, that great English philosopher John Locke, is also the father of modern empirical science. Both democracy and empirical science ideally eschew dogmatism, intolerance, and so-called received truths. Although these aberrations intrude in both systems from time to time, it is more usual for these systems to demand that all sides of an issue be explored and put to the test of experience. Disciplined dissonance is the music of both endeavors seeking progress in their own arenas of inquiry. By "disciplined" I mean, in democracy, that conflicting ideas should be bandied about within the framework of parliamentary procedure, and not settled by gangs of toughs in the streets or by dictatorial fiat. In the case of science, I mean that truth and reality should be sought within the framework of the canons of scientific methodology, and not by ideology, reputation, and authority. Out of any clash of contending ideas should emerge a tentative harmony. This process stands in contradistinction to ideologists of any persuasion, whose conclusions precede their inquiry—if indeed there *is* an inquiry.

The value of love, as such, is only an *implicit* principle of democracy. Although the theme of altruistic love runs below the surface of the writings of many of the philosophers of democracy who laud the "common man," freedom is the preeminent theme. Arnold Toynbee, one of the great historians of our century, has said that we are free to the extent that we follow the highest law of God—the law of love.[13] But this law of love, in the sense that it is a constructive, cohesive, and altruistic bond with our fellows, demands freedom for its general expression. The lack of freedom—oppression in its many forms—is the political expression of lovelessness. It is a blatant contradiction to assert that we can love those whom we oppress and to whom we deny the possibility of creative growth. Where there is coercion there is no love; where there is love there is freedom. This is true whether we are talking about married couples or whole societies.

Altruism, an unselfish, positive regard for the interests of others, is a form of love. If there is any distinction to be made between love and altruism, it is perhaps in the greater intensity implied by the former, a difference in degree rather than in kind. Some modern, biologically oriented thinkers believe that there is a genetic basis for altruism. Warder Allee is one evolutionist who feels that the evidence points to stronger tendencies toward altruism in human nature than toward any "dog-eat-dog" egoism. The evolutionary reasoning is that the fruits of hunting and gathering in humankind's first "societies" had to be shared more or less equally among members of the group or band if the band was to survive as a social unit. Since humans are social animals, the survival of the band meant the survival of each individual in it. Any member of the band who did not show social impulses toward altruistic cooperation would have been denied access to the cave and the gene pool.[14] If too many members of the band refused to share food and shelter with other members, the band would cease to exist as such. This is the fate that befell the unfortunate Ik. Because no primitive band, clan, or tribe could survive without cooperation, cohesion, and altruism, and because no individual can long survive outside a social grouping, altruism has been selected for the biology of Homo sapiens.

However, the logic of this proposition necessarily limits the notion of altruism to the small kinship constellation. It was toward kin, clan, and tribe that individual altruism was directed, because these were the groups and individuals most likely to reciprocate. Outsiders had no stake in one's survival; in all likelihood, the very opposite was true. Perhaps the fear of strangers (xenophobia) also has its origins in those prehistoric ages when life was difficult and short. The more one avoided contact with humans outside of one's circle, the more likely one was not to be harmed or killed. Avoiding contact outside of one's circle must have inevitably strengthened the attachment to those within it. This form of selective altruism takes place in the emotional limbic brain, unaffected by the reasoning of the neocortex. Its survival is mindless tribalism, which today is expressed in the form of flag-waving nationalism and patriotism.

From any reading of history or the social sciences, it is impossible not to conclude that we humans regard the interests of others in direct proportion to the closeness of the ties we share with them. This would appear to be a sort of law of diminishing return of the Golden Rule. The Chinese philosopher Mo-tzu described the nature of tribal altruism more than four centuries before the birth of Christ:

> A thief loves his own family and does not love other families, hence he steals from other families to benefit his own family. Each grandee loves his own clan and does not love other clans, hence he causes disturbances to other clans to benefit his own clan. Each feudal lord loves his own state and does not love other states, so he attacks other states in order to benefit his own state. The causes of all disturbances . . . lie herein. . . . it is always from want of equal love to all.[15]

How compelling is this statement of Mo-tzu's. Whenever humans set themselves apart from others and speak of "us and them," we tend to see a general increase in in-group attachment coupled with an increase in outgroup indifference or cruelty. During times of maximum differentiation, such as wartime, a nation will draw together, and we usually see a significant reduction in anti-social behavior within the nation. On the other hand, the "enemy" is systematically set apart from "us" to such an extent that it seems quite natural to behave in a beastly fashion toward it. The domestic equivalent of rampant nationalism is racism. Both racism and nationalism rest at bottom on a sharp distinction between "us" (who are superior) and "them" (who are inferior). It is a sign of social maturity when a society condemns racism; when we rise above nationalism, it will be a sign of species maturity.

What has this to do with democracy? Alexis de Tocqueville, an aristocratic Frenchman who admired the young American democracy, was perhaps the first to note that altruism becomes more generalized as societies become more democratic, with less rigid distinctions being drawn between categories of people. It does so because as others come to be considered more like ourselves, the more readily we are able to understand and empathize with their concerns and suffering. De Tocqueville made the observation that in no country was criminal justice administered with more mildness than in the United States of the 1830s. He attributed this mildness to the equality of conditions existing in white America at that time.[16] (The treatment of slaves was not counted because at that time they were, both by law and custom, still considered less than human—not "us.")

Nineteenth-century French sociologist Emile Durkheim also recognized that as nations become more democratic their systems of justice move progressively away from retribution to restitution. Whatever the shortcomings of the penal codes of democratic nations are said to be, there is little doubt that they are administered with more fairness and concern for the accused than in nondemocratic nations. It seems to go against the grain of human nature to be overly harsh with those whom we perceive to be similar in many ways to ourselves. Some hold that the feeling of beneficence extends beyond national boundaries, for it is a fact of history that no two democracies, qua democracies, have ever gone to war with each other. As de Tocqueville so presciently put it: "Those tendencies to pity which are produced by the equality of conditions [tend to] quench the military spirit. . . . amongst the civilized nations, the warlike passions will become more rare and less intense in proportion as social conditions shall be more equal."[17]

The fact that no two democracies have ever gone to war with each other, a striking testimony to de Tocqueville's 150-year-old insight, is an extremely powerful statement. No other fact or conglomeration of facts could attest more forcefully to the moral superiority of democracy. Democracies generally allow their own citizens to know, grow, and love themselves. In the knowing of our own needs and lovableness we come to know the needs and lovability of others. The struggles for equality and dignity for minorities and women that can only occur in a democracy constitute grounds (and practice) for recognizing the equality and dignity of others beyond our national boundaries.

The full integration of women into the political sphere of democracies (yet to be accomplished, but in motion) will perhaps further humanize the political process in the same way that women humanize their menfolk. The Greenham Common women in Britain and the Peace Camp movements in the United States and West Germany are examples of female commitment to peace and sanity in the world. Recall that subjugation of women was one of the defining characteristics of Fine's culture of hate.

The altruism of predemocratic humans is intense and sacrificial, since the intensity of their altruism is in inverse proportion to the range of perceived kinship (the narrower the range, the more intense the feeling of "us-ness"). The fanatical suicide fighter pilots of Japan in World War II and the guerrillas called terrorists in present-day Islamic countries are but two examples of the coupling of intense in-group loyalty and intense out-group hatred. The pure altruism of democracies is generally far less intense and personal, because it is more broadly focused and less particularistic. (De Tocqueville noted that men in democracies rarely sacrifice themselves for one another.)

If democracies produce men less willing to sacrifice themselves, they may also—at some times—produce men less willing to sacrifice others in the name of some fatuous doctrine or another. I don't want somebody to sacrifice his or her life for me, thereby signifying that that life is less valuable or worthy than mine. What I do want, however, is not to be a sacrificial lamb for ignorant people who despise me because they see me as different from them. Respect me, appreciate me, and accept me as a fellow citizen of the world for all my differences. If we don't extend this feeling of "we-ness" to all humankind, we will continue the divisiveness that has characterized human history.

Someone once said that the world is in a mad race between education and disaster. Democracy is a difficult form of government because we have to make ourselves intelligent if we are to function in freedom. Perhaps the assumption of human rationality and intelligence is democracy's strength and self-fulfilling prophesy. Wouldn't it be marvelous if we could establish a new world based on the values of love, freedom, equality, and intelligence? Aldous Huxley, author of *Brave New World*, a book that engulfs us in the horrors of a world built on hatred, oppression, hierarchy, and ignorance, provides us with his recipe for a better world and the values it must embrace:

> The value, first of all, of individual freedom, based upon the facts of human diversity and genetic uniqueness; the value of charity and compassion, based upon the old familiar fact, lately rediscovered by modern psychiatry—the fact that, whatever their mental and physical diversity, love is as necessary

to human beings as food and shelter; and finally the value of intelligence, without which love is impotent and freedom unattainable.[18]

Democracy is by no means a perfect system of government; it has a long way to go to realize Huxley's dream. Nevertheless, it has gone further toward it than any other form of government. If we add up the profits and losses of democracy, we will find it very definitely in the black. Red ink here and there is outweighed by the dignity and camaraderie among equals that it engenders.

MARXISM, CAPITALISM, STALINISM, AND CHRISTIAN LOVE

We who wax positive about democracy are its native sons and daughters, so we must be careful not to fall into the "us/them" trap decried earlier. With this caveat in mind, let's briefly examine democracy's most powerful, though steadily weakening opponent, in the modern world.

Unlike democracy, Marxism is a sociopolitical system with a philosophy that *explicitly* extols love as the organizing force in human affairs. Countries labelled socialistic or communistic claim adherence to the humanistic tenets set forth by its founder, Karl Marx. While a young student in Trier, Germany, Marx set forth a principle that was to be the guiding motif of his life:

> The main principle . . . which must guide us in selection of a vocation is the welfare of humanity, our own perfection. Man's nature makes it possible to reach its fulfillment only by working for the perfection of his society. Then we experience no meager, limited egoistic joy, but our happiness belongs to millions, our deeds live on quietly but eternally effective and the glowing tears of noble men will fall on our ashes.[19]

Marx, ever the pragmatic philosopher, could never rest content to illuminate a principle and then leave it. It is evident from the body of his works that he felt love to be the greatest good; humanity had to actualize it by struggling toward that end. Love to Marx was not viewed as some syrupy theological entity apart from humanity; it was not a spiritualized essence that simply existed but rather a totally human accomplishment for which mankind must strive. Marx and Engels railed against the spiritualization of love, because this form of love endows it with an independent existence outside of those of us who experience it. Such a view of love, said Marx and Engels, contributes to our alienation from ourselves and from our fellows.

Marx anticipated Freud in positing a physical basis for love. He saw love infusing the young organism with libidinal energy and giving it the ability to abstract itself from the rest of existence. "Love first really teaches man to believe in the objective world outside of himself, which not only makes the man an object, but the object a man."[20] Becoming an object to oneself, in the sociological sense, means the ability to take the role of the other, to empathize and sympathize with the emotional and cognitive reality of others. Those who are deprived of love, as we have seen, lack this ability. Love means security, and a sense of security enables one to become autonomous enough to reach out and embrace others, rejoicing in, rather than fearing, the differences that separate the ignorant and unloved.

In light of what we have just said, listen to what political sociologist Seymour Lipset has to say about the antidemocratic character.

He [the anti-democratic personality] is likely to have been exposed to punishment, lack of love, and a general atmosphere of tension and aggression since early childhood—all experiences which tend to produce deep-rooted hostilities expressed by ethnic prejudices, political authoritarianism, and chiliastic transvaluation religion.[21]

On an individual level, Lipset's description of the antidemocratic personality is very much like Fine's description of hate cultures; both highlight the link between the personal experience of love and positive social attitudes and structures.

In a capitalist mode of production, reasoned Marx, human beings are not secure, and therefore they are not loving or autonomous. They are alienated from their work, from themselves, and from others because capitalism generates conditions that objectify human relations. By "objectifying" human relations, Marx meant that under capitalism human needs are subordinated to material things, and relationships are mediated by economic considerations—the "cold cash nexus." Relationships thus mediated are inauthentic; they are "it-it" connections rather than the "I-Thou" attachments of Martin Buber.

There is truth in Marx's criticism of capitalism, for we surely sacrifice human authenticity and spirituality if we lose ourselves in a vortex of acquisitiveness, particularly when laws are passed to ensure the means of acquisition to a few, at the expense of many other citizens. American sociologist Neil Smelser sees the emphasis on personal success in a capitalist society leading to a displacement of familial commitment by occupational obligations—and thus to a less-loving society.[22] This is probably true to some extent; after all, we have only so much time and psychic energy to devote to various tasks. But we have to ask ourselves if the condition is so severe or so terminal as to demand a "solution" as drastic as a Leninist or Stalinist dictatorship in which, Leon Trotsky predicted, "all would rise to the level of Aristotle, Goethe, and Marx"? It did not happen, but it has not in democracies either.

In Shakespeare's *Taming of the Shrew*, Kate complains bitterly that Petruchio, her husband, inflicts all manner of suffering and indignities upon her "i' th' name of perfect love." Claiming to operate in the name of Marx's "perfect love," whole societies are seen to have humiliated and oppressed their citizens. It is painfully obvious that communism has not become a liberating or positive alternative to capitalism. Marx's clarion call for universal love and brotherhood has been turned into petrified dogma, just another form of totalitarianism. The governments where communism triumphed before 1989 turned Marxism into a caricature of Marx's ideas, and its members became antirational catechists: "Who made you?" "The Soviet state made me." "Why were you made?" "I was made to struggle for the inevitable victory of the proletariat."

In practice, Stalinism's assumptions about human nature are the antithesis of Marx's. If one would grasp the essence of the Soviets' and their imitators' view of human nature, one could do no better than to read Fyodor Dostoyevsky's exposition of what his beloved Russia was or perhaps would become, in his *Brothers Karamazov*, more specifically, in the chapter entitled "The Grand Inquisitor."

The Grand Inquisitor was a wizened old cardinal of the Roman Catholic church in Spain at the height of the Spanish Inquisition. One day he chanced across the resurrected Jesus Christ walking the streets of Seville. The Inquisitor had Jesus arrested and proceeded to lecture him on the medieval church's conception of human nature, and then to castigate him for returning and jeopardizing that conception. The Inquisitor boasted that the collusion of church and state had at last "vanquished freedom and [had] done so to make men happy." Frightened, selfish, sinful, and unintelligent men can only be captivated by "miracle, mystery, and authority." If this does not satisfy, they can be placated "with children's songs and innocent dance" (and, of course, the Inquisition).

The Inquisitor further berated Jesus for his foolishness and lack of compassion for humanity, evidenced by his refusal to accept the Devil's offer of the purple of Rome and his refusal to demonstrate his divinity by casting himself from the topmost pinnacle of the temple. Had Jesus done so, reasoned the Inquisitor, humans would have had unequivocal proof that he was the savior, and he would have assured himself of humanity's love and devotion and stamped himself with myth, mystery, and authority.

The scene could just as well have been played in any other center of absolutism where humanity is considered weak and inadequate, with minds too fragile to handle the clash of contending ideas. The private property most hated by a soviet-type regime is the possession of a private mind. The evils of capitalist exploitation pale into insignificance when placed alongside those committed by totalitarians in the name of the good of the state or society—which in reality means the good of themselves at the head of it.

Whatever the price, as the Grand Inquisitor informed Christ, it is worth it because it is necessary for the happiness of humanity. The old Inquisitor genuinely believed this to be so, and the Stalinists, with the same sort of sincere but twisted logic, would so inform a resurrected Marx, who surely would rail against their chains of gulags if he could return to earth.

What of Jesus's decision not to accept the Devil's offer? Dostoyevsky seems to be telling us that Jesus was respecting humanity's freedom by refusing to capture its devotion or love in such a manner. The beloved actualizes love in response to his or her worthiness. Had Jesus accepted, he would have become an object in which "love" was "compelled," in effect, for who could not help "loving" one so demonstrably powerful? But would the onlooker's or follower's emotion be love? Dostoyevsky thought not. Fear, awe, reverence, commitment, but not love, since the impetus would have been "forced" upon the onlooker, so to speak. Jesus refused to take advantage of our susceptibility to myth, mystery, and authority because, unlike the old cardinal and his followers, he respected human freedom and dignity.

Jesus wished for reasoned love from the hearts of free human beings, the respect desired of citizens by democracies. Absolutist states, as well as authoritarian religions, demand obedience from its captives or adherents by nationalizing affection or worship and turning it into state narcissism or dictated behavior. Such states attempt to capture the minds of their people by generating mindless tribalism through the use of militaristic anthems, parades, flag worship, and pledges of unconditional allegiance. In any evaluation of which brand of devotion is most in accord with human nature, one cannot ignore the walls erected to contain those who abhor herd mentality and look beyond the pasture yearning to be free. We cannot ignore the jubilance witnessed in Berlin when one such wall came tumbling down.

Let us not leave this soulless, antirational system of tyranny without an evaluation from a true believer. For those who may have believed that communism is institutionalized and politicized altruism, hearken to the words of Mao Tse-Tung, a man who should know what he is talking about: "Communism is not love. Communism is a hammer which we use to crush the enemy."[23]

THE MIDDLE WAY

Marxism and Leninism were not so much a reaction against democracy as they were against capitalism, albeit a form of capitalism that has for the most part ceased to exist. "Pure" capitalism is inimical to a loving society. As Ayn Rand, a supporter and philosopher of unfettered capitalism, put it: "Capitalism and altruism are incompatible; they are philosophical opposites; they cannot exist in the same man or the same society.[24]"

Yet, some form of capitalism appears to be a necessary bedfellow of democracy. Even Marx wrote eloquently in *The Communist Manifesto* of capitalism's role within his own lifetime in the advancement of science, the abolition of slavery, the beginnings of universal political suffrage and mass education, and an increase in general wealth. To be sure, these things were not intended consequences of capitalism, but capitalism made—or permitted—them to happen nonetheless. Capitalism, tempered by democratically imposed constraints, usually brings with it a general increase in the wealth of the citizenry and freedom from a dulling want. It is only when we are free of scratching for food that we are free to extend our psychic energies outwards to embrace others. Much of the Soviet-led world is today cautiously moving toward capitalism, and hopefully will become freer because of it. It was, and is, the excesses of unfettered capitalism that are decried by so many social philosophers.

The levelling tyranny of Stalinism and the oppressive inequalities of capitalism have led many social thinkers to curse both their houses. The thinking seems to be that the amelioration of one disagreeable situation can only be accomplished by substituting the other. This is only true if we accept the absurdity of simple negation, that is, of believing that if something is evil only its polar opposite can be good. The price of freedom does not have to mean untrammeled exploitation of the "masses" by the privileged, nor does achieving equality have to mean imposing state ownership of property and personal powerlessness on everyone. We must stop thinking of freedom and equality, those two beacons of political experience, as polar opposites. Freedom need not be purchased at the expense of social justice, nor need equality devour precious freedom. Freedom and equality are as compatible as love and rationality, for they are the political embodiment and expression of those qualities. Freedom without equality is unloving, and equality without freedom is unreasoned.

Some theorists are pessimistic about the prospect of generating an atmosphere of love within the modern urban society. They believe that such an atmosphere is only possible within a close-knit community. The erosion of the old sense of community and the corresponding onward rush of mass society has been a favorite topic of philosophers and sociologists since the Industrial Revolution. The German sociologist Ferdinand Tönnies idealized "community" (*Gemeinschaft*) and placed it in opposition to "society" (*Gesellschaft*). Community was humanity's natural living arrangement, providing for all our natural psychological needs in an enduring network of common values, mutual care and obligations, emotional ties of blood, neighborliness, friendliness, and an organic sense of belonging in which, Tönnies asserted, "one lives from birth on bound to it in weal and woe."[25]

Tönnies considered *Gesellschaft,* on the other hand, to be an artificial mode of human living. Human bonds in *Gesellschaft* are weak and rationally goal-oriented rather than emotional; its principle is struggle rather than concord. Rational market principles are substituted for emotional reciprocity, and atomized individuals live for themselves in a state of tension and competition with others similarly situated. We should not be surprised, then, that many people living in *Gesellschaft* societies fall victim to social pathologies. Unfortunately, these pathologies are part of the price we pay for freedom.

Urbanized societies are here to stay, for better or for worse; there will be no "withering away of the state." Tönnies' rhapsodizing about *Gemeinschaft* is a glittering generality, but like Oscar Wilde's mackerel in the moonlight— it glitters, but it stinks. When we value the individual over the community, the community does suffer, but the individual with talent and/or money and good health is left alone to develop as he or she will. The so-called permissive societies of the West certainly have their casualties, but a tight community can be repressive, and a repressive society has many more casualties. Having the dignity and freedom of self-determination, many, it is true, will plow the wrong field, but many more will rise far above the inhabitants of more traditional and tightly bound societies. If people love in a free society they do so because they chose to, not because they must. Nonetheless, we still have a duty to those who do not love to help them find the loving path by means of love-centered education and social programs such as paid parental leave, well-financed day care, etc. Through these means we can perhaps rediscover some of the emotional benefits of *Gemeinschaft* without sacrificing individual freedom in the process. In the final analysis, who among us would exchange life under democratic capitalism for a stultifying existence in a "workers paradise"?

On a positive note, many nations appear to be edging to the conclusion that freedom without equality is not altruistic and not acceptable and that equality never really was produced in the U.S.S.R. We have witnessed increasing equality in capitalist countries over the last 100 years, and communist systems in Europe toppled in 1989–1990. Fear of what is best in the other system, or so it appears to me, has been the prime mover of change in both systems. There is no doubt that the capitalist United

States is much more egalitarian than it was in the days of the robber barons. Conservative economist Milton Friedman, albeit with a certain amount of distaste, points out that almost the entire economic platform of the American Socialist Party in the 1928 election—for example, unemployment relief, child labor laws, hour and wage legislation, social security benefits, and ten other planks—are accepted features of American society today. Surely the United States is a more altruistic society than it would otherwise have been had it not adopted socialist ideas of social justice.[26]

The Soviet Union enjoys more freedom today than anyone would have ever imagined possible prior to *glasnost* and *perestroika*. The remarkable events in Eastern Europe during the last few months of 1989 bear striking testimony to people's desires to be free and to have the same standard of living achieved under democratic capitalism. Despite decades of repression and brain-washing, the brave people of the Eastern-bloc countries rose up to embrace democracy and capitalism when the opportunity presented itself. Their leadership appears to be taking seriously the droll Russian definition of communism as "the longest and most painful route from capitalism to capitalism." Let us hope this trend toward greater altruism and rationality continues in both hemispheres.

How far might we reasonably expect this trend to go? Grace Cairns concludes her study of the great cyclical theories of history in oriental and western thought by stating: "All the philosophies of history we have examined emphasize Love as the constructive and cohesive bond through which human societies grow and flourish; a world Global Society can grow and flourish on the basis of the same bond of love."[27] This is a beautiful thought, but it *is* debatable whether humans have the capacity for emotional engagements with social groups of any and all sizes up to and including a "world Global Society."

Cynics would argue that to believe that such is possible is maudlin sentimentality. *Liking* all humanity is humanly impossible, because it is plainly not within our power to like everyone. However it *is* within our power to be kind or unkind, to respect or disrespect the basic humanity of all people. Altruistic love is not an intensification of liking, as hate is an intensification of disliking. We can love even those we don't particularly like; that's why the ancient religions exhorted us to love rather than like our neighbors.

We have to have faith that the highest goals of humanity are possible. I have always been impressed that the three giants of the behavioral sciences, Sigmund Freud, Karl Marx, and Abraham Maslow, despite radically different concerns and theoretical orientations, had faith in the human capacity for the growth of social love.[28] History itself shows that we have extended fellowship from family to band, tribe, province, and nation, as we have come to reject the artificial barriers separating "them" from "us."

It's only one more step to extend human sympathies to all the races and nations of the world.

DEMOCRACY AND ROMANTIC LOVE

That special feeling of complete emotional involvement with one unique individual, which we call romantic love, has probably been a feature of our species since we began to walk upright. The exquisite joy of love has its origins in human biology, but the forms that it takes differ considerably from culture to culture and from age to age. For most of human history, romantic love did not have the same meaning that it does in today's Western cultures. In the Introduction we saw that throughout much of history and across a great number of cultures, romantic love has been considered potentially disruptive to the social system. This attitude, quite strange to our way of thinking, did not mean that people who held it were cold and heartless robots who did not enjoy or value romance. Our ancestors recognized the awesome power of love, as the definition of love offered by the twelfth-century French writer Andreas Capellanus makes clear: "Love is a certain inborn suffering derived from the sight of and excessive meditation upon the beauty of the opposite sex, which causes each one to wish above all things the embrace of the other and by common desire to carry out all of love's precepts in the other's embrace."[29]

But it was the very power of romantic love that made it so dangerous. Who would marry whom had great importance in premodern history (and still does in some cultures)—not for the individuals concerned, but in terms of the practical, political, social, and economic concerns of the family, tribe, or state to which the betrothed belonged. The new social units formed by the marriage of men and women were supposed to fit comfortably into the neat, hierarchical, communal patterns characteristic of traditional societies. The needs and feelings of the individuals concerned were of no importance. Indeed, the idea of individualism had very little meaning in those societies and in those times. The term *individual* meant "indivisible" or "inseparable," and to describe an individual was to describe the group to which he or she belonged. Respect and appreciation of the uniqueness of the separate human being was an alien concept, both practically and philosophically. This was the *Gemeinschaft* of which Tönnies was so enamored.

Young men and women were married off by others for purposes other than their own. If young people were allowed to make their own decisions about whom they would marry, love, not reason (defined in the terms of those making the arrangements), would motivate their decision. Love was exciting but unreliable, and a love marriage might eventually prove to be valueless and troublesome to the individuals concerned and to their social grouping.

Many premodern love stories contain a common theme of passion in conflict with family or politics, as well as the tragedies that inevitably befall young men and women irrational enough to fall in love with "unsuitable" partners. The love stories of Tristan and Iseult, Lancelot and Guinevere, Heloise and Abelard—and perhaps most fully expounded in the tragic story of Romeo and Juliet—are considered to be tales of great love and courage by modern readers. To the readers in the past, however, the moral of such stories might well have been "beware of foolish, antisocial love entanglements." It was taken for granted by early readers of these tales that if love was to arise in a relationship, it was meant to grow after a man and a woman were firmly tied in their matrimonial vows.

If arranged marriages were to be functional and unproblematic, methods of controlling the powerful emotion of romantic love had to be institutionalized. The sociologist William Goode lists a number of institutions by which this control was achieved.[30] The most prevalent was, and is, child marriage. The objective here is to cement the marriage commitment before any potential love attachment could develop between any pair whose marriage would run counter to family, tribe, or state purposes. This was a pattern common in India, in preliterate societies, and among the nobility of Europe.

Another common pattern was strict segregation of the sexes, which also made love attachments improbable (except perhaps between members of the same sex). This pattern was common in China, Japan, and Muslim countries. Yet another, and more enjoyable pattern, was that of "free love." In this pattern, youngsters are encouraged at an early age to engage freely in sex play with members of the opposite sex. (Drs. Prescott and Fine would surely approve.) Pair-bonds were expected to be brief and nonexclusive, the variety and brevity of relationships being designed to minimize feelings of intimacy and attachment to any one person. The system was also supposed to prevent jealousy and to impress upon youngsters that any marriage partner chosen for them was as good as any other.

While romantic love was controlled to various degrees, it was forever in the background waiting to burst forth. The rich and well-born have always been able to indulge their romantic urges with relative freedom. The consummate historical example of such indulgence is surely Henry VIII of England. When one has the power Henry enjoyed, one bends and breaks social norms to suit oneself, which is exactly what he did. The nobility and lesser aristocracy of any country were able to dabble in romance with paramours, chambermaids, and even with their wives. Without the unpleasantries of manual labor, they were able to enjoy an esthetic and amorous life.

The peasantry lived an entirely different life. Like the twentieth-century Ik, all their mental and physical resources were mobilized in the task of avoiding starvation. Under such conditions, romantic love was a luxury generally beyond the imaginations of the great mass of folk: "Poverty lacks the means to feed up love," wrote a seventeenth-century commentator. For the untitled, romance, like so many other of life's enjoyments, had to await a general rise in the economic standard of living.

With the advent of industrialism and the free market came the possibility of romantic love, as even Marx and Engels agreed. Romantic love was not on the conscious agenda of industrialists and capitalists. The social, political, and economic systems that evolved in the western world provided a context that made romantic love possible, perhaps inevitable. Most sociologists take it as a given that industrialism and the general wealth and leisure it engenders is a necessary, if not sufficient, condition for the emergence of romantic love as a pursuit open to all. As two early twentieth-century sociologists, Sumner and Keller, phrased it: "Capital . . . as a store of supplies relieving men from anxiety about maintenance, sets free the imaginations to find attraction in the human form and so awakens sex emotion of a more refined order."[31]

Riding on the coattails of these evolving socioeconomic systems was a growing respect for the individual, as well as the philosophical conviction that each person had the right to enter freely into individual contracts. The beginning of democracy marked the beginning of the end of traditional relationships based on considerations apart from those of the parties concerned. People became free to make their own contracts and commitments, including those of love and marriage.

In a free-market democracy the state has no need or desire to control the marriage market. It is true that until quite recently some southern states in the United States legally forbade interracial marriages, but it was psychological fear, rather than social and economic fears, that motivated these proscriptions. Just as democracy leaves individuals alone to develop and pursue their economic inclinations, it leaves them alone to follow their emotional inclinations. It is true that marriage decisions are still determined to some extent by many practical, nonemotional considerations as well as by love. But the important thing to note is that whatever these considerations may be, they are the private considerations of the individuals involved. Free individuals may make unwise decisions in love and marriage just as they do in careers and business enterprises. Modern marriages are notoriously frail and brittle, indicating that many poor choices are being made. But who of those involved in any kind of romantic relationship would give up the freedom to make their own choice, for good or for ill?

NOTES

1. Ronald Rohner, *They Love Me, They Love Me Not: A Worldwide Study of the Effects of Parental Acceptance and Rejection* (New York: Hraf Press, 1975), pp. 166–173.
2. Colin Turnbull, "The Mountain People," in *Anthropology 82/83*, ed. E. Angeloni (Guilford, Conn.: Dushkin, 1982).
3. Ibid., p. 36.
4. James Prescott, "Body Pleasure and the Origins of Violence," *Bulletin of the Atomic Scientists* 31 (1975): pp. 10–20.
5. E. Adamson Hoebel, *The Cheyennes: Indians of the Great Plains* (New York: Holt, Rinehart and Winston, 1960).
6. James Prescott, "Body Pleasure," p. 13.
7. Ibid., p. 19.
8. Sigmund Freud, *Civilization and Its Discontents* (New York: Norton, 1961), p. 48.
9. For interpretations of Freud's Eros concept, see D. Morgan, *Love, Plato, the Bible, and Freud* (Englewood Cliffs, N.J.: Prentice-Hall, 1964), and R. Osborn, *Marxism and Psychoanalysis* (New York: Dell, 1965).
10. T. Berry Brazelton, "Why Is America Failing Its Children?" *New York Times Magazine* (September 9, 1990): pp. 44ff. (italics added).
11. Reuben Fine, *The Meaning of Love in Human Experience* (New York: John Wiley, 1985), p. x.
12. Erich Fromm, *The Sane Society* (New York: Fawcett, 1955), p. 71.
13. Arnold Toynbee, *A Study of History*, 12 vols. (London: Oxford University Press, 1934–1961), vol. 7, p. 416.
14. Warder Allee, "Where Angels Fear to Tread: A Contribution from General Sociobiology to Human Ethics," in *The Sociobiology Debate*, ed. A. Caplan (New York: Harper and Row, 1978).

A "genetics" of altruism may not sit well with those readers who are aware that genes do not directly code for behavior. They code for physiological processes that indirectly affect behavior by influencing structures in the brain and the nervous system. A study by J. Philippe Rushton and his colleagues at the University of London Institute of Psychiatry, England, using 573 twin pairs (296 identical and 277 fraternal pairs), found a heritability coefficient for altruism of .51. What this means is that 51 per cent of the altruism variance in the sample is attributable to nonenviromental (genetic) variability. Because females and older individuals were significantly more altruistic than males and younger individuals, regardless of genetic relationship, this figure reflects adjustments for age and sex. Rushton and his colleagues hypothesize that gonadal hormones such as testosterone predispose toward aggressiveness, which in turn decreases nurturance and altruism. Because females and older males have lower levels of testosterone, it is believed that genes influence altruism via gonadal hormone secretion patterns. See J. Philippe Rushton, Davd Falker, Michael Neale, David Nias, and Hans Eysenck, "Altruism and Aggression: The Heritability of Individual Differences," *Journal of Personality and Individual Differences* 6 (1986): pp. 1192–1198.

15. Mo-tzu cited in Pitirim Sorokin, *The Ways and Power of Love* (Boston: Beacon Press, 1954), p. 459.

16. Alexis de Tocqueville, *Democracy in America* (New York: Mentor, 1956), pp. 72–77.

17. Ibid., p. 274.

18. Aldous Huxley, *Brave New World,* quoted in Grace Cairns, *Philosophies of History* (New York: Citadel Press, 1964), p. 474.

19. Karl Marx, *Writings of the Young Karl Marx on Philosophy and Society,* trans. and ed. L. Easton and K. Guddat (Garden City, N.Y.: Doubleday, 1967), p. 39.

20. Karl Marx and Friedrich Engels, *The Holy Family, or Critique of Critical Critique* (London: Foreign Language Publishing House, 1956), p. 32.

21. Seymour Lipset, *Political Man* (New York: Doubleday, 1963), p. 114.

22. Neil Smelser, *Theory of Collective Behavior* (New York: The Free Press, 1962), p. 63.

23. Mao Tse-Tung, quoted in Anthony Walsh, *Human Nature and Love: Biological, Intrapsychic and Social-Behavioral Perspectives* (Lanham, Md.: University Press of America, 1981), p. 318.

24. Ayn Rand, *For the New Intellectual* (New York: Random House, 1961), p. 54.

25. R. Herberle, "The Sociological System of Ferdinand Tönnies: 'Community' and 'Society,' " in *An Introduction to the History of Sociology,* ed. E. Barns (Chicago: University of Chicago Press, 1947), p. 228.

26. Milton Friedman, *Free to Choose* (New York: Avon, 1978), pp. 299–300.

27. Grace Cairns, *Philosophies of History* (New York: Citadel Press, 1962), p. 472.

28. Anthony Walsh, "Love and Human Authenticity in the Works of Freud, Marx and Maslow," *Free Inquiry in Creative Sociology* 14 (1986): pp. 21–26.

29. Andreas Capellanus, *The Art of Courtly Love,* trans. J. Parry (New York: Unger, 1959), p. 28.

30. William Goode, "The Theoretical Importance of Love," *American Sociological Review* 24 (1959): pp. 38–47.

31. Sumner and Keller cited in V. Grant, *Falling in Love: The Psychology of the Romantic Emotion* (New York: Springer, 1976), p. 157.

Part Three

In Love

8

Romantic Love: Its Origin and Purpose

Between two people, love itself is the important thing, and that
is neither you nor him. It is a third thing you must create.
—D. H. Lawrence

IN THE BEGINNING WAS THE FEMALE

"Male and female created He them," says the Book of Genesis. Most of
us are eternally grateful for this dual creation, but the authors of Genesis
got it backwards. The basic being is female; Adam, not Eve, is nature's
afterthought. For each human being is the product of the union of a woman's egg and a man's sperm. The egg carries only the female X chromosome and is therefore wholly female. Spermatozoa can be male (carrying
a Y chromosome) or female (X chromosome). The X chromosome is a
giant compared to the male Y, and it carries more genes. The egg itself
is about 85,000 times larger than the single sperm that will penetrate and
fertilize it. That single sperm has won a frantic race with about 250,000,000
of its brothers and sisters for the privilege of fusing with the waiting egg
to form the human zygote (from the Greek, "yoked," or "joined together").
Male spermatozoa are slightly more vigorous than their female counterparts,
so slightly more males are born. The ratio of male to female babies is about
52:48, although this ratio more than reverses itself over the lifespan, due
to the greater mortality rate of males at all ages.

The X or Y chromosome contained in the single sperm that impreg-
nates the female determines whether the zygote will differentiate as female
or male. If the embryo carries two X chromosomes, female ovaries will
form about six weeks after fertilization. If the embryo carries a Y chromosome, the male testes will form during the same period. With testes formed,
the male embryo starts to secrete the male androgens. A "complete" male
differentiation requires the presence of both the Y chromosome and the
secretion of androgen; the differentiation of a fertile female depends on

the presence of two X chromosomes and the absence of androgen action on the brain during this period.[1]

While the genes on the Y chromosome govern sensitivity to androgen via a histocompatible antigen called the H-Y antigen, a small proportion of XY fetuses are androgen insensitive. In such cases, the genetic male will develop female genitalia. Likewise, a genetic XX female fetus which experiences an excess of androgen will develop the external genitalia of a male, but with internal gonads. The androgen appears to operate by interacting with genetic material at the target cells by binding with receptors designed to accept it. The hormone is then carried to the nucleus of the cell, where it changes those cells from the basic female form to the male form.

With the testes secreting androgens there comes a modification of the male brain. The so-called "androgen bath" bathes the limbic system, making it androgen-sensitive. An androgen-sensitive or masculinized brain simply means that the threshold for firing the neurons governing characteristic male responses to stimuli is lowered. For instance, we saw in chapter 2 how testosterone (the most important of the androgens) lowers the firing threshold of the amygdala to produce male aggression (and also the sex drive). It may also be the androgenization of the brain that is responsible for the greater laterality of the male brain. Whatever else the androgen bath may affect, it is plain that it represents some addition to or modification of the basic human being. There is no analogous chemical "feminization" of the female brain that is governed by the ovaries. Sexual differentiation of a fertile female depends on *the absence of androgen*.[2]

The greater male tendency toward extremes and abnormalities of all kinds may be viewed in part as a function of the male's departure from the "standard" human being. Among females, any abnormality, whether positive or negative, that may be recessively present on one of the X chromosomes can be offset by its dominant partner on the other X chromosome. Hemophilia is an example of this process. Females carry the recessive gene for hemophilia, but it is usually only males who suffer from it. For a female to suffer from hemophilia she would have to be the daughter of a female carrier and a hemophiliac father—a rare occurrence. If a male inherits the gene for hemophilia from his mother, he lacks the second X chromosome to counteract it.

This is another example of nature's "bias" in favor of women. It seems that there is less departure from the norm in females in either direction, because they are too valuable to the species for nature to experiment with. Since there is greater possible variability in the male genetic package because of the XY pattern, nature has been freer to experiment with males. We see more geniuses among men but also more fools, more madness, more criminality, and more deviant behaviors of almost every kind.[3]

THE ORIGIN OF SEX

Nature loves symmetry; it arranges things in pairs. If we envision Adam and Eve in their primitive spendor cavorting in the Garden of Eden, we see two eyes and two ears behind which are two frontal lobes. Each has two arms, two legs, two kidneys, two lungs, and Eve has two breasts; Adam has two vestigial breasts, and two testicles between his legs. It is between the legs that nature departs from symmetry, providing Adam with a penis and Eve with a vagina. But Adam and Eve themselves are a pair just as necessary to one another as, say, the two frontal lobes each of them possesses. The penis and the vagina are the instruments that restore an apparent departure from symmetry to make male and female parts in a complementary whole.

Why do humans come in pairs? Why aren't we complete in ourselves as individuals? Why the perennial search for our "better halves," a search that generates a lot of jealousy, anger, depression, anxiety, and even murder, as well as joy and pleasure? It is not simply that sex is necessary for reproduction, because it isn't. Asexual reproduction abounds in nature, and it is more efficient than sexual reproduction. Earthworms, for instance, house both sexes in a single body. To reproduce themselves, earthworms simply do what unfriendly types use a four-letter word to tell us to do when they get mad at us—they fertilize themselves.

The answer to why we reproduce ourselves sexually lies in the *necessity for evolutionary adaptability and variety* in the human species. This can only be achieved by the scrambling into new permutations of genetic material from two genetically unrelated human beings. It is the constant shuffling of genes between men and women generation after generation that is the engine of human evolution. There would be no biological improvement if we reproduced asexually; each reproduction would be a carbon copy of the self. Amoebas simply divide like Plato's spheres, and that is why a "modern" amoeba, with the exception of changes brought about by random mutations, is no different from an amoeba of 500,000,000 years ago. An amoeba doesn't need to love in order to complement itself; it is complete in itself. This must be very boring, but I don't suppose amoebas care. Men and women do need one another to reproduce, and love may be considered a byproduct of the sexual reproductive imperative.

FALLING IN LOVE

While reproduction is nature's imperative, it is not the sole raison d'etre of sex. In fact, the means for accomplishing nature's reproductive design are so pleasurable that the end constitutes only a rare motive for exercising the means. People hardly ever consider nature's "grand design" or "higher goal" when male and female bring their genitals into intimate juxtaposition. We are aware of it, however, and usually take steps today to subvert nature's plan by using birth-control devices when partaking of our sexual pleasures. Nature made us smart as well as horny. Nevertheless, the sheer number of sexual encounters assures the species of more than enough births.

If reproduction were the sole purpose of sex, we would not see the diversity of elaborate courtship rituals throughout the world, which have nothing to do with reproduction. Sociobiologist E. O. Wilson notes that if reproduction were the sole biological function of sex, "It could be achieved far more economically in a few seconds of mounting and insertion."[4] (I can imagine a legion of cynical females responding to Wilson, "Do you mean that there's more?").

In species where pair bonding does not exist, insemination is in fact accomplished without ritual and foreplay in a few brief seconds. No emotion accompanies the frenetic mating among lions, dogs, chickens, etc. After accommodating the cock, the hen nonchalantly shakes her ruffled feathers and resumes pecking her feed. Among western human beings, probably only the prostitute/john relationship is as emotionally cold as animal copulation. Frequent and prolonged (relative to other species) sexual intercourse facilitates and cements human pair bonding, and that's the second grand design that nature has fashioned from sex.

The uniquely human pattern of mating probably has a lot to do with the evolution of love and human sociability. In comparison to humans, most mammal species are extraordinarily individualistic. Their short dependency periods and their survival instincts make them much less reliant on others and more complete in themselves. Even among the most social of nonhuman mammalian species, members resemble more the rugged Yankee individualist than the Parisian bon vivant. For most of the year the nonhuman male is supremely uninterested in the female, and vice-versa. This lack of interest dramatically changes when the female sends out olfactory signals that she is "in heat" and ready to accommodate the male sexually. Nonhuman mammals become much more "social" during these periods of *estrus*, and feathers, fur, and blood fly as males compete for sexual favors. Females may make up for their former asexuality by copulating (depending on the species) with up to 40 males in a single day. Once the female is impregnated, she ceases to be receptive to further copulations, and years may pass before she again goes into estrus.

In contrast to nonhuman animals, the human female is sexually receptive at all times. She is the only mammalian female who has lost the period of estrus. Although her sexual desire does wax and wane slightly according to her monthly cycle, it is never an "all or nothing" situation. This continual receptiveness makes the human female continuously attractive to the human male. The evolutionary advantage conferred by long-term intersexual attraction may be to a great extent responsible for the human loss of estrus. Evolutionary biologist Richard Morris explains that there was certainly a time in human history when females, like all other primates, went through estrus. Some females, he goes on to speculate, must have enjoyed longer periods of sexual receptivity than others. Males would naturally be more solicitous of such females, providing them with extra food and protection. These females would be more likely to survive, as would their offspring. Over time, natural selection would spread the genes for longer receptivity throughout the population, eventually leading to the disappearance of estrus altogether.[5]

This is a plausible and widely accepted speculation for the human loss of estrus. It has been noted among monkeys that males are far more attentive to females, and more generous in sharing food with them, when females are in estrus. (It seems that erotic, after-dinner expectations are not limited to the tuxedoed "naked ape"). Why is it then, given the benefits accruing to receptive females, that other species have not lost estrus? I would argue that they have not done so for two reasons. First, the females of other species are not so dependent on male protection and food sharing because the short dependency period of their offspring soon leave mother and infant free to forage for themselves. Second, human females are intelligent and are aware of the advantages of continual male support and protection. They were able to make the connection between their sexual receptiveness and the attention they received when they were. They were then able to turn this awareness to their advantage, and to the advantage of their children. It is not difficult to imagine prehuman females "faking" estral signals and copulating with an ever-willing male in exchange for continued support. After all, the literature tells us that it is not uncommon today for females to pretend receptivenss and orgasm for much the same reason.[6]

So far, we have pair-bonding between men and women because each offers the other some concrete advantage: for him, guaranteed sex, for her, guaranteed protection. But what has this businesslike quid pro quo to do with love? We certainly would not deem a couple to be in love today if their only reason for being together was for mutual back-scratching, even though it appears to be the basis for many marital couplings. We know that love can exist without sex. Some of the great loves in history and literature were unconsummated, and certainly the so-called sexual revolution of the late sixties and early seventies showed (if it was ever doubted) that sex can be totally divorced from love.

But let us be aware that the cultural evolution of love occurs rapidly from age to age, and has essentially very little to do with the biological evolution of love. The biological evolution of love can only be understood in terms of the environments encountered at its dim beginnings. The recorded history of love is overlaid by social forces. Unconsummated love may have been the result of social prescriptions and proscriptions about who may marry whom, the code of courtly love and chivalry, or poetic romanticism in which the sweet agony of unrequited love seemed somehow spiritually superior to consummated love.

How the mutually advantageous exchange led to that deep emotion we call love must necessarily involve a great deal of speculation, but it almost surely must have had something to do with human intelligence. According to the speculations of the zoologist Desmond Morris, the available physical anthropological evidence suggests an intimate relationship between the evolution of intelligence and the evolution of love. Morris speculates that about 25 million years ago our ancestors faced an ecological crisis as the African forests receded to give way to the grassy savanna. The savanna was a dangerous place for such physically puny animals as our homonid ancestors were. Having to keep their wits about them as they trudged through the tall grasses, it became advantageous to evolve into an upright bipedal animal. Assuming that the natural selection for bipedalism was taking place coterminously with the gradual loss of estrus, sight would have slowly replaced smell as the impetus to mating. Upright males and females could now view one another in their full splendor face to face.[7]

Assuming our ancestors liked what they saw and given the change in bodily configurations accompanying an upright stance (genitals to the fore), the uniquely human practice of face-to-face intercourse could not be far behind. Frontal intercourse involves far more skin contact between lovers than the old impersonal method of seizing the female from behind and staring out into space. Because of the intimate connection between the brain and the skin, humans find tactile stimulation most pleasing—the more skin contact the greater the pleasure. For our ancestors sexual intercourse increasingly recalled the pleasures lovers once found in their mothers' arms. The sucking of the lover's breasts, the warmth of skin-to-skin contact, eye gazing, and the feeling of security and that all is right with the world—all evoked deep memories of the mother/infant bond, the template of all loving. As British writer Jill Tweedy puts it: "Face-to-face intercourse became essential to strengthen the bond over and above the ordinary promiscuous sexual drive because only by looking into the face while fucking could you mimic and capitalize on the mother/child bond and begin to know the individual from, as it were, the faceless bottom of old-style mounting."[8]

Face-to-face intercourse involves more of the senses than are involved in belly/buttocks coupling. Noses are nuzzled, lips covered, tongues are mingled, and eyes are gazed into. Lovers are now communicating their pleasure to one another through their bodies. The evolution of human language enabled lovers to translate their physical and visual pleasure into words and to name each other. The human intellect now cannot help recognizing the unique features of the lover. He or she is no longer merely a set of genitals that looks and smells like every other set; he or she is now a distinct and separate individual who captures and holds the imagination. Human imagination allowed our ancestors to replay previous sexual encounters with their lovers and to anticipate future ones. This reflection made for the wedding of emotion and intellect, a ceremony that perhaps took place in Paul Chauchard's "brain of the heart"—the late-arriving prefrontal brain—to produce that exhilarating experience we call love.[9] Sexual intercourse in its highest form is the ultimate celebration of love.

We have already seen that evolution exerted different selection pressures on the males and females of our species. We can briefly recapitulate by making eight points:

1. Due to the variability of environments and experiences confronting protohumans, adaptability and intelligence were being selected for in their repertoire of traits.

2. The brain of an animal whose primary defining characteristic is its intelligence is larger in relation to the rest of its body than the brain/body size ratio in lower forms of life.

3. The size of the human cranium housing such a brain would be too great to pass through the birth canal, so human infants are born before the brain is fully developed relative to the infant brains of nonhuman mammals.

4. This seemingly "premature" birth of the human infant brings with it a developmental lag, and hence the longest dependency period of all animals.

5. This long dependency period means that the human infant must have someone to administer to its needs fully and unconditionally while it is helpless.

6. Fully and unconditionally administering to the needs of another is a definition of love, and this kind of love was selected into the behavioral and emotional repertory of women.

7. While the female was busy administering to her infant's needs, she required someone to administer other needs, and those of her child, for food, shelter, and protection.

8. The male, less prone to unconditional love, became willing to exchange care for the mother and infant for continued and exclusive sex-

ual favors from the mother. Rather than proceeding to the next sexual conquest, the male had to somehow "pairbond," to develop an emotional attachment to the mother of his child. It is suggested that the evolutionary processes of selecting for the female loss of estrus, upright bipedalism, and intelligence had a lot to do with the develoment of romantic love.

This is the story so far. We can now explore male/female romantic love separated from considerations of maternalism and paternalism, and from speculations about its origin.

THE CHEMISTRY OF FALLING IN LOVE

What happens when we fall in love? The very word *fall* seems to imply that the process is quite irrational, something beyond our cognition control. I am reminded of a song by Nancy Sinatra that was popular during the 1970s in which she admits, "We got married in a fever." How else can we explain people marrying one another when everyone except the parties involved knows the marriage will be a disaster? Having spent some time in the corrections field, I have seen many apparently well-adjusted women who volunteer to befriend and counsel prison inmates fall in love and marry the most appalling of criminal psychopaths. They can even admit that intellectually they know what they are doing is not wise: "But I love him!" Romantic love can turn the wisest of us into irrational gonadal reactors. This is probably the kind of love the English wit Samuel Jonson must have had in mind when he defined love as "a disease best cured by marriage."

Falling in love is something that happens to us, not something we make happen. Sometimes it even happens when we least expect and want it, at least on a fully conscious level. It is different from being *in love*, which is an ongoing process involving rational as well as emotional components. Falling in love is a discrete event; loving is a series of events taking place over time. I do not mean to imply that "love at first sight" is a common phenomenon, although I suppose it does happen. "Falling in love" is most often preceded by a steady buildup of acts, thoughts, gestures, imaginations, and delicious fantasies. We meet someone, and somehow his or her unique characteristics begin to have an anabolic effect on what scientists unromantically call our hypothalamic-pituitary-gonadal axis. For a woman, it may be a man's power, his intellect, and/or maturity (policeman, professor, politician), the way he smiles, his confidence or athletic prowess, his gentleness with children, his exotic foreign accent, or simply because he is nice and courteous. For the male, more prone to visual than emotional stimuli, it may be the way her ski-slope nose turns up, the delightful way her buttocks undulate as she walks, the creamy silkiness of her skin, the whiteness of her teeth set between fleshy red lips, or, again, simply because she is nice and courteous to him.

No matter what the particulars leading up to the event might be, when it happens it happens with a bang (often literally as well as figuratively these days). The Russian writer Ivan Turgenev likens falling in love to a revolution in its intensity: "First love is exactly like a revolution: the regular and established order of life is in an instant smashed to fragments; youth stands at the barricade, its bright banner raised high in the air, and sends its ecstatic greetings to the future, whatever it may hold—death or a new life, no matter."[10] Like the French Revolution, falling in love will often suffer a Thermidorian reaction, but we will discuss this bleak prospect later.

The anabolic chemical reactions to the stimuli presented to us by our love objects do arouse us to a kind of biological revolution. When we see, touch, or most of all, make love with our lovers, our senses of sight, smell, and touch send messages to the limbic system. The pleasure centers in the limbic system process the flood of information that we may collectively call desire or passion and send it on to the *hypothalamus*, the part of the limbic system that, among other things, synthesizes hormones and activates sexual behavior. The hypothalamus gets excited and releases a peptide called *adrenocorticotrophin*, releasing a hormone (ACTH) from the pituitary gland. ACTH is then transported through the bloodstream to receptors at the adrenal gland, which then releases a substance called *corticosterone*. This substance increases the metabolism of glucose, which results in the classic symptoms of feeling love and/or sexual excitement: flushed skin, sweating, heavy breathing. In short, our lovers' gonads are on "Go!" You may have noticed, by the way, that this whole process is biochemically identical to the stress response.

Romantic love, then, is an intense emotional state precipitated by the stimuli presented to us by the love object. It is perhaps the strongest of all emotions experienced by human beings; at the very least, it is the strongest of all positive emotions. When it strikes us, we become *different* people. Our perceptions are drastically altered, the world revolves around the loved one, and little else besides him or her seems to matter very much. If love is returned, the world seems to be a finer place, we smile at strangers, we search for superlatives to describe the beloved, and foreign phrases and pet names gush forth: "Szeretlek my Nampa Nymph," "Te amo mucho, Fair Grace."

In love's progression we discover reservoirs of poetic expression. Rivers no longer simply flow, they court and lap the shores; mountains, once "just there," now stretch their peaks to embrace the heavens; and trees fondle one another with their sinuous boughs. Sheer euphoria threatens to turn us into giggling schoolchildren at the same time that it makes us feel more confident, competent, attractive, capable, hopeful, and optimistic. We feel boundless energy within, and we feel less need for food, sleep, and our other ordinary pleasurable diversions.

If this description sounds very much like a description of a drug-induced high, that's because it is. Stimulant drugs such as cocaine and amphetamine have much the same effect as love—love is a natural high. Whether we fall in love or take a stimulant drug, the upshot is increased limbic-system activity in the form of increased neurotransmitter activity. This observation should not diminish our humanity or the marvels of romantic love. Rather, it should comfort us to think that nature has wired us to respond to other human beings with such pleasure. Natural highs, such as the "runner's high," are positive highs that are beneficial to us. They are nature's way of bringing some joy into our lives. It is precisely because some people experience so little joy mediated by the brain's own internal chemicals that they resort to artificial chemicals that briefly mimic pleasure, and soon become physically addicted.

Scientists have not yet discovered neurocenters specific to exogenous stimulants such as amphetamine, but we can hypothesize that they affect the brain indirectly by prompting the release of excitatory transmitters such as dopamine and norepinepherine and blocking their reuptake. Psychiatrist Michael Liebowitz has speculated that the experience of romantic love is chemically mediated by a naturally occurring amphetaminelike substance called phenylethylamine (PEA).[11] PEA does have an amphetaminelike effect on laboratory animals, and a decreased level of PEA has been shown to be associated with depression among humans. While its relationship to romantic love may be speculative for the moment, there is little doubt that PEA is an important emotion-regulator. When we are in love our brain secretes increased amounts of PEA and we feel grand. Each time we see or anticipate seeing our lover, the whistle blows at the PEA factory and we get another fix.

Why should our brains respond this way to the presence of a loved one? Liebowitz believes nature has wired our brains to "light up" strongly when we are in proximity to members of the opposite sex who we consider to be receptive to us. It is a device that has slowly evolved in our species and it appears, says Liebowitz, "to be nature's way of ensuring that we seek out and form relationships that last at least long enough to reproduce the next generation.,"[12]

We have seen that Liebowitz might be somewhat remiss in his conclusion that love must endure only "long enough to reproduce the next generation." Such a single-minded strategy would make every woman fall into every sailor's willing arms, making every mother just a mother, and marking each weaning with a new pregnancy. Love must go beyond and mean more than simple sexual attraction for reproductive purposes. Men and women fall in love today because ancient couples with the propensity to do so stayed bonded together long enough to allow for their offspring to survive and pass on that propensity. Couples who simply copulated and parted were less likely to have any issue of that brief union survive. Evolution selected love as a way of insuring that men would stick around long enough to assist women to care for the children.

We have social institutions, such as welfare, these days to assume the responsibilities of fathers who cannot or will not assume them themselves. Male presence is therefore no longer the survival imperative that it once was. It is perhaps because of this modern lack of necessity for the male presence, indicated by an ever-rising divorce rate, that romantic love is viewed more and more today by the cold-hearted as an irrational process. But love as experienced today, I must again emphasize, can only be understood when we consider the conditions under which it originally emerged and evolved, as well as its original adaptive consequences. Surely there is nothing more rational than the survival of the species.

The "lighting up" of the brain in response to stimuli presented by the love object is a chemical high that makes us feel so good that we find a real need to expose ourselves to the stimuli repeatedly. After a period of time, which varies greatly among individuals, the same stimuli fail to produce their former effects on the brain's chemical factory. When a drug user's drug of choice fails to produce its former effects he or she is said to have developed a *tolerance* for the drug. Drug tolerance is the adjustment of the body to a constant dosage, and explains why addicts have to increase the amount of the drugs they take in order to produce the same effects. If love is a high chemically analogous to a cocaine or amphetamine high, we can expect lovers to develop a "tolerance" for one another over a period of time (the Thermidorian reaction).

This is not a far-fetched speculation. We develop a tolerance for many of the pleasant things that happen to us if they happen regularly. We get used to those things and begin to experience a sort of ennui. My first journal article and first book sent me into a kind of ecstasy as I fondled the pages and reread every precious word. A new publication, although still a pleasant experience, has nowhere near the impact on my pleasure centers that the early ones did. The point I am making is that we can develop a tolerance for chemicals released naturally in response to pleasures derived from people and things just as we develop a tolerance for the drugs we ingest.

When the magnetic effects of pure attraction dissipate, something else must occur if the pair-bond is to endure. Lovers must become attached to one another after the delights of sheer attraction are only sporadically or dimly felt. If lovers *like* one another, then, with maturity and familiarity, they may find the quiet security of companionate love more emotionally satisfying than the mad, gonadal helter-skelter of the attraction phase, just as they come to prefer the harmonious beauty of Beethoven over the crotch-raw cacophony of Bon Jovi. (This doesn't mean that attached lovers can't indulge in a little Bon Jovi from time to time.) This smooth and quite normal transition is most likely when lovers enter into relationships with heads not too fuzzied by PEA-induced euphoria.

The euphoria of the initial love attraction seems to increase in proportion to the idealization of the loved one. We all know that there is a tremendous tendency to idealize the love object during the early mad days of falling in love. Our lover's positive attributes are magnified beyond all reason, and their faults are denied or downplayed, if they are even perceived at all. Sexologist John Money of Johns Hopkins University Medical School likens the idealization process to the Rorschach inkblot test, in the sense that lovers project their own images of perfection onto one another. Money emphasizes that these projections should not stray too far from the reality of the partner's actual attributes if the relationship is to endure.[13] The more reality is distorted during the courtship period, the more difficult it is to deal with after the blinders are removed. It is the same phenomenon seen among drug abusers: the more intense the high, the more devastating is the crash. A lover can no more become the image we have projected on him or her than a Rorschach inkblot can actually become a butterfly. It often happens, though, that the butterfly image metamorphosizes into an image less appealing, such as a bloood-sucking bat, if the initial image did not approach reality.

When such a drastic change of images occurs, we tend to interpret the love experience as infatuation. I used to believe that what is called infatuation was simply love that didn't work out. A love that somehow endured was "true" love, whereas a love that died was infatuation. The difficulty in differentiating between love and infatuation is that it can only be done retroactively. *Infatuation* comes from the same root word as *fatuous*, meaning "silly" or "foolish." To become infatuated is to become foolish. But becoming somewhat foolish or irrational when we fall in love is common to the experience regardless of the outcome. The same chemicals whirl in the limbic system regardless of whether we later call the experience infatuation or love.

I would seriously doubt your love, however, if there were not some element of idealization of the object you are attracted to. People tend to idealize their parents, children, and countries to varying extents without any ill effects, unless let down very badly. Idealization is the motivator of enthusiasm, and enthusiasm is the stuff of love. We could hardly share hopes, plans, and dreams unless we enthusiastically believed in the possibility of their fruition. Moreover, the idealization of the loved one may in fact result in his or her conforming more to the idealized image than was formerly the case. After all, love is supposed to be a growth-enhancing process, and there are such things as self-fulfilling prophesies. The only caveats are that we do not insist on conformity to our idealizations as a condition of love, and that we not carry our idealization to unreasonable and self-deceptive extremes.

I now believe, following Liebowitz's lead, that it is more useful to think of "true" love as attraction plus attachment, and what we call infatuation to be attraction minus attachment. Attraction is active, intense, and exciting; attachment is quiet warmth, comfort, and security. Liebowitz feels that attachment is also a chemical process with an evolutionary history. His basic idea is that attachment involves narcotic-like substances in the brain, more specifically, the *endorphins*. When people are in situations described as secure and comfortable, the brain secretes endorphins that produce the feeling of well-being.[14] Close involvement with another human being is one situation producing a feeling of well-being; we have seen earlier how contact comfort with the mother raises an infant's level of endorphins and secures its attachment to her. Few things, if any at all, make us feel so warm and secure as the knowledge that we are needed and loved.

Attachment also has its roots in evolutionary history. We have seen in previous chapters how maternal separation is an extremely negative experience. In human and nonhuman primates it results in fear, anxiety, depression, and even a suppression of the immunological system. All these reactions are, of course, mediated by brain chemistry. The adaptive value of the separation response lies in the long dependency of human beings. Because of this, children have to learn to become independent, to leave the nest now and then, and to learn to bond with age-peers. However, when they are hurt, afraid, hungry, or sick, a strong attachment between mother and child assures them that she will be available on their return to comfort them and take care of their hurts and needs. Having an attachment response such as this genetically wired into us has obvious survival value. If the child's needs are met lovingly upon returning from exploration and play, he or she will feel comforted and secure in the knowledge that mother is always there when needed.

According to mental-health professionals, this knowledge provides a trusting foundation that allows the child to develop his or her independence and to develop attachments to others in later life. Children who are denied such a stable base from which to branch out and form other attachments continue to suffer separation anxiety and become fearful "clingers." They do not venture out to learn independence because their little minds reason that mother may not be around when they come back. A neglected child who is rebuffed when presenting its mother with the fears and injuries of play and exploration will tend to limit such activities. He or she will then have fewer opportunities to form attachments with others outside the family. Such is the origin of an abiding fear and mistrust of the external world and of other people. Fearful children will have difficulties making attachments to others later in life. Such children have learned to mistrust others and their environment rather than to trust. Parents must provide their children with a sense of security, with roots, but they must also provide them with a set of wings with which to soar in this beautiful world of ours.

The implications of failure to form secure attachments or, conversely, to become overly dependent on a single clinging attachment should be clear. Those individuals without attachment experience will probably flit from one infatuation (attraction minus attachment) experience to another. They very much enjoy the mad excitement and novelty of a new lover, but when ennui sets in and they no longer experience a high with the lover, they seek a novel love to start all over again. "Attraction junkies" is the term Liebowitz uses to describe such individuals. They are so addicted to the attraction experience that becoming attached presents an impediment to their lifestyle that they would rather avoid. They would rather avoid it not only because it militates against further attraction experiences but also because they fear attachment. These are the people who learned during childhood that they couldn't rely on anyone to be there when needed. Rather than risk the pains of separation, they do not allow themselves to become attached.

Remaining with the drug-addiction analogy, a similar strategy is seen in the drug addict who takes a short respite from drugs so that the brain can become "unhabituated." By taking a rest from drugs, the addict's brain lowers its threshold of excitement so that small doses can again regain their former power. Taking a break from one's lover, meeting an old flame again, or being reunited with a spouse after a long separation also tends to rekindle the passions of attraction because the separation has lowered the brain's threshold for excitement. Absence does make the heart grow fonder, up to a point. The "newness" of the reunion is a powerful aphrodisiac, as is the newness of an illicit affair. The intensity of most extramarital affairs is probably attributable to the combination of sexual passion, frequent separations and clandestine meetings, and the thrill of the forbidden. Such a triple stimulation, all other things being equal, means that the limbic system has pumped out chemicals functioning synergistically to intensify the pleasures of both the passion and the thrill.

Just as attraction junkies are addicted to their stimulant high, attachment junkies become overly dependent on a single established relationship. Of course, a deep attachment to one's love-mate is a necessary and positive feeling; becoming completely dependent for one's well-being and feeling of self-worth on one's lover is not. Such intensity of attachment is pathological and turns the addict into a possessive, jealous, and untrusting bore. Husbands refuse to allow their wives any independent social life; wives search their husbands' pockets and sniff their shirt collars. Even negative evidence fails to assuage the fear that the spouse will leave him or her for another. Being so paralyzed by anxiety, there is tremendous reluctance to allow the spouse any freedom at all. Thus "love" turns into a stifling, growth-inhibiting oppression.

I am sure you have noticed that the attachment junky's behavior is identical with the care-eliciting behavior and deficiency-love exhibited by neurotics described in chapter 5. Excessive attachment behavior is neurotic in the sense that the individual's subjective, internal world rather than objective reality guides his or her responses to the spouse. The spouse is not valued for his or her self, but rather as a vehicle to fill the emptiness in the D-lover's own life. If or when the spouse may leave, the D-lover is all but devastated. He or she suffers many of the symptoms suffered by the narcotic addict undergoing withdrawal, since the comforting endorphins are no longer being secreted. The nineteenth-century novelist Stendhal sums up what love and its loss means for the addicted D-lover: "Love is always haunted by the despair of being abandoned by the beloved and of being left nothing but a dead blank for the remainder of life."[15] Most of us are saddened by the breakup of a romantic relationship if that relationship meant anything to us at all, but if such a parting threatens to leave us "dead blanks" the rest of our lives, we had better reassess our relationships and ourselves.

A number of popular books, such as *Letting Go* and *How to Fall Out of Love*, have recognized the difficulty of becoming unaddicted to this kind of neurotic love. These books offer some imaginative behavioral-therapy techniques to assist the addict. The trouble is that before anyone can take steps to conquer the addiction, he or she must not only recognize the destructive nature of the relationship but also have the courage to do something about it. Just as narcotic junkies will suffer gladly all the indignities of addiction as long as they have their supply of chemical comfort, the attachment addict will remain in an undignified and otherwise unsatisfying relationship to avoid the pain of withdrawal. Psychologically and chemically, both addictions are similar.

We don't like to think of love in terms analogous to drug addiction. But it has been characterized as "just about the most common, yet least recognized form of addiction."[16] On the other hand, Ruth Winter and

Kathleen McAuliffe assure the incurable romantics among us that science will never be able to reduce physical attraction and love to a series of chemical reactions. There are many cognitive, interpretive, and idiosyncratic goings on in the "mind's eye" to be considered; and there are enough of them to assure that romantic love will retain much of its mystery. Nevertheless, Winter and McAuliffe are excited about the discovery of what they call "Mother Nature's love potions [phenylethylamine and the endorphins] and the sorcery she uses to get us hooked on each other." I hope you consider love important enough to share their enthusiasm.[17]

THE PUZZLE OF HOMOSEXUAL LOVE

It is fashionable to consider men the less romantic sex, despite the fact that the vast majority of love poems have been written by men, sometimes to other men. The most moving love story in the Bible is that of David's love for Jonathan. Men and women in all ages and in all cultures have been sexually and romantically attracted and attached to members of their own sex. These same-sex love affairs have occurred and endured in cultures where homosexuality has been severely punished, as well as in cultures where it has been approved of. Given that nature's aim is the survival of the species, it is puzzling that homosexuality has become an established pattern in the sexual repertory of human beings. It is even more puzzling to realize that exclusive homosexuality, an enduring emotional and sexual preference for members of the same sex, appears to be found only among human beings. Homosexual behavior has been observed in other animals in unusual circumstances, but there is no documented evidence for same-sex preference as an abiding trait appearing in any other species.[18]

Since the famous Kinsey reports of 1948 and 1953, sexual orientation has been considered a continuous trait rather than a dichotomous either/or one. Kinsey's sexual orientation continuum is measured on a seven-point scale ranging from 0 for exclusive heterosexuality to 6 for exclusive homosexuality, with various degrees of bisexuality and incidental homosexuality in between. As with many other statistically deviant behaviors, more males than females had experienced homosexuality. Kinsey reported that 37 per cent of American males and 20 per cent of American females have experienced at least one homosexual encounter, and that about 4 per cent of males and 2 per cent of females were exclusively homosexual.[19] These figures predate gay liberation and the emergence of many homosexuals from the closet. The figures are probably on the low side today. Whatever the actual figures may be, in all societies male homosexuality is far more common than lesbianism.[20]

Most homosexual behavior is episodic or deprivation homosexuality. It occurs in prisons, on board ships, in boarding schools, and in other circumstances where heterosexual outlets are unavailable. Many men engage in impersonal homosexual encounters in adult bookstores and in restrooms simply to satisfy immediate sexual urges as an alternative to masturbation. No emotional intimacy is desired or offered, and these men easily perform heterosexually when the opportunity presents itself. Homosexuality in this context is "next-best-thingism." We may consider such episodic homosexuality to be normal, perhaps even biologically advantageous, to the extent that it relieves sexual frustrations. We may consider it normal because it has been observed across species and because it has even been perhaps the preferred mode of sexual expression in some cultures (for example, in ancient Greece, and among the Siwans of Africa and the Sambia of New Guinea).

Even in those rare cultures where homosexuality is rife, respected, and robust, a minimal amount of heterosexual intimacy is necessary to maintain the culture. The ancient Greeks married, had female concubines, and enjoyed the pleasures of the *hetairai* (geishalike courtesans), and the *pornai* (prostitutes of a lower order). After all, it was the face of a woman, Helen of Troy, that "launched a thousand ships upon Ilium," if we are to believe Homer. Despite King David's love for Jonathan, he kept a number of wives and concubines to copulate with from time to time and to provide him with offspring. The ancients were more "joyously bisexual" than homosexual, their preference for homosexuality perhaps being more a function of the oppression and seclusion of women than anything else. ("What sensible thing are women capable of doing?" asks Cleonica in Aristophanes' *Lysistrata*.) Although we have no supportive statistics, it is not likely that the percentage of individuals in homosexually oriented cultures who were or are exclusively homosexual significantly exceeds the Kinsey figures for the United States. It is the presence of the primary homosexuals that constitutes the puzzle of homosexuality. How can we account for a form of love that has no apparent survival benefit to the species?

Accounting for the presence of homosexuality is not problematic as long as it is considered learned behavior, a simple deviation of a basic sexual aim. After all, the basic sex aim among heterosexuals is directed preferentially toward different types of men or women according to learned fancies. Most homosexual encounters are the consequence of learned behavior. We all find stimulation of the genitalia to be intensely pleasurable and seek ways to obtain such pleasure. Most of us seek to obtain it with socially approved partners; others seek it without prejudice in respect to gender. To the extent that alternative means of obtaining organ pleasure are visible and to the extent that these means become less unacceptable, if not exactly approved, more people will experiment with them. (Freud is reported to have said that in a cultural vacuum males would attempt to mate with anything.) If we do decide to experiment with alternative sexuality and find it to be rewarding, we may repeat the experiment from time to time and possibly come to prefer it to heterosexuality for various reasons.

According to sociologist Laud Humphreys, not the least of these reasons is the quick and easy access to impersonal homosexual encounters in the public rest room circuit, dubbed the "tea room trade."[21] Many bisexual men are fond of saying that not only is it easier to obtain homosexual satisfaction but also that "a man can give me something a woman can't." This is an anatomically undeniable fact, and those who subscribe to such a philosophy are able to experience both ends of the stick, so to speak, by effectively doubling their potential sources of sexual satisfaction.

But learning is not a sufficient explanation for primary homosexuals, many of whom knew from early childhood that they were sexually "different." These are individuals who always preferred the company, playthings, and paraphernalia of the opposite sex, who felt trapped in the body of the wrong sex. These preferences and feelings endured into adulthood despite social prescriptions to the contrary. How can we account for such apparently "born homosexuals?"

It is difficult to advance a genetic theory of homosexuality since homosexual love is not procreative. If homosexuals do not procreate, any combination of genes that may contribute to their sexual proclivities would soon be culled from the gene pool. There can be very little doubt that there is a strong evolutionary bias against homosexuality and a strong bias in favor of heterosexuality. As biologist Philip Applewhite wittily remarked: "Most women are attracted to something that looks like a plucked turkey neck surrounded by hair, and men are attracted to a furry hole and bumps on the chest—it must be genetic!"[22]

But even individuals placing themselves very much on the homosexual end of Kinsey's sexual preference scale do experience occasional heterosexual intercourse, if only to keep up an appearance of "respectable normality."[23] So a genetic theory is not entirely precluded, and some researchers have claimed to find fairly high concordance rates for homosexuality among identical twins.[24] A high concordance rate points to, but does not definitely establish, a direct genetic influence. Concordance rates may be a function of the intrauterine influences experienced and shared by twins rather than of their shared genetic inheritance. It is the intrauterine experience that currently seems to be the best biological explanation for primary homosexuality.

We know that during the critical period of fetal development in the womb genetic XY males undergo an androgenization of the developing brain. The process goes beyond simple differentiation of the male and female genitalia. The androgenization of the brain also sets the stage for the male pattern of hormone release at puberty, which in turn constitutes a biological readiness to receive sexual messages from females. When a genetic male embryo is deprived of the proper level of androgen the brain will retain the "standard" form—a feminine brain in a masculine body. Likewise, if a genetic XX female embryo is exposed to high levels of androgen, her brain takes on a masculine pattern—a male brain in a female body. This is not an all-or-nothing process, but is more a matter of degree. According to this theory, homosexuality is the result of a botched neurochemical process during a critical fetal period in which sexual differentiation conforming with the sex determined by genes is supposed to occur. More things can go wrong in the male brain, so this is perhaps the reason why there appears to be more primary homosexuality among men than among women.

Most of the pioneering work in the area of the prenatal origins of primary homosexuality has come from the laboratory of East German endocrinologist Gunter Dörner. By experimentally manipulating hormone levels during the critical sex-differentiating period among rats, Dörner found that, as adults, male rats deprived of androgen and female rats exposed to excess androgen were preferentially excited by members of their own sex.[25] The same deprivation of androgen (or injections of estrogen) in males in adulthood, or injections of androgen in females in adulthood, does result in the acquisition of some secondary characteristics of the opposite sex, but the tilting of the hormonal balance does not alter sexual orientation. Similarly, high doses of testosterone administered in adulthood to male homosexual rats (or for that matter, to human male homosexuals) does not result in heterosexual activity. If it does anything at all, it leads to increased libido and increased homosexual activity. Thus, we have evidence among one breed of mammal that a basic sexual orientation develops prenatally deep within the hypothalamic nuclei and cannot be changed.

While the evidence for Dörner's theory is strongest where rats are involved, he and his colleagues have also performed retrospective studies among human beings. He reasoned that if the brains of male homosexuals were in fact feminized, then they should evidence the female pattern of response to the luteinizing hormone (LH) if estrogen is artificially administered to them via injections. Ovulation is triggered in postpubescent females by natural surges of estrogen. Estrogen, produced by the ovaries, first actuates the secretion of a neurohormone called *luteinizing hormone-releasing hormone* (LHRH) from the pituitary gland. As its name implies, LHRH stimulates the release of LH, which then stimulates the ovaries to ovulation and further estrogen secretion. The levels of estrogen, LHRH, LH, and another hormone called *follicle-stimulating hormone* rise and fall during the 28-day female cycle in what endocrinologists call a "positive feedback response." By way of contrast, LH stimulates the production of testosterone in postpubescent males in a continuous, rather than a cyclical, pattern.

The interesting thing about all this is that when homosexual males are injected with estrogen, LH levels rise as though it were trying to stimulate a phantom ovary, indicating the female positive feedback response. The same estrogen injections given to heterosexual males results in a drop in LH or no hormonal response at all. Males who occasionally engaged in homosexual activity (bisexuals) showed a response identical to that of exclusively heterosexual males. This last finding suggests that homosexuality is more a learned behavior among bisexuals than a condition that has a hormonal basis.

While no scientist disputes Dörner's finding about rats, scientific and ideological objections are raised in respect to humans. The (West) German Society for Sex Research has even accused him of advocating "endocrinological euthanasia of homosexuality," despite the fact that Dörner's findings were instrumental in the legalization of homosexuality in East Germany.[26]

Ideological considerations aside, Dörner's findings have been replicated in pristinely scientific fashion in the laboratory of American psychoneuroendocrinologist Brian Gladue.[27] Gladue and his colleagues selected for their study homosexual and heterosexual males who represented the polar opposites of Kinsey's spectrum of sexual orientation; their subjects were either exclusively homosexual or exclusively heterosexual. Also included in the study were heterosexual females.

After artificially administering estrogen to the three study groups, it was found that the secretory pattern of LH in the the homosexuals was intermediate between that of the females and the heterosexual males. All three groups significantly differed from one another in observed LH levels. They also found that testosterone levels were depressed for a significantly longer period in the homosexual men than in the heterosexual men, although baseline measures of testosterone were virtually identical in both groups. Since LH stimulates the production of testosterone in males, and since LH levels were significantly higher in the homosexual males, one might have expected the homosexual males to reach baseline testosterone levels more quickly. That they did not is perhaps further indicative of the failure of brain masculinization among primary homosexuals.

In addition to naturally occurring hormonal accidents during the critical period of sexual differentiation, steroid hormones given to women during at-risk pregnancies may produce the same results. Psychobiologist June Reinisch, now director of the Kinsey Institute for Sex Research, conducted a study of 84 children whose mothers were given steroid hormones during the first trimester of pregnancy. She administered a series of personality tests to the children, whose average age at the time of testing was 11.8

years. Regardless of gender, children whose mothers had been primarily on the steroid *progestin* (chemically similar in action to androgen) scored significantly higher on traits such as self-sufficiency, independence, and individualism. Children primarily exposed to estrogen were more group-oriented and group-dependent. Similar results were obtained when steroid-exposed children were compared with unexposed siblings within their families. Progestin-exposed children were found to be more "inner" or "self" directed than their unexposed siblings, and estrogen-exposed children were more "outer" or "other" directed than their unexposed siblings.[28]

Reinisch's findings have nothing to say about homosexuality per se, since her subjects presumably were not yet sexually active. Nevertheless, her study shows that prenatal exposure to sex hormones affects personality and temperament in characteristically male or female directions regardless of the genetic sex of the exposed fetus. Her work fits into Willard Gaylin's assertion that females have a primary drive for attachment, while males have a primary drive for work and mastery, and with Paul Pearsall's observation that the male brain is more "self-centered" and the female brain more "other" and "us" centered.[29]

The realization that primary homosexuals are born rather than made should lead us to a more benign attitude toward them. They have not made naughty choices in violation of our circumscribed sexual mores any more than heterosexuals have made the "right" choice. Nor are they "fixated" at an infantile stage of development and therefore pathological and neurotic, as some would have it.

Homosexuals have made an unusually great number of contributions to civilization, especially in literature and the arts. Scientists such as Sidney Mellen and Edmund Wilson have even speculated that the greater sensitivity and emotionality they attribute to homosexual males have contributed to human altruism and a less brutally aggressive species. Vern Bullough's monumental book *Sexual Variance in Society and History* informs us that in cultures where homosexuality has been accepted as normal, homosexuals have occupied valued social roles.[30] Love is a many-gendered thing, and homosexuals live and love just like the rest of us, albeit somewhat more promiscuously in the case of males. That they direct this love toward their own sex does not diminish the value of that love one iota. Love is love.

NOTES

1. J. Money and A. Ehrhardt, *Man and Woman, Boy and Girl: The Differentiation and Dimorphism of Gender Identity from Conception to Maturity* (Baltimore: Johns Hopkins University Press, 1972).

2. A. Ehrhardt and H. Meyer-Bahlburg, "Effects of Prenatal Hormones on Gender-related Behavior," *Science* 211 (1981): pp. 1312–1318.

3. Glen Wilson, *Love and Instinct* (New York: Quill, 1981), p. 42.

4. Edward Wilson, *On Human Nature* (Cambridge, Mass.: Harvard University Press, 1978), p. 141.

5. Richard Morris, *Evolution and Human Nature* (New York: Avon, 1983), pp. 139–140.

6. Shere Hite found that 53 percent of 1664 females in her study admitted to faking orgasm, some "infrequently," some "always," most "sometimes." Shere Hite, *The Hite Report* (MacMillan Publishing, 1976), p. 154.

7. Desmond Morris, *The Naked Ape* (New York: Dell, 1967).

8. Jill Tweedie, *In the Name of Love* (New York: Pantheon, 1979), p. 89.

9. Paul Chauchard, *Our Need of Love* (New York: P.J. Kennedy & Sons, 1968), p. 30.

10. Ivan Turgenev, *Spring Torrents*, trans. L. Schapiro (New York: Penguin, 1980), p. 100.

11. Michael Liebowitz, *The Chemistry of Love* (New York: Berkley Books, 1983), pp. 37–38.

12. Ibid., p. 49.

13. John Money, *Love and Lovesickness: The Science of Sex, Gender Difference, and Pair Bonding* (Baltimore: Johns Hopkins University, 1980), p. 65.

14. Liebowitz, *The Chemistry of Love*, pp. 136–137.

15. Stendhal, *On Love* (New York: Liveright, 1947), pp. 156–157.

16. Stanton Peele and Archie Brodsky, *Love and Addiction* (New York: Taplinger, 1975), p. 17.

17. Ruth Winter and Kathleen McAuliffe, "Hooked on Love," *Omni* 6 (1984): p. 82.

18. Sydney Mellen, *The Evolution of Love* (San Francisco: W.H. Freeman, 1982), p. 211.

19. Kinsey's figures on incidence of homosexuality cited in James Coleman and Donald Cressey, *Social Problems* (New York: Harper & Row, 1987), p. 318. Most people who have looked at Kinsey's research methods have concluded that he overestimated the percentage of homosexuals in the United States. Morton Hunt, for instance, found that only 1 per cent of the males and .05 per cent of the females in his sample were homosexual, although he admits that these figures are on the low side. Morton Hunt, *Sexual Behavior in the 1970's* (New York: Dell, 1974), p. 310. Perhaps the actual figures fall somewhere between these two sets of estimates.

20. Ira Reiss and Gary Lee, *Family Systems in America.* (New York: Holt, Rinehart and Winston, 1988), p. 118.

21. Laud Humphreys, *Tearoom Trade, Impersonal Sex in Public Places* (Chicago: Aldine, 1970).

22. Philip Applewhite, *Molecular Gods: How Molecules Determine Our Behavior* (Englewood Cliffs, N.J.: Prentice-Hall, 1981), p. 191.

23. A. Bell and M. Weinberg, *Homosexualities* (New York: Simon and Schuster, 1978).

24. F. Kallman, "Twins and Susceptibility to Overt Male Sexuality," *American Journal of Human Genetics* 4 (1952): pp. 136–146.

25. Dörner's seminal work in the neuroendocrinology of sexual behavior and sexual orientation is spread over many publications, including: Gunter Dörner, *Hormones and Brain Differentiation* (Amsterdam: Elsevier/North-Holland Biomedical Press, 1976); "Hormone Dependent Differentiation, Maturation and Function of the Brain and Sexual Behavior," *Endokrinologie* 69 (1976): pp. 306–320: G. Dörner, W. Rohde, and D. Schnorr, "Evocability of a Slight Positive Oestrogen Feedback Action on LH Secretion in Castrated and Oestrogen-primed Men," *Endokrinologie* 66 (1975): pp. 373–376. For an excellent overview of Dörner's many publications in these areas, see Robert Goy and Bruce McEwen, *Sexual Differentiation of the Brain* (Cambridge, Mass.: MIT Press, 1980), pp. 64–73. For an overview written for the layperson, see Linda Murray, "Sexual Destinies," *Omni* 9 (1987): pp. 100–128.

26. Linda Murray, "Sexual Destinies," p. 104.

27. B. Gladue, R. Green, and R. Hellman, "Neuroendocrine Response to Estrogen and Sexual Orientation," *Science* 225 (1984): pp. 1496–1499.

28. June Reinisch, "Prenatal Exposure of Human Foetuses to Synthetic Progestin and Oestrogen Affects Personality," *Nature* 266 (1977): pp. 561–562.

29. See note 15 (Gaylin) and note 26 (Pearsall) in chapter 3.

30. Vern Bullough, *Sexual Variance in Society and History* (Chicago: University of Chicago Press, 1976).

9

Romantic Love: How Do I Love You?

Love is a sudden sensation of recognition and hope.
—Stendhal

LOVE AS EXCHANGE AND BARTER

We do not have to be told that males and females differ considerably in their attitudes and behavior relating to love and sex. We all know that they exist, but we are not so sure why they exist. To simply say that the observed differences are derived from a different biology or from a different upbringing is to beg an awful lot of big questions. To begin with, there are more similarities between the sexes than there are differences. Both males and females need to love and be loved, and the vast majority of both sexes enjoy the experience of giving sexual expression to that love. But differences, certainly in terms of the present topic, are often more interesting than similarities.

Popular stereotypes of women portray them as being romantically impulsive and foolish in matters of the heart, easy prey for the manipulative cad. On the other hand, the male is seen as a sober and rational lover in easy control of his romantic, if not his sexual, urges. Stereotypes aside, which of the sexes is the most romantic? The answer to this question depends on whether we are talking about the rapidity or the robustness of romance. A large research literature indicates that men tend to fall in love more quickly than women, but love is more intense and lasting for women. Social psychologists Kanin, Davidson, and Scheck designed a study around the question of which of the sexes is most romantic. They concluded that males tend to experience feelings they interpret as love earlier in the relationship than do females. On the other hand, once females define what they are feeling as love, they tend to indulge themselves more in its euphoria. At the more intense levels of involvement, females are also more prone to idealization of their lovers.[1]

What possible advantages might this romantic asymmetry between the sexes have for males and females? We don't need any surveys to tell us that males have an abiding propensity to seek multiple sex partners, and that they are much more ready and willing (even if less able) to abandon themselves to urgent sexual needs than are women. Women, on the other hand, are more prone to value long-term, exclusive sexual relationships with one partner. Given a seductive situation, a male's biological desire for intercourse is easily aroused. It is not difficult to imagine many males immersed in such a situation interpreting sexual urgency as love. This is not necessarily a misinterpretation, for males generally place a higher value on the physical aspect of love than females do. For the male physical intimacy usually precedes the emotional feelings of love, while for the female the opposite sequence is usually the case. Putting it another way, men tend to see sex as a means to *develop* a relationship while women tend to view it as a way to *express* a relationship.

Being more visual/spatial than verbal animals, men are much more likely than women to choose a partner on the basis of physical attributes. Men seek women with wrinkle-free faces, pointed breasts, firm round buttocks, and who are properly powdered, painted, douched, depilated, and deodorized. Since sex appears to be the primary animating factor in seeking out female companionship, it's easy to see why males should be more immediately attracted to comely facial features and well-formed figures than to personality or intellectual attributes. (In one of his television shows, British comedian Benny Hill said he'd trade "25 IQ points for a good pair of knockers any day.") The unfortunate upshot of this is that men are forever searching for those anatomical features most likely to be found adorning younger females. This search is as old as history itself. Will Durant writes of it in ancient Greece: "Those men who yield [to laws forbidding bachelorhood] marry late, usually near thirty, and then insist upon brides not much older than fifteen. 'To mate a youth with a young wife is ill,' says a character in Euripides, 'for a man's strength endures, while the bloom of beauty quickly leaves the woman's form.' "[2]

The situation today in the United States is not much different, and both men and women are well aware of it. A study conducted by psychologists Albert Harrision and Laila Saeed makes this clear. They examined 800 advertisements in "lonely hearts" columns to find out what men and women typically want from a prospective mate and what it is that they emphasize about themselves as selling points. They found that women were much more likely to emphasize their physical attractiveness, while men tended to emphasize their financial security. These attributes—female attractiveness and male solvency—are the sex-differentiated coin of the marriage mart. Some buyers enter the market, alas, with little more than pocket change, while othes enter flush with assets. The lonely-hearts advertisers realistically demand from a prospective mate what they consider affordable after reviewing their assets. The more attractive female advertisers considered themselves to be, the more likely they were to be explicit about their desire for a man who was financially secure. Similarly, the more financially secure men said they were, the more likely they were to demand youthful physical attractiveness from any prospective respondent.[3] Similar findings have been found consistently by other researchers from the examination of the "personals" and other such marriage and dating forums.

Another interesting finding of this study was that not only were men looking for women younger than themselves but also women were looking for men older than themselves. Apparently, when women see older men they see experience, sophistication, intellectual maturity, and security. When men see older women they don't allow themselves to see much more than wrinkles and sagging breasts. Fortunately, there *are* men who find a special kind of beauty in a mature woman that greatly surpasses that of the teenybopper. Older women are also more sexually experienced and interesting and far more intellectually and emotionally satisfying. Nonetheless, there can be little doubt that both sexes are aware of what the other sex is looking for in a relationship and of the "shopping list" element in romantic love.

This awareness is not merely an American phenomenon. British psychiatrist Anthony Clare's review of marriage bureaus in a number of different countries led him to conclude: "Men tend to want young and physically attractive women while women prefer men several years older than themselves."[4] This is further substantiated by the International Mate Selection Project, a 1989 study of 10,000 people of both sexes from 37 different countries ranging from modern urban societies to rural third-world societies. No matter what the nationality, men want mates who are young and pretty, and women want mates who are somewhat older than they and who are financially secure, or have prospects of becoming so. According to this study, Western European and North American men were least likely to demand large age differences between themselves and their mates, and British, Dutch, and Zulu women were least concerned with their mate's prospects.[5]

While these sex-differentiated preferences appear to be universal, those who are somewhat less than perfectly endowed physically or those who are on the wrong end of the income distribution may also take heart from this study. Mate selection is more than, to put it crudely, her ass and his assets. The study found that men and women of all cultures value kindness and intelligence in their partners more than physical attractiveness or financial prospects. The only fly in this soup is that those lacking in the latter attributes may never get the opportunity to display the former attributes to the most desirable members of the opposite sex. Attractiveness and financial solvency may be viewed as attributes that gain one a head start in the marriage race, while intelligence and kindness assert their influence only after the race is under way.

The preference of older men for younger women and of younger women for older men generates a lot of frustration and loneliness for older, less-attractive women and for younger men who are competing for attractive females. As Glen Wilson points out, marriage bureaus and dating services have surpluses of older women and younger men among their clientele, and have great difficulty finding suitable partners for them.[6] Anthropologist Sydney Mellen refers to the male preference for youth as "perhaps the supreme example of the absence of justice and compassion in nature."[7] Unfortunately, nature is only concerned with species survival, and any means justifies this end as far as it is concerned.

The age-discrepancy preferences of both sexes, as well as differences in the rapidity and robustness of love observed in men and women, probably have their origins in what biologists call "sex-differentiated reproductive strategies." While gladly assenting to the undeniable fact that love is an extremely complex affair and that the motives of lovers are sometimes unfathomable, the evolutionary biologists view human beings as they view any other animal. Individual human beings exist, when all is said and done, to make other human beings. We are all a part of nature's reproductive system and are endowed with species traits developed over eons of time and designed to maximize reproductive success. But not even the most mechanistically minded evolutionary biologist today views mating and reproduction as obeying the adaptive purpose of the species in any way that is independent of individual purpose. The reproductive purpose of the species lies in our genes, but nature has provided individual human beings with a brain capable of molding—and even subverting—our genetic impulses. Nevertheless, while culture and individual experience shape our love lives to an enormous extent, we each feel in various degrees the tug exerted by our evolutionary legacy.

Let us take the male preference for younger women as our first example of this innate legacy. It has often been claimed that the reason American males prefer younger women is that our culture glorifies youth and all it implies. If this glorification of youth were simply an American cultural invention, we would also see older women in hot pursuit of younger men. While some may do just that, it is a far cry from the norm. America didn't invent the lust for nubile young women; history and anthropology, as well as the International Mate Selection Project, tell us that the male preference for youthful women is an abiding one across time and place. Standards of beauty vary greatly from place to place and from time to time, but regardless of any cultural standard by which it is measured, men prefer young women and more often associate youth with beauty. The very power of culture to direct perceptions of female beauty in any and all directions (while in no known instance has a culture generated a preference for older women) is itself a powerful argument for the biological basis of the male preference.

Although most men are not aware of it—and most would give every reason but this one—*the reproductive fitness of younger women* is the biological reason why men prefer younger women. A social scientist would heap scorn on such an explanation, asserting that the acquisition of a beautiful wife or girlfriend confers social status, prestige, and admiration on the man. It is a symbolic affirmation of his standing as a successful member of society, and it is this psychic reward that propels most males to seek young women. A 50-year-old male with a woman half his age on his arm undeniably evokes envy and grudging admiration from other males. Such an explanation, while quite accurate as far as it goes, begs the question of why the "possession" of a young and beautiful woman is unquestionably accepted by other males as symbolic of male success. I submit again that the underlying mechanism is biological in origin and reflects the greater reproductive fitness of younger women generally. This silent inner urging remains a biological motivator even when having a child by a beautiful woman is the last thing in the world a modern male may have on his mind.

It is biologically indisputable that younger females produce the most robust babies. By the time a human female fetus is 15 weeks old she will have all the eggs she will ever possess (about 400–500). Subjected to a variety of chemical environments and to radiation throughout the lifespan, these eggs are more likely to deteriorate in quality the longer they are around. For instance, the likelihood of a teenage mother giving birth to a Down's-syndrome child is less than 1 in 2,000. The probability of such a birth rises with each passing year, and is about 1 in 40 after the age of 45. From this simple biological fact, we can readily discern that the optimal reproductive strategy for a male, one that assures him of the largest number of healthy surviving children to push his genes into the coming generations, would be to seek mates among younger females. Protohuman males with a preference for youthful females would be more likely to pass on their genes, including those guiding the preference for youth. Males without such a preference would be somewhat less likely to pass on their genes.

Youthfulness of the male has no similar reproductive advantage. Male sperm is not subject to deterioration by aging because it is constantly being replenished by the billions. Although somewhat less numerous, the sperm of a 50-year-old man is qualitatively on a par with that of a 17-year-old boy. Since male youthfulness does not confer any reproductive advantage in terms of the ability to produce robust offspring, the female preference for men older than themselves is not a function of reproductive fitness in the sense of quality and quantity of offspring. The advantage offered is that an older, more mature man is a better prospect as a provider for her and her children, thus increasing her chances of pushing her genes into the future.

From studies of the romantic personals, and from many other sources, it is apparent that women are more interested in security than in the esthetic appeal of the youthful form. It's not that women are unresponsive to the vigor and beauty of younger males. The heroes of the romantic novels so beloved by many women are always handsome and dashing (but just about always considerably older than the heroine). Yet, a muscular body and a handsome face just doesn't turn on many women, when these qualities are stacked against social position, financial security, wisdom, experience, and maturity. These are the qualities that are most likely to result in a secure nest for the woman and her offspring, and these are the qualities most often found among older men. They are the qualities that provide women with evidence of a male's fitness for the role of father, protector, and provider, and that motivate her selection whether she realizes it or not.

As we have seen, whether a woman is successful or not in realizing a favorable reproductive strategy depends on what she has to offer in the marriage market. This observation is equally true for men. In terms of socioeconomic status and marriage, most marriages occur within the same class. When mobility does occur across class lines, women are more likely to marry into a higher social class than their own, and men are more likely to marry down the social class ladder. Women are especially more likely to marry into a higher social class if they have what males are looking for—youthful beauty.[8]

The reason that we observe opposite directions in male and female mobility is the different distributions of male and female marriage assets. Female attractiveness is more or less evenly distributed across class lines; the young women on the assembly line at the local factory will be as beautiful as the young ladies at Radcliffe College. The more successful, higher-class males can "raid" the factories and other such places for beautiful marriage mates, where they will find many interested young women. On the other hand, the qualities desired by a woman in a prospective partner are, by definition, concentrated in the upper classes. Lower-class males will have very little success if they attempt to seduce the young ladies of Radcliffe.

One of the consequences of all this, in general, is that women who are left out of the marriage game are the most successful career women, and men who are left out may be among the least successful—the so-called cream of the crop and bottom of the barrel, respectively. Consider a woman who spends ten years getting a Ph.D., M.D., or something similar, and also a man on the same career track. By the time they are settled into their careers they may both be about 30 years old. If both are not married at this time in their lives, they are on what sociologists call an "opposite marriage gradient." His marriage prospects are terrific, bags of money and prestige to spare. He will be able to pick and choose among women who will be, on average, about five years younger.

She will find things a lot more difficult for a variety of reasons. First, there are very few eligible males around who are older than she is. If there are, they probably want someone younger. Second, some men do not like the idea of a wife whose attainments surpass their own, nor do women particularly want a mate less accomplished than themselves. A male Ph.D. can marry a high-school teacher, or a male physician a nurse, but we rarely see females "marrying down" like this.

The opposite marriage gradient is plainly visible in the results of the Carnegie Commission Faculty Survey of 326,306 faculty members in U.S. colleges and universities. The survey found that while only 8.5 per cent of male Ph.D.s never married, fully 46.4 per cent of female Ph.D.s never made it to the altar. Male marriage prospects decline with a decline in the prestige of the degree earned, while female prospects *increase* with a *decline* in the prestige of the degree. Among the males with masters and bachelors degrees, 12.6 and 15.9 per cent, respectively, were never married. The corresponding figures for female faculty were 41.6 and 32.6 per cent.[9] A small number of these women may have chosen the single life, but reseach findings show the great majority to be unhappy and exasperated about the situation.[10]

Let's get back to the mating strategies of females with better prospects. The generally more pragmatic selection process of females in their choice of mates fits nicely with research findings indicating that males identify their feelings for a particular woman as love earlier than women do.[11] A man's susceptibility to "imprint" on some physical stimulus presented by a woman is more spontaneous. After all, physical attributes are immediately perceived and evaluated in a way that character and maturity are not. Further, a man can afford to "love at first sight;" he doesn't have to bear and care for any children that might spring from what he may later interpret to be mere infatuation.

Not only can the male afford to love, he insists on it as a requisite to marriage. A survey of 1,000 young people by sociologist William Kephart asked: "If a boy (girl) had all the other qualities that you desired, would you marry this person if you were not in love with him or her?" Two-thirds of the males replied with a resounding "No!" Conversely, more than

75 per cent of the females equivocated, stating that they either would marry that person or that they were undecided.[12]

Since a woman has more invested in parenthood—she must bear and care for children—she requires more time and takes more care in selecting and falling in love with a potential father of her children. This biologically based propensity survives even after parenthood has long ceased to be a consideration. Her concern in choosing a mate is not so much the intensity of the feelings she has for him but rather the intensity of the male's feelings for her. It requires time for her to gauge the prospective mate's feelings for her, as well as to evaluate his fitness to provide for her and her child. She is more concerned, in other words, with being loved than her own romantic urges. Once the choice is made, the female can "manage" her emotions so that they conform to the expectations of love.[13] Kephart took note of the male-female differences in romantic orientation and illustrated it with a quote from one of his female respondents: "I'm undecided. But if a boy had all the other qualities I desired, and I was not in love with him—well, I think I could talk myself into falling in love."[14]

OTHER DETERMINANTS OF ROMANTIC LOVE

Just as romantic love is not always just a hormonal shot in the dark, neither is it always simply a rational decision based purely on instrumental considerations. A successful businessman may forsake a dozen gorgeous young women and fall in love and marry a "plain Jane" because of her inner beauty. A beautiful, witty, and clever young woman may marry a gypsy truckdriver with bulging muscles when she could have had an orthodontist with a bulging wallet because the truckdriver better conforms to her ideal of what a "real man" is. The genes governing our reproductive strategies have us on a chain, but it is a very long chain. Evolutionary biologists expect a fit between the reproductive strategies that evolved eons ago and the human psyche operating in its modern cultural context, but this is not necessarily a particularly tight fit. For instance, 83 per cent of the women and 77 per cent of the men sampled in a 1974 Roper poll insisted that they got married purely and simply because they were "in love." Notwithstanding the social pressures to answer in this way, and the unspoken and perhaps unrecognized instrumental reasons underlying those decisions, these are large percentages.[15]

Let's take the respondents to the Roper poll at their word and explore romantic love from a psychological point of view. What is it apart from the natural imperative to love and mate that draws particular individuals to other particular individuals? The closest thing psychology has to a law is the proposition that people strongly tend to repeat behavior that has rewarding consequences and not to repeat behavior that has negative consequences. It follows from this that the desire for repeated and intimate close encounters with a loved one flows from an excess of rewards over punishments. As a general statement this is true but not very useful. We have to determine what it is that lovers specifically find so rewarding in each other.

Similarity of interests, attitudes, and outlooks is a good candidate for the glue that bonds. This certainly holds true in friendship relationships. We like people who reward us in words and deeds, and grow angry or cold toward them if they stop rewarding us. In this tit-for-tat world, our friends will grow cold toward us too if we no longer make them feel good about themselves. It is also trite but true that we tend very much to like those who like us. It is therefore quite obvious in common sense terms that having things in common is a hallmark of a fruitful relationship—"birds of a feather flock together," and all that. If similarity is useful in determining liking and friendship patterns, it should also be useful in determining love patterns. While it is true that romantic love is not simply an intense form of liking, it certainly cannot hurt to like the one we love. Literally hundreds of studies have documented the fact that husbands and wives are more similar to one another in many characteristics than we would expect by random chance.

An interesting study conducted by George Levinger and James Breedlove casts some doubt on the meaning of this body of love-and-similarity literature. By asking husbands and wives to indicate their own attitudes and beliefs on a variety of topics, they too found a great similarity. However, they also asked the husband-and-wife teams to report the attitudes and beliefs of their spouses. When they compared self-reports with the reports provided by spouses, they found a rather large discrepancy between attitudes and beliefs that respondents actually held and the attitudes and beliefs that their spouses *thought they held*. This finding led Levinger and Breedlove to suggest that spouses tend to stress similarities in order to avoid potential sources of conflict and that a great deal of misconception exists in a lot of marriages.[16]

An interesting and sophisticated study of happiness in marriage conducted by Raymond Cattell and John Nesselrode found that the happiest couples had opposite rather than similar personality traits—"opposites attract," and all that.[17] A spouse who is nurturing, for instance, would be happy with someone who enjoys being nurtured, one who is dominating would get along well with one who is submissive, and so on. Personal growth is made more possible when two people in an intimate relationship have different friends, interests, and pleasurable pursuits. He can introduce her to jogging, Beethoven, and Oriental religion; she can introduce him to Agatha Christie, the piano, and Mexican food. If both parties are open to new experiences, they have both contributed to the creative growth of the other, which is Ashley Montagu's definition of love.[18]

Psychologist David Lewis offers an interesting twist to the "opposites-attract" thesis. He invites his readers to make a list of their attributes and aptitudes, both favorable and unfavorable. This list constitutes the "real self." He then asks them to make another list of the attributes and aptitudes they don't possess but would like to. This is a list describing the "ideal self." He suggests that many of us seek marriage mates who possess the qualities we list under the "ideal self" heading.[19] For instance, if the ideal self is creative, intelligent, and assertive, we are likely to feel drawn to people whom we see possessing these qualities. By attaching ourselves to such a person and loving him or her we are essentially loving our ideal selves. We can bask in the reflected attributes of the lover and vicariously live up to the goals of the ideal self. In pursuing such a strategy we have complemented ourselves, and perhaps an extended relationship with the "ideal other" may result in our acquiring some of the qualities we admire so much in him or her.

It seems obvious, however, that differences in interests cannot be too extreme. A party-going extrovert is not likely to be very compatible with a bookish homebody. The distance between two such personalities would seem so great as to preclude any rewards accruing from attempts to partake in each other's favored pastimes. (I wonder how much latent hostility has been generated in women who have sat through endless TV football games because it pleases their husbands or who have done things alone if their husbands are unwilling to budge from the weekend games.)

It would seem that opposites have a better shot at an enduring love relationship if their differences are first filtered through a "consensus sieve." That is, a minimal degree of similarity in the relationship seems to be necessary. These similarities are most useful to a relationship when they involve similarities of background and interests rather than personality traits. Similarity is comforting; we understand those who are quite like ourselves. We know what to expect, and that makes life easier. Only after we perceive a foundation of similarity do we let ourselves partake in the excitement of the different and unknown. Romantic love would seem to thrive best on a foundation of basic similarities around which is built an edifice of interesting and even exciting differences.

STYLES OF LOVING

Thus far we have looked at love and loving from the perspective of the attributes of those toward whom love is directed. The other half of the love equation involves personal *differences in the way we love.* We do not all love similarly. Just as people differ in styles of liking, hating, playing, and working, they differ in the way they love. One theory of romantic love, that of Canadian sociologist John Lee, assumes at least six different orientations toward love. He calls these the eros (passionate), ludus (game-playing), storge (companionate), mania (neurotic), pragma (rational), and agape (selfless) styles. These styles are "pure types," with most people loving in different combinations, and also with the same people operating under different styles at different times in their lives and with different lovers.[20]

Eros. The erotic lover is somewhat akin to what Liebowitz calls the attraction junkie. They "imprint" very quickly on the physical attributes of others and they are "love-at-first-sighters." They immerse themselves in the life of the beloved, are ever ready to reveal their souls to their lovers, and expect the same in return. They are usually self-assured enough to make themselves vulnerable by self-disclosure. They wish to make themselves and their lovers transparent, and thus develop a great deal of emotional rapport. They tend not to be overly possessive and jealous (an indication of their self-assurance). The erotic lover wants sex very early in the relationship, since there is a great desire to possess the physically attractive attributes that caused the emotional *Sturm und Drang.*

The erotic lover loves transiently, however. Lee found that the purer the erotic type a person was, the less likely he or she would be involved in a lasting relationship. A test of Lee's theory by Bailey, Hendrick, and Hendrick found that males were significantly more likely than females to exhibit this style of loving. They also found that the more stereotypically masculine the males were, the more they engaged in erotic love. Consistent with the estheticism and romanticism of this type of lover, erotic lovers were much more likely than any of the other types to hold the attitude that sexual intercourse is "a form of human communication and the joining of two persons in close physical and spiritual harmony."[21]

Given the physiological differences between the sexes that we have discussed, this is the pattern one would expect. It was indicated in chapter 6 that males have an average of about 20 per cent less MAO than females and that low MAO is associated with sensation-seeking of all kinds. The erotic lover may be in love with love, or more correctly, with the sensations associated with being in love. When such individuals reach the inevitable tolerance threshold they must seek out a fresh partner with whom to experience more PEA-induced euphoria.

Ludus. Ludic lovers are also attraction junkies. They view love as a game—"anyone for love?" Unlike the erotic lover, who is deeply, if often briefly, committed, the ludic lover plays the game of love with several partners simultaneously in order to minimize commitment. The enjoyment for these ludic Don Juans is not so much the prize as the pursuit. They never reveal the self as do the erotic lovers; sex is for fun not for emotional fulfillment. Given the nature of the game as they play it, it's not surprising that ludic lovers are rarely possessive or jealous. Extreme ludics tend to report less happy lives than average and that their childhood experiences weren't that great. A man or woman who falls for a ludic lover—and many do fall prey to their carefully cultivated charm and sexual expertise—is destined for heartache. In the Bailey study, ludic love was found to be positively related to masculinity (the more masculine the man, the *more* likely he is to be a ludic lover) and negatively related to femininity (the more feminine a woman, the *less* likely she is to be a ludic lover).

I cannot help seeing something of the psychopath in the ludic lover. Like the psychopath, the ludic lover appears to lack the ability to form intimate relationships. He uses women simply to satisfy his urges and then discards them to their misery. He is a sensation seeker, although he doesn't seem to get the same kind of high from love activities as the erotic lover. He is also disinhibited and very susceptible to boredom. The fact that he moves faster than the erotic lover from woman to woman may well indicate that he has lower MAO levels than the erotic type. The correlation between the ludic love style and permissive sexual attitudes was by far the highest of any of the groups, as was the attitude that sex is simply a pleasurable pastime. Both the ludic and the erotic love styles are associated with extroversion, which is associated with stimulus seeking, which is associated with low MAO. It would be very interesting and instructive to design a study in which the various styles of loving were identified and in which MAO levels of each of the groups were determined and correlated.

Storge. The storgic lover makes a good companion. He or she loves peacefully, securely, and affectionately, but not with much passion or intensity. Storgic lovers seem to forego Liebowitz's attraction phase and slide slowly but surely into the attachment phase. Sex is not too important to storgic lovers and tends to take place quite late in the relationship. According to Lee, marriage between two storgics has the best chance of lasting.[22] Unlike the ludic, whose lack of passionate intensity is intentional, the storgic lover does not seem to have the capacity. Love evolves slowly for the storgic lover, who does not seem to comprehend the tumult implied by "falling" in love. This is the kind of love that some refer to as "mature" love, as differentiated from the infatuation, passion, and sentimentality of other love styles. Storgic lovers yearn for marriage and the settled existence; the passion of the erotic or the game-playing of the ludic seems uncivilized to them. No sex differences were found in the Bailey study on storgic love, although it indicates that previous studies have found females to be more storgic than males. Storgic love was significantly negatively correlated with sexual permissiveness and sexual game-playing.[23]

Mania. Manic love is full of alternating agony and ecstasy. It is the kind of possessive, obsessive, jealous love that Freud had in mind when he wrote about neurotic love. No one has described manic love with more insight than Shakespeare, in Polonius's account of Hamlet's experience of love. Hamlet, says Polonius:

> Fell into a sadness, then into a fast,
> Thence to a watch, thence into a weakness,
> Thence into a lightness, and, by this declension,
> Into the madness wherein now he raves.

Lee sees manic love as a combination of erotic and ludic love, walking a tightrope beneath a cauldron of intimacy and detachment. Manics feel the same intimacy as the erotic lover, but they are more jealous and more readily crushed by disappointment. The manic lover seeks constant reassurances of love: "Tell me that you love me!" "Where have you been?" "Is there anyone else?" They lack confidence and self-esteem, being the only group in the Bailey study with significant negative self-esteem. Another test of Lee's theory found, not surprisingly, that manic love is associated with neuroticism.[24] Manic lovers are the kind of individuals who will fall in love with people, even knowing that they will be left unsatisfied and hurt. The wife who does not leave an abusive husband and the husband who is insanely jealous are examples of manic love in action.

Manic love was found to be significantly related to femininity in the Bailey study, but not with masculinity. This fits with previously discussed data indicating that women are more likely to indulge in the euphoria of love but that they also experience greater degrees of depression when love goes awry. Next to the erotic lover, manics showed the strongest correlation with the "sex as communion" attitude.

Donald Klein, a psychiatric colleague of Michael Liebowitz, has coined a term to describe his patients who are extremely manic in their orientation to love. This term, *hysteroid dysphoria,* emphasizes the hysteric and dysphoric ups and downs of the manic's experience. He treats such patients with MAO-inhibiting drugs. These drugs have the effect of relieving depression, reducing the patient's sensitivity to rejection, and reducing the craving for romantic entanglements by retarding the breakdown of phenylethylamine.[25]

Pragma. Pragmatic lovers seek compatibility in love. They choose only partners with similar backgrounds, ones who enjoy the same kind of activities. Lee considers the pragmatic lover as a mix of the storgic (the need for a comforting similarity) and the ludic (a conscious manipulation to find the "right" partner). Once the right partner has been found, intense love can develop, especially with another pragmatic type. Marriage between two pragmatics tends to last, and we can view this as a vindication of sorts of the widely prevalent old custom of arranging marriages based on rational criteria. Femininity, but not masculinity, was found to be significantly related to pragmatic love in the Bailey study. This finding conforms with the notion that female reproductive strategy requires a woman to be more discriminating in love than males. Pragmatic love was significantly correlated negatively with attitudes of sexual permissiveness.

Agape. Agapic love is the traditional Christian ideal of selfless and spiritual love. It is the altruistic giving of the self to the loved one without conditions. Predictably, Lee found no pure agapic types in his study; few of us are saints. The Bailey study did find, as we might expect, that females were significantly more agapic than males.[26]

I want to emphasize once again that these styles of loving are "pure" types, and that few, if any of us, can be characterized as a single type. If we always operated with the same style we would not experience that state of affairs known as "mixed emotions." Any relationship between human beings is a chemical mix that may blend or explode. Although we all have a primary style of loving, we can experience other styles, depending on our partners' styles and when, during our lives, we experience them. We can experience different styles simultaneously or sequentially. For instance, a naval officer may select a wife *pragmatically* according to her "suitability" as a navy wife. He may love her *storgically* and genuinely while simultaneously carrying on a number of *ludic* affairs with other women. One of his affairs may be with a *manic* female whose passionate attachment to him results in his becoming a romantic *erotic*. With "mixed emotions," he may sever the relationship after a while because a divorce may affect his promotion opportunities and/or because he decides to sacrifice his own romantic interests for the sake of his wife's. That would involve an element of *agape.*

From this brief discussion of love styles we see that love means different things to different people. Understanding this should help us to understand and perhaps modify our expectations of love and of our partners. We have a tendency to believe that the way we feel and act toward love is the way everyone feels and acts (or should). We feel hurt when our lovers conform to their own love styles rather than to ours. It would be a lot more comfortable psychologically if we all loved alike, but a lot less interesting. Let's take a further look at these differences in love styles with reference to sex differences in monogamous/polygamous behavior.

MONOGAMY AND PROMISCUITY

Eminent psychoanalyst Theodor Reik has written that his years of clinical practice led him to the conclusion that "love does not mean the same thing to men and women. . . . sexuality has a different emotional place in their lives." A voluminous amount of research from Kinsey onwards has confirmed Reik's conclusion, which is what most of us have long suspected.[27] On the whole, men tend to seek sex, both intimate and impersonal, with multiple partners. The female's strategy, on the other hand, is to seek that one, special, meaningful relationship with a particular male. The Bailey study on styles of loving arrived at the same conclusions that evolutionary biologists reached long ago. Males are sexually permissive, they play games, and they are oriented to the goal of sexual consummation. Females are more relationship-oriented, practical, and dependent.[28] Yul Bryner, as the King of Siam, summed it up for us more poetically when he sang in *The King and I*: "A woman is like a blossom, with honey for just one man. A man is like a honey-bee and gathers all he can."

Although men and women love one another, they do not understand one another very well. The lack of understanding is due in large part to this rather fundamental difference in the romantic and sexual propensities of the two sexes. This difference has been the cause of so much pain in love relationships and is the basic reason for that long-standing state of affairs we know as "the battle of the sexes." Both sexes would benefit by a dispassionate attempt to understand the love styles of the other. If sex differences could be realistically and sympathetically appraised, perhaps men and women would more readily accommodate them without recrimination and rancor. Males, more prone to the erotic and ludic love styles, can understand the female's biological need for commitment and stop looking at efforts to forge one as a "trap." Females, more prone to storgic and pragmatic love, can understand the male urgency for sex and stop calling it "game playing" and "animal lust."

According to Fredrick Naftolin, professor of obstetrics and gynecology at Yale University School of Medicine, the different love strategies of males and females arose out of their different physical reproductive mechanisms.[29] The female reproductive pattern is periodic; she sheds one or more of a finite number of precious eggs (ova) at a certain time of the month. For her to reproduce requires the synchronization of the availability of a fertile egg, sexual receptivity, and the proper uterine environment. If the male's reproductive pattern were also periodic, sperm shedding, sexual receptivity, and the aggression needed to fend off competition would have to be synchronized with the female cycle of receptivity. Such a synchronicity, according to Naftolin, would be difficult to accomplish, and too many ova would be wasted. The biologically efficient strategy required that males constantly produce fertile sperm and be constantly ready to utilize them. Such a strategy is wasteful of sperm, but it serves to minimize the loss of the much scarcer and more precious ova.

The evolution of our reproductive mechanisms thus provides us with clues regarding male/female differences with regard to monogamous and promiscuous sexual behavior. Endowed with cheap and plentiful sperm, and relatively free of responsibility for the care of offspring, the visual/spatial and aggressive male was free to spread his genes as far and as wide as his capabilities and good fortune would allow. Those males with the ability to attract as many females as they could service were assured of pushing more of their genes into the next generation than less aggressive and less promiscuous males. Morality aside, sexual promiscuity would seem to be the optimal reproductive strategy for the male to pursue. He has done this with relish from time immemorial, and he is not likely to change just because moralists find it to be distasteful.

Females are better served in their reproductive strategy by being more monogamous. Had protofemales been as sexually active as protomales, they would have certainly been able to attract numerous partners, but they would not have been able to form long-term attachment relationships with a single partner. Sexual exclusivity on her part would be more likely to assure care and protection by a jealous mate than would promiscuity. Any malelike propensity toward easy sexual arousal at the mere sight of a handsome male body among females would have played havoc with their reproductive strategy. More than one observer has pointed to the female ability to work night after night in massage parlors without experiencing sexual arousal as evidence of the continued influence exerted by evolutionary selection for the optimal female reproductive strategy.[30] Needless to say, males would be highly aroused by this sort of impersonal visual and tactile kneading of the flesh of the opposite sex.

It would be unfair and untrue, however, to infer from the massage-parlor data and from the other evidence outlined above that women are not interested in sex. Women are active, curious, and passionate in the bedroom *when sex is meaningful* rather than mechanical. But it is true that as a theoretical prospect many women are less interested in sex than most men. A case in point is a study conducted by sociologists Cameron and Fleming. They asked a representative sample of people of both sexes ranging from 18 to 55 years of age to rank-order 22 pleasurable activities on a five-point scale. Among males aged between 18 and 25, sex shared the number one spot with music. Among females of the same age group, sex ranked fifth, after music, nature, family, and traveling. Among males in the 26 to 29 age category, sex sat unabashedly at the top of their list of pleasurable activities. Females of the same age group listed sex and their jobs tied for fifth. Jumping to the 40 to 55 age group, sex gets something of a bashing. Males listed it behind family in joint second place (with nature). Females in this group listed sex 15th, behind such mundane pleasures as sleeping, attending church, watching TV, and even housework![31]

If this is typical, it means that a midlife housewife would rather fire up the vacuum cleaner to tease the carpet than fire herself up to tease the old man's libido. But then perhaps his preference parallels hers, if the truth be known. The women's responses in this age group may also represent a sexual lifetime of poor sex offered by the men they slept with.

Enough of these depressing statistics. Let's return to the more youthful years in which both sexes are warmed by the fires of love. The female tendency to withhold sexual favors until ties of intimacy are formed and until she has certain guarantees of love reassures not only the female but also the male. The male's difficulty in obtaining his mate's sexual favors provides him with some assurance that she will not fall prey easily to some other male and that she has formed an intimate bond of affection with him. It is imperative to the male to know that he is "the only one." If males are reasonably sure of their mates' fidelity, they are then reasonably sure of their own paternity if a child should be produced in the relationship. Women cannot be cuckolded, but males certainly can. If females mated as promiscuously as males, the odds would be against a man knowing the paternity of his mate's child, and no man could be expected to stick around to care for a child that might not be carrying their genes. The female reproductive strategy has thus operated to make her more restrained, conservative, and discriminating in her sexual activities.

The differential reproductive strategies of males and females have led to justifiable charges that a sexual double standard exists for men and women. Not only is the double standard a reality but both sexes seem to subscribe to it. It may even be more widely accepted by women. In Morton Hunt's randomly selected national sample of over 2,000 respondents, 82 per cent of the males and 68 per cent of the females thought that pre-marital coitus was acceptable for males if accompanied by love. The corresponding acceptance of the same behavior for females was only slightly lower (77 and 61 percent, respectively).

The gap between the sexes widened considerably when these respondents were asked to indicate their acceptance of premarital coitus for males and females in situations where strong affection was missing. Sixty per cent of the males and 37 per cent of the females considered premarital coitus without love to be acceptable for males, and 40 per cent of the males but only 20 per cent of the females considered this acceptable behavior for women.[32] Both sexes appear to believe that "boys will be boys, and girls will be virgins" before marriage. While this is true in the abstract, fewer and fewer men appear to care if their prospective mates have lost their virginity—as long as they've still got the box that it came in.

If further evidence is required that males and females differ with respect to love and sex, consider the historical evidence. Dating and mating is a competition for scarce resources. When there are more women than men in society, such as in the 1920s and the 1960s through 1970s, men call the mating shots and create a licentious environment. SO MANY WOMEN . . . SO LITTLE TIME is a popular bumper-sticker slogan announcing such a male-favoring environment. Following their reproductive strategy, men flit from bed to bed and resist romantic entanglement for as long as possible. Marriages become scarcer, and divorces more common. Women have to accommodate the male strategy or face being left out in the cold.

When there are more men than women of marriagable age (the 20 to 30 age group), as is the case today, the love and sex game does a slow flip-flop. Women become the scarce resource, and men must then accommodate the female strategy or face a mateless future. The love game becomes less lusty and more romantic, relationships become more stable, and divorce more rare. Men start serious courting as women gain the luxury of picking and choosing from a wider range of suitors.

The effects of changing male/female ratios on the customs and mores of society are so lawlike that demographers can predict marriage and divorce patterns from it, physicians can predict venereal-disease rates, and economists can predict the health of the floral, jewelry, restaurant, and travel markets. All other things being equal, when the female reproductive strategy predominates, society is a kinder and gentler place. SO MANY MEN . . . WHICH ONE WILL I LOVE? might become a slogan adorning the bumpers of women's cars in the near future.

The whole business of differential sexual strategies is summed up for us by America's foremost evolutionary biologist, Ernst Mayr:

The male has little to lose by courting numerous females and by attempting to fertilize as many of them as possible. Anything that enhances his success in courtship will be favored by selection. The situation is quite different in the case of the female. Any failure of mating with the right kind of male may mean total reproductive failure and a total loss of her genes from the genotype of the next generation.[33]

MALE AND FEMALE ORGASM

Again, none of this should be taken to mean that females do not enjoy giving sexual expression to love or that they are less capable of enjoying it than males. In truth, women are capable of greater orgasmic capacity than males.[34] The fact that the male penis and the female clitoris are formed from the same embryonic, sexually undifferentiated genital tubercle does not mean that female sexual pleasure begins and ends at that strategic spot. Erectile tissue is spread throughout the woman's entire vulvar area, while for males it is concentrated in the penis. Unlike the penis, which has excretory and reproductive functions to perform, the only function of the clitoris is sexual pleasure.

Even though she is fortunately endowed with such a marvelous love organ and *possesses considerably more orgasmic potential than the male* (which would have come as news to Freud and other male denigrators of women's orgasmic potential), the female does not realize it as often as the male does during sexual intercourse. (Recent evidence shows that females can achieve orgasm just as fast as males using clitoral masturbation.)[35] A survey of 100,000 females by Tavris and Sadd found that in their premarital sexual encounters only 6.7 per cent of females experienced orgasm "all the time," and an astonishing 34.2 per cent never experienced orgasm at all. However, things improve considerably in marital sex, with 15 per cent reporting that they do "all of the time," and only 7 per cent reporting that they never do.[36] Similar results have been reported from other large surveys. This would seem to indicate that orgasmic pleasure is best realized for women in the context of a stable relationship in which she feels loved and wanted.

Unless encumbered by the dreaded "brewer's droop," orgasm for the male is a foregone conclusion every time. As is the case with many activities in modern society, the focus for men is in the *product* of the activity rather than the *process*. Orgasm is the product of male sexual activity, a kind of quantifiable "unit" of sexuality: "I had sex four times last week" ("I've published 40 articles," "I make $60,000 per year," "I can run a mile in six minutes"). Sexual arousal is like a tension in males that has to be relieved as soon as possible, within the boundaries of sexual etiquette and adequate "performance," of course. Just as the male ethos of performance demands one more article, another $1,000 added to his salary, or 30 seconds shaved off his mile, he seemingly cannot tolerate not adding to his climax score for very long once he is sexually aroused.

One of the problems with the female lack of orgasm is that the male is finished before the female is on the starting block. The male is like a sprinter: off the mark with lightening speed as soon as the gun goes off, frantic pumping until the finish line is reached, and then semi-exhaustion. According to Kinsey's research, about 75 per cent of males reach orgasm within two minutes, although research published in 1981 shows the average duration of sexual intercourse in the Western world to have doubled since Kinsey's time to four minutes.[37] (Yet another quantification of male performance!)

A woman sexually is like the marathon runner: a slow, almost casual start, a slow build-up to a comfortable stride, periods of mild tiredness followed by second and third winds, and a decently paced canter home. She tends to focus on the *process* of the activity. For her, sexual activity is less a "task" to be brought to "completion" by climax than it is a pleasurable interlude in which she seeks psychic as well as physical pleasure—a time for closeness and reassurances of love. Happily, with increasing sexual experience these different speeds moderate to a more equal pace, with men slowing down and females speeding up. As far as the ability to satisfy their mates goes, "nice guys finish last."

Even though we hear much talk about an increasing awareness among women of their sexual capacities and of their dissatisfaction with the traditional "two-minute wonder," orgasm does not seem to be so terribly important to many women. When women were asked in the Tavris and Sadd study: "Of all aspects of sexual activity, which one do you like best?" only 23.1 per cent chose "orgasm." "Feelings of closeness to my partner" was chosen by 40.3 per cent of the women, and 20.8 per cent chose "satisfying my partner." The remaining women chose among four other categories: foreplay, oral sex, masturbation, anal sex.[38] While we don't have comparable figures for males, is there any doubt that the response ratings would be radically different? It seems clear that men and women attach different but overlapping meanings to love and sexuality.

Female orgasm is irrelevant to the reproductive process and is therefore less biologically important than male orgasm, without which, of course, there could be no reproduction. There is no evidence that nonhuman female primates achieve orgasm in their natural state, although orgasmiclike responses from female monkeys have been observed after prolonged stimulation of their genitals by scientists in the laboratory. Since female orgasm is irrelevant to reproduction, one wonders why female orgasm exists at all, other than to decongest the vaginal area after intercourse. (Maybe God or nature intended them to have pleasure too!)

In a reproductive sense, just as it would have been counterproductive for females to be as readily arousable as males, it would be almost as counterproductive for females to reach orgasm with the same general speed as males during intercourse for two reasons. First, there is a strong tendency to terminate intercourse when orgasm is achieved. If females reached orgasm before males, nature's reproductive purpose may have been thwarted on too many occasions. Second, the blood-congested vagina acts to stop the outflow of semen after male orgasm. Because female orgasm decongests the vagina, there is a greater probability that semen would escape from the vagina of a woman whose orgasms came before those of her mate's. Since it does not appear to have much evolutionary value in reproductive terms, female orgasm may be viewed as a biological capacity that is differentially realized just as is the human capacity to run, lift weights, and sing on key.

It seems that female orgasm is almost as much a product of the female mind as it is of the clitoris. The potential is there in all females, as we have seen, but things have to be "right" to actualize the potential. There are cultures (usually highly religious and sexually repressive ones) in which orgasm is unknown, even in theory. (I suspect, however, that many women in such cultures have discovered its delights and partake of it in solitude.) In times or cultures where sex is considered sinful, dirty, and simply "male lust," not to be enjoyed but rather to be endured by women (such as among the Manu of New Guinea and many Arabic nations), anxiety and learned distaste will prevent autonomic nervous system responses to sexual stimuli in women. "Lie back and think of England," advised the Victorian mother, and many of the daughters appeared to have done just that.

There are other cultures, such as the Trobriand islanders and the Marquesans, in which female orgasm is highly valued and expected with each sexual encounter. Where the potential for female orgasm is recognized and valued, a man in love with his woman will want to help her to achieve it. In this sense, female orgasm is a "higher cultural" invention in places where females are valued for themselves, and in which men are concerned about their mates' pleasure as much as their own. It is a psychophysiological "reinforcer" that urges women to participate in repeated sexual communion with as much delight as their lovers. It is a sign for both sex partners that love exists between them.

Orgasm is quite possible for women with partners they do not love. There have been cases in which women have had orgasms with men they hated, despised, or were indifferent to, such as women subjected to rape or women performing as prostitutes. Nonetheless, it is much more likely to be achieved with regularity in the context of love. We might say that physiologically an orgasm is an orgasm but psychologically its appreciation varies with the context in which it takes place. Women who engage, like many men, in casual sex are the least likely to achieve orgasm according to the Tavris and Sadd survey.[39] It is almost as though female orgasm is a "reward" for monogamy, for engaging in the sexual strategy that best assures her genetic survival.

From an evolutionary perspective it makes sense that nature rewards women for engaging in behavior most likely to contribute to species survival. Maternal as well as monogamous behavior is rewarded by an increased propensity for orgasm. Pelvic vasocongestion increases with each pregnancy, and vasocongestion is directly related to the intensity of pleasure that women obtain from coitus.[40] The relationship between maternalism and sexuality is further emphasized by the fact that *oxytocin* (the mother-love intensification hormone) is released in greater quantities the more intense the sexual excitement is for the female.[41] It is clear that female sexual and reproductive physiology is designed to increase personal sexual gratification to the extent that she cooperates with the grand design of species survival. Mother Nature is indeed clever.

If orgasm is a pleasure best achieved and enjoyed in love, it follows that it will be more common in cultures where women are valued for themselves rather than as property or chattel. Men who love their women will enjoy the pleasure of "giving" their women orgasms as much as they enjoy giving other tokens of affection. If men are to do this, they must learn to view sex more as a process than as a product, a slow and beautiful process centered in the mind and spirit as much as in the genitals.

In cultures where women are valued only as baby-makers, cooks, and as a means to relieve male sexual tension, efforts are often made to severely limit female sexual pleasure. In many Islamic countries, female adultery is punishable by death, whereas, technically, a man may have four wives. In certain African cultures the practice of *clitoridectomy* (the removal of the clitoris) and *infibulation* (the scraping of the vaginal walls so that they fuse in the process of healing) is widespread. Such cruel practices indicate a total devaluation of women, hardly a condition in which love can blossom. Thus we return to the theme that only when all human beings of both sexes are considered equally worthwhile and valuable is love possible.

NOTES

1. E. Kanin, K. Davidson, and S. Scheck, "A Research Note on Male-Female Differentials in the Experience of Heterosexual Love," *Journal of Sex Research* 6 (1970): pp. 64–72.

2. Will Durant, *The Life of Greece* (New York: Simon & Schuster, 1939), p. 304.

3. Albert Harrison and Laila Saeed, "Let's Make a Deal: An Analysis of Revelations and Stipulations in Lonely Hearts Advertisements," *Journal of Personality and Social Psychology* 35 (1977): pp. 257–264.

4. Anthony Clare, *Lovelaw: Love, Sex & Marriage Around the World* (London: BBC Publications, 1986), p. 38.

5. David Buss, "Sex Differences in Human Mate Preferences: Evolutionary Hypotheses Tested in 37 Cultures," *Behavioral and Brain Sciences* 12 (1989): pp. 1–49. These age preferences are reflected in actual marriage-age differentials, with men being an average of 2.5 years older than their wives at first marriage (27 per cent being 5 or more years older). Age differences increase with second marriages. J. Ross Eshleman, *The Family*, 5th ed. (Boston: Allyn and Bacon, 1988), pp. 259–261.

6. Glen Wilson, *Love and Instinct* (New York: Quill, 1983), p. 90.

7. Sydney Mellen, *The Evolution of Love* (San Francisco: W.H. Freeman, 1981), p. 202.

8. Randall Collins, *Sociology of Marriage & the Family: Gender, Love, and Property* (Chicago: Nelson-Hall, 1986), p. 131.

9. M. Faia, "Discrimination and Exchange: The Double Burden of the Female Academic," *Pacific Sociological Review* 20 (1977): pp. 3–20.

10. Christine Doudna and Fern McBride, "Where are the Men for the Women at the Top?" in *Single Life: Unmarried Adults in Social Context*, ed. P. Stein (New York: St. Martin's Press, 1981), pp. 21–34. Many of the women responding to Doudna and McBride's questions indicated that they felt particularly chagrined at having to adopt the male dating/mating strategy, saying that it left them feeling used, dirty, and degraded.

11. See note 1: E. Kanin, K. Davidson, and S. Scheck.

12. William Kephart, "Some Correlates of Romantic Love," *Journal of Marriage and the Family* 29 (1967): pp. 470–474.

13. Constantina Safilios-Rothschild, *Love, Sex, and Sex Roles* (Englewood Cliffs, N.J.: Prentice-Hall, 1977), p. 72.

14. William Kephart, "Some Correlates of Romantic Love," p. 473.

15. A. Pietropinto, "Current Thinking on Selecting a Marriage Partner," *Medical Aspects of Human Sexuality* 14 (1980): pp. 81–83.

16. George Levinger and James Breedlove, "Interpersonal Attraction and Agreement: A Study of Marriage Partners," *Journal of Personality and Social Psychology* 3 (1969): pp. 367–372.

17. Cattell and Nesselrode, cited in David Lewis, *In and Out of Love: The Mystery of Personal Attraction* (London: Methuen, 1987), p. 19.

18. Ashley Montagu, *Growing Young* (New York: McGraw-Hill, 1981), p. 106.

19. David Lewis, *In and Out of Love: The Mystery of Personal Attraction*, p. 20–22.

20. John Lee, *The Colours of Love: An Exploration of the Ways of Loving* (Don Mills, Ontario: New Press, 1973).

21. William Bailey, Clyde Hendrick, and Susan Hendrick, "Relation of Sex and Gender Role to Love, Sexual Attitudes, and Self-Esteem," *Sex Roles* 16 (1987): pp. 637–647. This study is one of a relatively large number of studies based on Lee's theory, with very consistent results.

22. John Lee, "The Styles of Loving," *Psychology Today* (October 1974): p. 48.

23. W. Bailey, C. Hendrick, and S. Hendrick, "Relation of Sex and Gender Role to Love," p. 642.

24. D. Lester and J. Philbrick, "Correlates of Styles of Loving," *Personality and Individual Differences* 9 (1988): pp. 689–690.

25. Michael Liebowitz, *The Chemistry of Love* (New York: Berkley Books, 1983), p. 179.

26. A study of mine, which is still in progress at the time of writing, is looking at sexual behavior referents of the six love styles in terms of number of coital partners. The 104 males so far included in my sample had an average of 10.56 coital partners, and the 131 females had an average of 5.65 coital partners. These averages fit closely with national estimates of 10 and 5 coital partners claimed by heterosexual males and females, respectively, reported by Glen Wilson, *Love and Instinct*, p. 203. Predictably, male ludic lovers averaged the largest number of coital partners (23.82), and the pragmatic females had the lowest average (1.0).

27. Theodor Reik, *Listening with the Third Ear* (New York: Pyramid, 1964), p. 97.

28. W. Bailey, C. Hendrick, and S. Hendrick, "Relation of Sex and Gender Role to Love," p. 638.

29. Fredrick Naftolin, "Understanding the Bases of Sex Differences," *Science* 211 (1981): pp. 1263–1264.

30. See J. Durden-Smith and D. deSimone, *Sex and the Brain* (New York: Arbor House, 1983), p. 232, and Glen Wilson, *Love and Instinct*, p. 105. It appears that males are quite put off by females who engage in malelike sexual activity. A national sample of 815 American males found that 67 per cent disliked women who made love on the first date, even though the male usually initiates such behavior. Carl Arrington, "A Generation of Men Grows Up," *Men's Life* (1990): pp. 64–70.

31. P. Cameron and P. Fleming, "Self-Reported Degree of Pleasure Associated with Sexual Activity across the Adult Life-Span," St. Mary's College of Maryland mimeographed research report, 1975.

32. Morton Hunt, *Sexual Behavior in the 1970s* (Chicago: Playboy Press, 1974).

33. Ernst Mayr, "Sexual Selection and Natural Selection," in *Sexual Selection and the Descent of Man 1871–1971*, ed. B. Campbell (London: Heineman, 1972), p. 91.

34. William Masters and Virginia Johnson, *The Pleasure Bond* (New York: Bantam, 1975).

35. R. Levin, "The Female Orgasm: A Current Appraisal," *Journal of Psychosomatic Research* 25 (1981): pp. 119–133.

36. C. Tavris and S. Sadd, *The Redbook Report on Female Sexuality* (New York: Delacorte, 1977), p. 165.

37. R. Levin, "The Female Orgasm."

38. C. Tavris and S. Sadd, *The Redbook Report on Female Sexuality*, p. 167. Another study of 2,000 married women asking them what they liked best about sex found the following rank-order: "feeling of closeness' (22 per cent), "orgasm" (21 per cent), "intercourse" (20 per cent), "foreplay" (19 per cent), "everything about sex" (9 per cent), "oral sex" (7 per cent), "other" (2 per cent). James Wagenwood and Peyton Bailey, *Women: A Book for Men* (New York: Avon, 1979), p. 144.

39. C. Tavris and S. Sadd *The Redbook Report on Female Sexuality*, p. 54. Tavris and Sadd indicate that only 33 per cent of promiscuous women reported that they usually achieved orgasm, whereas 87 per cent of the strictly monogamous women did so most of the time. Many sexually permissive women have indicated to me in interviews that they do not particularly like or get much pleasure from their sexual behavior. Their primary motivation appears to be a desperate attempt to gain some form of closeness in the only way they know how. These women tend to have had a very negative childhood. In my ongoing study of love styles and sexual behavior, I've found a rather robust correlation of -.51 between quality of childhood relationship with parents and number of coital partners. In other words, the more negative the childhood, the greater the number of coital partners.

40. Alice Rossi, "A Biosocial Perspective on Parenting," *Daedalus* 106 (1977): p. 17.

41. R. Berde, *Recent Progress in Oxytocin Research* (Springfield, Ill.: Charles C. Thomas).

10

Romantic Love:
Its Problems and Possibilities

Love one another, but make not a bond of love. Let it rather
be a moving sea between the shores of your souls.
—Kahlil Gilbran

THE OBJECTIFICATION OF LOVE

The preference of males for younger women and their dabbling in impersonal
sex with multiple partners has led to justifiable charges that men view women
as objects. If men can experience feelings they interpret as love by being
exposed to visual stimuli without any knowledge of the "real person" within,
in a very real sense they are responding to objects rather than to unique
individuals with minds and emotions as well as bodies. The female objects
men respond to are esthetically pleasing and utilitarian, meaning they look
good and they can be used to satisfy sexual urges. The sexual objectification
of women is echoed in the familiar female lament, "You only want me
for my body," or in the male adage, "If you can't be with the one you
love, love the one you're with."

The initial male fixation on female face and figure is not necessarily
a dark and deplorable strategy that men purposely and consciously engage
in. From the data on brain hemisphericity we know that males have brains
designed for processing visual information to a greater degree than women
and that women have brains more designed to process the emotional content of stimuli to a greater degree than men. We should not be surprised,
then, if these two different but greatly overlapping methods of processing
information affect the processing of romantic and sexual information. This
difference is readily observed, for instance, in the reading material of the
males and females on these subjects. Pornography, usually of a visual kind,
is almost exclusively purchased and used by males, while romantic novels

are almost exclusively bought and read by women. The preferred reading material of each sex holds little or no interest for the opposite sex.

There is abundant evidence all around us of the male's greater tendency to objectify. Research conducted by Diane McGuiness and Karl Pribram among young children has shown that males have a great tendency to objectify from the very earliest years of life. Males respond to a greater degree than females to what is visually exciting in their environments. When male children are asked to draw a picture, they tend to draw objects, such as cars and trucks, rather than people. Girls respond much more to people than to objects, and their drawings reflect that preference. It has also been found that while female infants will respond with pleasure only to human faces, male babies will respond with coos equally to faces and to mechanical objects.[1] This apparently inborn tendency to objectification remains with males throughout their lifespan.

During adolescence and early adulthood, many young men are apparently overcome with the desire to express their sexual objectification by scrawling on bathroom walls. Wherever human behavior is manifested, be it in laboratory or lavatory, you can be sure that some behavioral scientist will feel the urge to study it. Some such hardy souls venture forth into public toilets to study graffiti. The study of male and female bathroom graffiti may be strange to some who may wonder what it could tell us about male and female attitudes about love and sex. The value of studying graffiti is like the value of studying the lonely-hearts personals. The most advantageous thing to this type of study is that it is unobtrusive. That is, the act of studying it does not affect the behavior being studied. Bathroom bards write only for themselves and for their sex-segregated audiences. They write anonymously in the privacy of their little cubicles, and therefore probably more freely than if they were responding to questionnaires and the like.

Graffiti researchers find the same sort of sex differences in bathroom prose that researchers in other areas find. In male toilets they find explicit references to masturbation, sexual intercourse, homosexuality, and other such topics, all described in obscene and vulgar ways, and often pornographically illustrated. Expressions of love and tenderness are rarely, if ever, on view in male toilets. As an occasional reader of this genre myself, I have yet to see a tender expression of love adorning the walls. Graffiti in female restrooms is almost directly the opposite. It contains few, if any, sexually explicit references. Female graffiti tends to be confined to expressions of love and yearning. If any "artwork" accompanies the prose, it is usually in the form of hearts and arrows surrounding statements such as "Jill loves Jack."[2]

All available evidence, then, indicates that to a far greater extent than women, men imprint and fixate on all kinds of objects in a sexual way. With the exception of the female use of vibrators (often introduced to them by males), the use of inanimate objects to arouse and enhance sexual pleasure is almost exclusively a male domain. Rubber, leather, shoes, underwear, enema hoses, and pornography of all kinds are overwhelmingly male "loves." Many men who are enamored of these so-called paraphilias often cannot function sexually in their absence. However indispensable these objects might be for sexual gratification to these men, there is no emotional attachment to them. If the underwear is lost, the enema hose broken, or the pornographic book torn, they are simply replaced. It is regrettable that some males also see women similarly as sets of interchangeable genitals.[3]

The objectification of a flesh-and-blood sex partner reaches its extreme in many male homosexual encounters. In such encounters the participants don't have to play games, since both partners know exactly what the other is looking for. Cruising bathhouses and "tea rooms," homosexuals are not looking for "a man," they are looking for a penis, which happens to be appended to a man. They don't have to falsely proclaim love, fidelity, security, or even be physically appealing in order to attract a partner. There is a popular saying that men give love in order to get sex, and that women give sex in order to get love. Homosexuals, both being men, get right down to the business at hand—sex.

An analysis of homosexual personals by Mark Strange showed that both the buying and the selling point focuses on the penis—the ultimate in objectification of a relationship. Little else other than the size, shape, and circumcision status seemed to matter very much in about one-third of the advertisements.[4] I cannot imagine a women advertising the topography of her genitals in heterosexual personals, nor a man getting any responses from a women if he were so crass as to advertise his. Contrary to the belief of many males, those few inches of turgid flesh hanging between the legs like Monday's damp washing are far down a woman's list of desirable male characteristics.[5]

Homosexuals can and do, of course, engage in deeply emotional love relationships with one another. But the evidence offered by the homosexual personals, and from the impersonal sex of the "tearoom trade," points to a real propensity to objectify relationships in which no genuflection has to be made to the differing emotional needs of the opposite sex. This observation doesn't point to the "moral superiority" of heterosexual males, who would doubtless behave in much the same manner as homosexual males were they not constrained by the dating and mating strategies of females. Heterosexual males have to compromise their sexual desires and strategies with those of females; homosexual males do not.

Differences in sexual objectification between men and women is seen even among men and women bisexuals. Blumstein and Schwartz, two sociologists, report that when basically heterosexual males engage in homosexual behavior they do so with strangers or male prostitutes. These bisexual men tend to conduct heterosexual and homosexual affairs simultaneously, and want nothing to do with their male partners after completion of the act. Bisexual males report that they are repulsed by the idea of having sex with males whom they know well. For females who have same-sex encounters the situation is reversed. For a female to be comfortable in a lesbian situation she has to have formed prior emotional attachments with her partner. Such women cannot imagine themselves having homosexual contact with strangers, and they tend to conduct their same-sex/opposite sex affairs at different times rather than simultaneously.[6]

If male homosexual behavior and bisexual behavior tell us a lot about the different attitudes of men and women toward love and sex, lesbian sexual behavior should enhance this understanding. Lesbians, too, are released from the constraints of having to compromise with the differing love/sex strategies of the opposite sex. As distinguished from male homosexuality, which he terms "sexually oriented and promiscuous," Willard Gaylin writes that "lesbianism, with its emphasis on caring and attachment, tends to minimize the sexual role. It tends to be extraordinarily devoted and monogamous, with warm and tender attachments prevailing over sexual needs."[7]

If males tend toward promiscuity and females toward exclusivity, we should see these tendencies magnified in homosexual and lesbian relationships. If we look at the average number of different sexual encounters of male homosexuals, male heterosexuals, female heterosexuals, and lesbians, the male homosexuals should have the most, the lesbians the least. This is indeed what we find. Estimates of the average number of male homosexual encounters over a lifetime are as high as 1,000, whereas for lesbians the estimate is two or three. Heterosexual men, who get less variety and novelty than they desire because of female restraint, average ten sexual partners over a lifetime, and heterosexual females, who evidently get more novelty than they want because of male insistence, average five sexual partners over a lifetime.[8] With tolerance for over-reporting (male wishful thinking) and under-reporting (female modesty) these are awfully compelling differences.

Social scientists like to tell us that sex-role socialization maximizes male and female differences. Males receive subtle and not so subtle messages that they are supposed to be studs. "Real men" are to sail the sexual seas and drop their anchors in any friendly port. On the other hand, females are told that "nice girls" keep their sails furled until such time as they are safely espoused. It is these messages, not biological proclivities, say social scientists, that best explain the different male and female sexual strategies. Such messages are certainly sent, but they are also received by men and women who are biologically receptive to them.

Messages to the contrary would find some receptive ears. (Witness the apparent sexual restraint of religious fundamentalist males or Erica Jong's "zipless fuck," long the shibboleth of the sexual liberation wing of women's lib.) But the vast majority of both sexes would be, and indeed are, deaf to them. The available evidence tells us that rather than sex-role socialization maximizing male/female differences with regards to love and sex, the process of socialization actually minimizes them, at least in terms of the number of novel sexual partners each sex encounters. In reality, and ironically, it is the sexually "deviant" males and females who best conform to our social image of what "real men" and "nice girls" should be sexually.

Even when we look at men and women in prisons we see this difference between male and female homosexual behavior. In male prisons, rape, promiscuity, and brutality is the norm. Rape is used to dominate and to humiliate as well as to relieve sexual tensions. On the other hand, coerced sexuality is rare in female prisons. Women tend to form close emotional relationships, get "married," and form "families." Often there is little sexual activity beyond holding hands and kissing involved, although more intimate forms of sexual contact are not infrequent. These behaviors in sex-segregated institutions add further credence to the proposition that males and females approach love and sex from different perspectives.[9]

Pointing out possible biological underpinnings for the male propensity to view women as objects does not by any means excuse it. It is a male sex-based trait just as aggression is. But not all men are aggressive, and some women are. It is the glory of the human species that we can alter our behavior altruistically and learn to look beyond the superficialities of the immediate to appreciate what lies beneath. Women, in their growing insistence that they not be viewed as objects, are beginning to require men to more fully and enthusiastically accommodate female feelings and concerns in a love relationship. It is not beyond the ability of men to do this, and more of them are becoming liberated from stereotypical masculinity and embracing their "better" natures.

Women, too, cannot escape the charge of objectification of love. They objectify themselves, first of all, by using their attractiveness as a means of "catching" a desirable male. "The use of sex by women to get what they want from men (money, status, prestige, or power) represents the ultimate dehumanization of sexual relations," writes Constantina Safilios-Rothschild.[10] While Safilios-Rothschild fails to see the evolutionary reproductive strategy at work here, she remains correct. The female propensity to search out the "right" man as a benefactor for her and her future children has an evolutionary history that benefitted the species in its struggle to survive. There is no more justice or morality in it than there is in the male's reproductive strategy.

While objectification of love is injurious to both sexes, it is more so for females. Women tend to be less happy than men in marital relationships. In a review of numerous studies by the sociologist Walter Gove, he found that almost all studies showed that wives were more likely than husbands to show symptoms of unhappiness and depression. On the other hand, when single men and women and divorced men and women were compared along gender lines, it was the man who was more likely to display these symptoms.[11] Other research has shown that the husband is perceived by both spouses to be the more loving of the two about twice as often as is the wife.[12] Furthermore, women tend to get progressively less happy with their marital lot as they age. A Gallup Poll conducted in eight European countries found that the percentage of "very happy" women fell from an average of 28.25 per cent at age 25 and under to 18.5 per cent at age 55 and over. For men interviewed for the same poll, increasing age tended to increase happiness slightly. Clearly, marriage is a more beneficial experience for men.[13]

At first blush these findings seem to fly in the face of research indicating that women are the more loving of the sexes, and that women, after a slow start, enter more euphorically into the love experience. Actually, these two bodies of research can be satisfactorily reconciled. It may be precisely because women are more loving that they fail to find happiness with men whose image of living and loving is somewhat different from theirs.

We have seen that women are less likely than are men to marry strictly for love because feminine love is bound tightly to considerations of reproduction and child-rearing. She is just as likely to accept a proposal of marriage from someone she doesn't love, but who loves her, and who shows great promise of becoming a successful provider, than she is to accept the proposal of a man she loves but who has poor prospects. Additionally, the female role as the pursued party, passively waiting for the pursuing male to initiate romance, often does not allow a woman the luxury of refusing a marriage proposal from a socially desirable man. After all, someone equally socially desirable whom she does love may never enter her life, and if he does, he may not be interested in marrying her. Having made a choice based on pragmatic considerations, many women then manipulate their feelings to convince themselves that they have married "Mr. Right" and that they truly love him. Sooner or later, this emotional manipulation and idealization are bound to hit the hard wall of reality.

Another reason why females become less happy with love and marriage is that the assets they entered the dating game with (youth and beauty) depreciate with age. Women may become more desirable with respect to many other attributes as they age, but the process inevitably takes its toll on youthful beauty. Men, on the other hand, tend to improve the assets that women value in them. As men grow older their financial position tends to improve, so they become more rather than less desirable as mates. As one feminist writer laments: "A man's wrinkles will not define him as sexually undesirable until he reaches his late fifties. For him, sexual value is defined much more in terms of personality, intelligence, and earning power than physical appearance. Women, however, must rest their cases largely with their bodies."[14]

Additionally, as men age they tend to become more emotionally open and secure in themselves, as well as becoming more attuned to the emotional and sexual needs of women. In comparison to the often sexual clumsiness and emotional insecurity of young males, these are changes that are viewed as desirable by many women. Under such conditions—subverting their own love feelings to those of the male, and the depreciation of their assets—it is understandable that women tend to be less happy in marriage as they age than do men.

EXTRAMARITAL LOVE

Extramarital love—adultery, if we are to call a spade a spade—cannot be excluded in any discussion of romantic love. Extramarital love is as old as marriage itself and has been engaged in by most men (and an increasing number of women) who have had the opportunity. Sexual exclusivity is a pious fiction for most people, as revealed by the "impious" behavior of a number of "You-can't-take-it-with-you-but-you-can-send-it-on-ahead-through-me" evangelicals from Billy Sunday to Jimmy Swaggart. Presidents George Washington, Thomas Jefferson, FDR, Dwight Eisenhower, JFK, as well as would-be presidents Teddy Kennedy and Gary Hart, have fallen to the allure of an adulterous affair. Adultery is not confined to one class, but as is the case with all life's little perks, it rises with rank and income.

The extramarital affair has been regarded both as destructive and as an elevation of love. Extramarital love affairs are only destructive if we consider that romantic love implies that sexual exclusivity should be observed. The idea that a man and woman should enter into a contract vowing never to love or have sexual contact with others "til death do us part" is a Western cultural idea strongly influenced by Judeo-Christian theology. This profoundly asexual tradition views extramarital love as absolutetly wrong and destructive in all cases. But then, the Christian tradition is none too sure about the sinlessness of marital sex either, the ideal love being selfless and sexless (*agape*), as St. Paul, St. Augustine, and others preached. Marital sex has been viewed by the church throughout much of its history as a regrettable necessity for the perpetuation of the race, not to be indulged in too lightly or too pleasurably.

Islam, while recognizing the male desire for variety, treats the expression of women's sexuality in anything but marriage as a grave crime. Adultery by men is also harshly punished, but then they are allowed four wives. Shia Islam even permits a *mut'a* "marriage," a form of legalized prostitution for married or unmarried males but *only* for unmarried females.

Other cultural traditions have been considerably more liberal in their acceptance of extramarital love. Among others, the Indians, Greeks, and Romans elevated and exalted illicit love as much as the Western Christian tradition has degraded and condemned it. Coleman and Cressey point to available studies indicating that only 10 of 190 nonwestern societies share our disapproval of premarital and extramarital sex.[15]

Some traditions have viewed extramarital love as more desirable, spiritual, and "real" than marital love. For instance, Hindu religious lore sees love as rising in a hierarchy that culminates in the purest form of love, that of the extramarital love affair. Other forms of love identified in this tradition—of a servant for his master, a friend for a friend, a parent for a child, and a spouse for a spouse, in that order—are instrumental. They are governed by reason, social propriety, a sense of duty, and norms of reciprocity, as well as by love.[16]

The illicit love affair is usually unencumbered by any practical tit-for-tat considerations or social or material gains. No reward is offered or expected other than the pure emotional enjoyment of the body, presence, and love of the beloved. Extramarital love, by its very nature, takes no note of status differentials. Whatever the respective status of the lovers may be outside of the romance, within it they are equals. Love between unequals, according to this line of thinking, is as flawed as a fine diamond set in tin; love between equals is love at its purest, a diamond set in gold.

The desire for sexual exclusivity is quite a normal and natural feeling when we are enveloped in the throes of passionate romantic love. During this period our love is so intense and all-encompassing that the attractive qualities of others barely phase us. In cultures where such passion is associated with marriage, mates are expected to retain the desire for sexual exclusivity after the passion has cooled, its place perhaps taken by the quiet security of storgic attachment. But, in no other choice we make in life is a commitment taken to mean "forever." Nathaniel Branden points out the lack of a reality base for such an expectation when he asks if we would view marriage as a lifetime commitment if a couple marrying in their twenties could expect to live and be healthy and sexually active for 500 years.

Life is a journey, and we can promise to share part of that journey with another individual. But to promise to share its entirety is quite radical according to Branden's thinking.[17] The promise "till death do us part" made sense when death came so much earlier than it does today for most people. In days past, many men and women had two or three "partings" due to the death of spouses, the women worn out by producing numerous offspring in dangerous and unsanitary conditions and the men dying from disease or war and leaving young wives who needed a new husband to help take care of her children.

The term *commitment* has become a sort of buzz-word of pop psychology. It has a quasi-legalistic air about it (I, party of the first part, do take you, party of the second part, . . ."). A commitment is a contract, not love, which is a passion. To be sure, the passion of love is often the motivator to enter the contract, but if you are in love you need no contract and if you need a contract perhaps you are not in love. Romantic love is a volitional act (to the extent that we have control over our emotions and/or the freedom to follow them); it is not a duty to be commanded by invoking nuptial oaths. In our insistence that we bind one another in a quasi-contractual commitment we are acknowledging the possibility that love can be transferred to a "party of the third part." We are, in effect, attempting to capture and imprison the volition of our lovers. The legal aspects of the marital arrangement, however, can be and should be viewed as duties and responsibilities that are morally binding, but my decision to love you is a commitment only to myself. I can promise to appreciate you, value you, respect you, to bring home the bacon to feed the kids, to defend you against the world, even to love you as a companion, but I cannot, even if it is now my deepest desire, promise you passionate love into perpetuity.

If our spouses do not maintain sexual exclusivity, we have a tendency to take their infidelity as evidence that they no longer love us rather than as evidence of a powerful drive for passion and novelty. This assumption may or may not be correct, but it appears to be more correct if it is a woman who is having the affair. According to the study of 100,000 married women discussed in the last chapter, 29.1 per cent of them had or were currently having an extramarital affair. The motivation for the great majority of these women who entered an extramarital sexual affair was much like their motivation for entering a premarital sexual affair—for love rather than lust.[18] This is not to say that women never enter affairs purely for sex, because of course many do. Nevertheless, of those women who rated their marriage "very good," only 19 per cent had extramarital sex, but 65 per cent of those who rated their marriage "very poor" had extramarital sex.

As we peruse these figures on extramarital sex among women, we should not take them as indicating there is very little difference between the sexes in their inclinations to engage in sex outside of marriage. Actually, there are very large differences between the sexes. Far more men have affairs, and men who have them have more of them. After reviewing a large number of studies relating to this issue, Annette Lawson estimates that between 50 and 65 per cent of married men have had at least one extramarital affair by the time they are 40. Further, she estimates that of the men who have had affairs about 40 percent have had four or more such affairs. Among women who have affairs, the corresponding percentage who have four or more affairs is 25.[19]

The difference between the sexes is magnified when we realize the differential opportunities to have affairs experienced by men and women. Almost any woman who desired extramarital sex could have it by simply smiling seductively at almost any man. The easy availability of readily arousable males makes the acquisition of extramarital sex unproblematic for females who desire it. If they don't take advantage of easy opportunities then it is because they don't want to. On the other hand, males tend to be prevented from having extramarital sex because of a relative lack of opportunity, not a lack of desire. Males desire frequently runs up against the wall of female reluctance and highly discriminating tastes. It is this coupling of lack of opportunity with strong desire that has made prostitution and rape such ubiquitous features of human history. Any comparisons of the rates of male and female marital infidelity must take into account these opposite trajectories of opportunity and desire.

It would be easy to infer from the above that men seek sex only for physical pleasure, and women only seek it for emotional pleasure. If you made this inference you wouldn't be too far off the mark—at least for younger men and women. Self-report studies among males and females aged 22 to 35 indicate that about 44 per cent of the males and 22 per cent of the females report that physical pleasure is their primary motivator for seeking sex. Thirty-one per cent of the males and 66 per cent of the females in this age category report love as their primary motivator.

As men and women age, however, the figures tend to become compressed, with love becoming more important for men and physical pleasure becoming more important for women. Fifty per cent of the males over age 36 reported that love and intimacy was their primary motivator, with the same percentage claiming that physical pleasure was primary. For women in the same age category, 43 per cent claimed that physical pleasure was their main motivation for sex, and 38 per cent claimed that it was love.[20] These are the findings we would expect if we take seriously the different reproductive strategies of males and females during the reproductive years. When the reproduction urge is strongest, male and female motivators for sexual activity should be most divergent. When the urge begins to wane, each sex can discover what the other sex previously found to be most satisfying about male/female relationships.

Returning to the issue of extramarital affairs: there does not appear to be any association between extramarital affairs and marital satisfaction for men. The greater propensity of men to separate love from sex means that men who are happily married seem to be just as likely to seek novelty as those who are unhappily married.[21] In fact, a study by Shirley Glass and Thomas Wright found that sexual experience outside of marriage contributed to happiness within it for males married 12 or more years.[22] Marcia Lasswell and Norman Lobsenz quote a 40-year-old engineer who insists that his affairs make his marriage happier. Note that this man's style of loving is a mixture of storgic and ludic love:

> I have had relationships with other women. My wife may have had lovers, too. But we both know that they could never cause us to break our primary tie to each other. . . . No one could ever take her place with me. But sometimes sex with someone else seems to happen naturally. I travel a lot and it's lonely on the road. If an occasional infidelity makes me feel happier, I'll be a better person for my wife to live with. She knows I would never want to share my life with anyone else, and that kind of thing makes a sex fling harmless.[23]

The Glass and Wright study augments the clinical insight of psychologists Howard Miller and Paul Siegel, who assert that a little adultery can be beneficial to a marriage if the marriage partners are secure in themselves and secure in their relationship with each other.[24] In case this be seen as a couple of men seeking to justify the sexual adventurism of their sex, a similar opinion is expressed by female sociologist Safilios-Rothschild: "exclusivity rules often made love and marriage suffocating and deprive people of rich and rewarding relationships. When there is a requirement that a love relationship must satisfy all needs for diversity, for companionship, and for understanding, love becomes stifled."[25] Safilios-Rothschild is echoing Plato's ancient warning against the expectation that any one individual can satisfy all of our emotional and physical needs.

Whatever our personal feelings about extramarital affairs, it is plain that they will remain an integral part of the love scene as long as men and women are attracted to one another. As either an injured or injuring party, we have to make decisions about how to handle them. Many wives know about their husbands' affairs and will ignore them if their mates are reasonably circumspect about them, and if they don't carry it so far as to threaten the marriage by falling in love with their paramours. To a pragmatic woman who values what her husband has to offer, or to an agapic woman who values her husband's happiness as much or more than her own, his odd bang at the old "Come and Go Motel" is not viewed as sufficient reason to sever the marriage relationship. Surprisingly few extra-marital affairs result in divorce. The great majority of affairs are not discovered, but when they are about half of the aggrieved spouses forgive or condone it.[26] We may assume marriages that survive infidelity are otherwise good marriages, but that infidelity provides the needed excuse to dissolve a poor marriage.

JEALOUSY

This is a good point at which to discuss jealousy, the emotion that Shakespeare called a "green-ey'd monster which doth mock the meat it feeds on." Jealousy is not necessarily as pathological as some people think; even the Almighty admitted to being a "jealous God." If we are in love with someone, it seems perfectly normal to feel jealous pain when that person displays an amorous interest in someone else. However, the fostering of dependence on one person as the primary or even sole source of emotional gratification, as in the case of monogamous pairing, often heightens jealousy beyond what might be considered "normal." (Interestingly, the God who is jealous is a god of a monotheistic rather than a polytheistic tradition.) I would certainly consider it pathological when a person is so ridden with possessive jealousy that he or she is constantly imagining infidelity where none exists, or who cannot bear the thought of his or her partner finding any sort of pleasure in the company of another member of the opposite sex.

While the total absence of jealousy in a relationship probably indicates a lack of value or strength in it, the depth of jealousy is not a measure of the depth of love. It is more a measure of one's sense of insecurity and inferiority. An insanely jealous person is allowing the real or imagined behavior of another to jeopardize his or her mental and physical well-being. The madly jealous person does not love the self, and therefore is incapable of loving anyone else. A mountain of studies has documented a strong correlation between jealousy and low self-esteem, and has also shown that excessively jealous persons have a malevolent attitude toward the world in general.[27] An individual with feelings of negative self-worth finds it difficult to believe that anyone else could find value in him or her. Consequently, that person is continually imagining that no one could really be faithful to such an undeserving soul. If a person feels this way about him- or herself, that atmosphere of insecurity, possessiveness, and accusations in such a relationship makes it more probable that the mate will eventually come to share the self-evaluation and go forth to seek someone more deserving of his or her love. If such an event does occur, it merely seems to vindicate what we've known all along—we're no good.

It is generally true that men confront the green-eyed monster more frequently and intensely than women.[28] Many theories have been advanced to explain this observation. Psychologists Miller and Siegel offer a classical Freudian explanation. They see the basis of adult sexual jealousy in the child-hood experience of losing the first love object (mother) to a more potent male (father). Adult jealousy is a psychic recapitulation of this traumatic infant experience whereby another, perhaps more potent, male is again competing for the beloved. For Miller and Siegel, a woman's jealousy is less intense because her early experience is somewhat different. A woman's first love object is also her mother, but the threat of loss in adulthood is not a true reenactment of her early experience, since her mother and her lover are of opposite sexes.[29]

An alternative explanation, first offered by Charles Darwin himself, is that jealousy played a key role in natural selection. This evolutionary perspective states that jealousy drove dominant males to secure and mate with as many females as possible, and to chase away any rivals. Jealousy provided the psychic and emotional motivation for minimizing the possibility of cuckoldry, that is, of a male providing care and support for infants not carrying his genes. The awful realization that children are always "mummy's babies and daddy's maybes" doubtless remains a powerful engine driving modern male jealousy. The specter of cuckoldry perhaps best explains the male tendency to abandon a love relationship in which jealousy-evoking events occur too frequently.

Female jealousy is less concerned with another woman stealing her husband's erection and sperm as it is with the other woman stealing his affections and economic resources. This concern goes a long way in explaining why some women are relatively "understanding" of their husbands' purely sexual affairs, but fight like hell if the affair involves love. It may also go a long way in explaining the typical female reaction to jealousy-evoking events. While the male tendency is to abandon the relationship, the female tendency is to preserve it by doing what she can to make herself more attractive. These responses are, of course, generalities: some males seek to preserve, and some females abandon.

Critics of the evolutionary line of thought may claim that it presupposes a recognition of the link between sexual intercourse and pregnancy on the part of our ancestors. Criticisms of this type reveal a lack of understanding of the mechanisms of evolution, and falsely assume its process to be both purposeful and necessarily progressive. But evolution is blind; it does not know what its optimum is. It simply selects that which aids species survival within a particular ecological setting at a particular time. The shorthand terminology of evolutionists has a lot to do with this misconception. When evolutionists talk to one another, it is understood that no evolutionary "purpose" is supposed, even if it is implied by their terminology. For instance, the term *selection* implies purpose, but the "selecting" is determined by nothing other than random chance—variations and mutations which are sometimes beneficial and sometimes harmful. For instance, the sickle-cell trait is a hemoglobin pathology, but it was "selected" into the gene pool of West Africans living in intensely malarious environments because the mutated red-blood cell protected against malaria. Now that malaria has been largely contained, the sickle-cell trait confers no benefits, only pathologies.

The selection for differential reproductive strategies, monogamy/polygamy, jealousy, and so on, are rather akin to this. While these traits were useful to reproductive success in the conditions under which they arose, they contain the seeds of much pathology in the entirely different cultural environments in which they are expressed today. Animals certainly make no intellectual connection between intercourse and pregnancy, but the males behave as though they do. John Money points out that in many species a dominant male is relatively indifferent to other males who sexually play with his mate when she is not ovulating. When she is ovulating, however, he guards access to her with all the power at his command.[30] Since the human female is continually receptive, the human male is continually jealous. Occasionally it may erupt into violence, murder, or suicide. Psychological and sociocultural variables, such as low self-esteem or the view of women as male possessions, can exacerbate the biological propensity. Of course, high self-esteem and an egalitarian view of women will have the opposite effect.

THE CAPACITY FOR ROMANTIC LOVE

Romantic love is a wonderful and natural thing. It is "caused" by many things: the biological necessity to reproduce, the pleasures of sexuality, the human need for affiliation and security, conformity to social expectations, the unique stimuli presented to us by the beloved (sights, sounds, smells, taste, touch), the need to feel worthwhile and wanted, and the need to complement the self. These are the important determinants; no doubt others could be enumerated. But what if, despite all these powerful motivators, we cannot love? "To be loved, be lovable," counseled the Roman poet Ovid. What if we're not lovable?

It has already been pointed out that psychiatrist William Glasser's theoretical backdrop for his reality therapy posits that all human beings have two basic needs: the need to love and the need to feel worthwhile to ourselves and to others.[31] These needs are intimately related. It is rare indeed to find a person who loves and is loved who does not have positive self-regard, and one who has this positive sense of self is usually one who loves and is loved. Since we are not born with a self-concept—all that a person thinks, feels, and perceives about the self—the love experience is temporally prior to self-evaluation.

The self-concept is the product of experience; we come to know what kind of persons we are by how others have responded to us. It is also the producer of experience. Nathaniel Hawthorne once said that how a person thinks of himself contains his destiny. A whole slew of academic studies have since verified this insight. If we think of ourselves as unlovable, it is difficult to accept that someone else could love us. If we believe that we are inherently lovable, we can gladly and joyfully accept the love of others. But how do we come to view ourselves as inherently lovable if we have not been loved? Let's turn Ovid on his head and say, "to be lovable, be loved," and explore the meaning of such a statement.

This observation brings us full circle to the early infancy and childhood experiences. The old adage stating that "the child is the father of the man," is perhaps nowhere more true than in the area of romantic love. Psychiatrist Otto Kernberg emphasizes the importance of infantile tactile stimulation ("skin love") to later romantic involvement:

> Two major developmental stages must be achieved in order to establish the normal capacity for falling—and remaining—in love: a first stage, when the early capacity for sensuous stimulation of erogenous zones (particularly oral and skin erotism) is integrated with the later capacity for establishing a total object reaction; and a second stage, when a full genital enjoyment incorporates earlier body-surface erotism in the context of a total object relation, including a complementary sexual identification.[32]

Taking the first of Kernberg's developmental stages, let us recall that in chapter 1 we spoke of how infants receive their first messages of their lovableness and worth through the medium of the skin. The pleasure received in mother's arms sent love messages swinging from synapse to synapse in the neuronal jungle to lodge itself in those special places in the brain reserved for it. The infant's neuronal "memory tapes" inscribed during this period may be reinforced later as he or she receives cognitive messages relating the same information. Lacking the maturity to do otherwise, children accept unquestionably the messages communicated by their parents. Information accepted unquestionably has a way of etching itself indelibly in our brains. The ease with which children learn basic information is why child-hood lessons, whether they be painful or pleasurable, have a way of intrud-ing into later behavior. If our later messages assure us that we are loved, we will feel worthwhile, and we will be able to extend that love to others. If those messages were in the opposite direction, we will not feel worth-while, and loving will be difficult for us.

Low self-esteem does not diminish the need for love. Indeed, low self-esteem individuals are starving for love. Being thus starved, they will be more receptive to the approval of others and perhaps more likely to "fall" in love than those with more secure personal identities. Such people will cling to anyone who shows the slightest hint of approval as a way of en-hancing self-esteem. But loving the source of approval is quite another mat-ter. The sources of approval and hoped-for love are used for what they provide, not for what they are. Energies are exhausted in eliciting words and actions of approval rather than loving. "Hungry" love is Maslow's D-love, or the Buddha's "love that leans," in contrast to "love that lifts." Leaning love is destined to quickly fail because of the constant strain on its human leaning post. Even two love-hungry souls locked in a mutual admiration society will soon tire of each other's incessant demands for reinforcement, for they forget that love is what you give as well as what you get.

The second of Kernberg's developmental stages toward romantic love involves the incorporation of "earlier body-surface erotism" into the context of romantic sexual eroticism. Returning to Harlow's poor deprived mon-keys, we noted that females deprived of love during infancy could not be induced to indulge themselves in the pleasures of the flesh, and had to be tied to rape racks to accomplish the reproductive purpose. Deprived males were shown to be similarly sexually inept. Deprived males did be-come aroused to normally raised females in estrus, but their social depriva-tion showed in their confusion as to how to copulate with them. They attempted to mate with the female's side, her face, and just about any-where but the right place. The females soon became impatient with all this bumbling and soon turned their attention to more adept males.[33] So early love deprivation not only renders peer-group relationships problematic but also sexual relationships. Romantic love is indeed a straight-line progres-sion "from skin love, to kin love, to in love."[34]

We have been called the "sexiest animals," and it does appear that we are programmed to enjoy sex more strongly than any other species. As intelligent and creative animals, we have many pleasurable activities to occupy our time. To compete with and maintain priority over other human pleasures, nature had to continually elaborate on the components of sexual pleasure until it reached its present unassailable position. Only feelings of love exceed the pleasures of sex, but when we make love we are often quite literally "making" (that is, creating) love. Since we have been able to divorce our sexuality from reproductive concerns, as far as we know, we humans are the only creatures who engage in sex solely for the pleasures it affords us. But the act of making love goes beyond the simple physical pleasures of the build-up and release of sexual tension. Sexual intercourse is the ultimate celebration of love; its sights, sounds, and feelings infuse our beings with a profound feeling of spiritual union with our partner. As Kernberg intimates, if we grow up alienated from our sexuality and lovableness, we will not create love in the process of making love: we will simply be fucking.

We know from many sources that abused and abusing (they usually go together) parents tend to report little joy in sexuality, and only a few such mothers report ever experiencing orgasm.[35] Recent experimental evidence indicates that neurons in the septum activate the orgasmic response, and we have seen that the septum and the amygdala may be competitors for emotional dominance during the most active phase of neuronal trail-blazing.[36] It is not too surprising, then, to find that women who were abused as children do not find much joy in the form of orgasm during sexual activity. It is clear that love is a conjunctive emotion we create anew when we move toward involvement with another. The way in which an infant first experiences need-gratification is critical to the later experience of romantic love. The foundation of romantic love is built upon the gratification of pleasure we experienced in our mother's loving arms. If that foundation is not well laid, we will have difficulty in loving.

Having stressed the importance of love to self-esteem, I should point out that the effects of love on self-esteem are experienced somewhat differently by males and females. I pointed earlier to Lord Byron's famous aphorism that while for men "love is a thing apart," for a woman it is her "whole existence." A woman is deeply embedded in the emotional life, revolving as it does around her intimate personal relationships. If love is indeed the vital core of the feminine existence, we should observe female self-esteem fluctuating more in sync with a woman's love experiences than would be the case among males.

This is exactly what a study conducted by Grace Balazs and myself found. We found that love was the most important factor among the several we looked at in determining self-esteem levels for both men and women. However, we found that love was approximately 2.8 times more important in determining self-esteem for women than it was for men. Women who were the recipients of very little love had much lower self-esteem than men in the same sorry love boat, but women who saw themselves deeply connected in their love relationships had significantly higher self-esteem than males who enjoyed the same high level of love.[37] So women have lower and higher self-esteem than men, depending on how well they love and are loved. On the whole, it appears that women put most of their self-esteem eggs in one basket, while for men the origins of self-esteem are considerably more diverse.

IMPROVING OUR LOVABLENESS

"There is nothing either good or bad, but thinking makes it so," wrote Shakespeare in Hamlet. The truth of this statement is a message of hope for those who have suffered from love deprivation. We have to believe that negative experiences are reversible in terms of the influence they have over present behavior. We do not have to let our memory tapes control our lives, although they certainly will if we don't believe in the possibility of change. We can begin to convince ourselves that we are individuals of worth, and hence worthy of love, despite our early conditioning. It is not an easy task to accomplish if our early experiences taught us otherwise. But no individual reading this book had experiences that were all negative; no one has had a life totally devoid of love. We can improve our loving and our lovableness. As Aristotle is reported to have said: "Assume a virtue and you have it."

One way of doing this is to embark on a systematic program of self-esteem enhancement. We cannot change our past love experiences, but we can work on how we feel about them and how we will respond to future love experiences. Just as love deprivation lies on a continuum rather than being an all-or-nothing experience, so does self-esteem. This book is not the place for a detailed discussion on improving self-esteem. However, I can recommend two excellent books to assist you in this endeavor. The first is How Do I Love Me? by Helen Johnson. This is an easily read, "how to" book, complete with self-esteem "workouts." The second is A New Guide to Rational Living by Albert Ellis and Robert Harper. This is a longer and more difficult book but well worth everyone's time. Merely reading these books will do nothing for you if you don't put the principles into practice any more than reading a book on body-building will give a man bulging biceps unless he exercises. You can improve your self-esteem if you work at it, just as a man can build his biceps. In the process of coming to love yourself you will come to love others. Johnson concludes her book by quoting Eric Fromm: "Love of others and love of ourselves are not alternatives. On the contrary, an attitude of love towards themselves will be found in all those who are capable of loving others."[38]

In the final analysis it remains to be said that we must love. Love is to the human being as rain is to the grass and sunshine to the rose. When we surrender ourselves to love, we do not lose the self, we discover a much larger, more beautiful, and more complete shared self. Love is the creative medium by which the self evolves in all sorts of directions, setting in motion a felicitous spiral of self-growth, lovableness, more self-growth, and more lovableness. When entwined lovers whisper that they need each other desperately, it is as much a biological fact as it is a romantic fantasy, for they are responding with all the emotional power of a million years worth of evolutionary pressure to feel that way. Pain and agony we also discover in love, for to love romantically is to become vulnerable. But as we bear any love-forged crosses, we can still glory in the knowledge that we are the only creatures in the universe who can grasp the meaning and joy of love.

NOTES

1. McGuiness and Pribram study cited in J. Durden-Smith and D. DiSimone, *Sex and the Brain* (New York: Arbor House, 1983), p. 60.

2. A. Arluke, L. Kutakoff, and J. Levin, "Are the Times Changing? An Analysis of Gender Differences in Sexual Graffiti," *Sex Roles* 16 (1987): pp. 1–7.

3. John Money, *Love and Lovesickness: The Science of Sex, Gender Difference, and Pair Bonding* (Baltimore: Johns Hopkins University, 1980), p. 84.

4. Mark Strange, *The Durable Fig Leaf* (New York: William Morrow, 1980), p. 74.

5. An unpublished survey conducted by the author asking 209 females to rank-order seven male physical attributes in terms of their appeal to these women found that the penis was ranked dead last by 98 per cent of them. The rank-ordering was face, buttocks, chest, height, arms, hair, penis. The highest ranking for the penis given by any women was fifth.

If any male reader is concerned with how he "measures up" in this department, a study of 2,436 males found that the average length of the erect penis was 6.15 inches for whites and 6.44 inches for blacks. The circumference of the erect penis was 4.83 and 4.96 inches for whites and blacks, respectively. J. Philippe Rushton and Anthony Bogaert, "Race Differences in Sexual Behavior: Testing an Evolutionary Hypothesis," *Journal of Research in Personality* (1987): pp. 538–539.

6. P. Blumstein and P. Schwartz, "Bisexuality: Some Social Psychological Issues," *Proceedings of the American Sociological Institute* (New York, 1976).

7. Willard Gaylin, *Rediscovering Love* (New York: Penguin, 1986), p. 199.

8. Glen Wilson, *Love and Instinct* (New York: Quill, 1983), p. 203.

9. Rose Giallombardo, *Society of Women: A Study of a Women's Prison* (New York: Wiley, 1966).

10. Constantina Safilios-Rothschild, *Love, Sex, and Sex Roles* (Englewood Cliffs, N.J.: Prentice Hall, 1977), p. 48.

11. Walter Gove, "The Relationship between Sex Roles, Mental Illness, and Marital Status," *Social Forces* 51 (1972): pp. 34–44.

12. C. Safilios-Rothschild, *Love, Sex, and Sex Roles*, p. 72.

13. Gallop poll cited in Sydney Mellen, *The Evolution of Love* (San Francisco: W.H. Freeman, 1981), p. 203.

14. I. Bell, "The Double Standard: Age," in *Women: A Feminist Perspective*, ed. J. Freeman (Palo Alto, Calif.: Mayfield, 1984), p. 256.

15. James Coleman and Donald Cressey, *Social Problems*, 3rd ed. (New York: Harper & Row, 1987), pp. 308–309.

16. Joseph Campbell, *Myths to Live By* (New York: Bantam, 1972), pp. 155–157.

17. Nathaniel Branden, *The Psychology of Romantic Love* (New York: Bantam, 1980), p. 183.

18. Carol Tavris and Susan Sadd, *The Redbook Report on Female Sexuality* (New York: Delacorte, 1977), p. 122.

19. Annette Lawson, *Adultery: An Analysis of Love and Betrayal* (New York: Basic Books, 1988), pp. 75–78.

20. L. Denworth, "Why We Want Sex: The Differences between Men and Women," *Psychology Today* (December 1989): p. 12.

21. Carol Tavris and Carole Offir, *The Longest War: Sex Differences in Perspective* (New York: Harcourt Brace Jovanovich, 1977), p. 70.

22. Shirley Glass and Thomas Wright, "The Relationship of Extramarital Sex, Length of Marriage and Sex Differences on Marital Satisfaction and Romanticism: Athanasio's Data Reanalyzed," *Journal of Marriage and the Family* 39 (1977): pp. 691–703.

23. Marcia Lasswell and Norman Lobsenz, *Styles of Loving: Why You Love the Way You Do* (Garden City, N.Y.: Doubleday, 1980), p. 158.

24. Howard Miller and Paul Siegel, *Loving: A Psychological Approach* (New York: John Wiley, 1972), p. 106.

25. C. Safilios-Rothschild, *Love, Sex, and Sex Roles*, p. 69.

26. Randall Collins, *Sociology of Marriage & the Family: Gender, Love, and Property* (Chicago: Nelson-Hall, 1986), p. 249.

27. R. Bringle and L. Williams, "Parental Offspring Similarity on Jealousy and Related Personality Dimensions," *Motivation and Emotion* 3 (1979): pp. 265–285.

28. P. Mullen and L. Maack, "Jealousy, Pathological Jealousy and Aggression," in *Aggression and Dangerousness*, ed. D. Farrington and P. Gunn (New York: John Wiley, 1985).

29. Howard Miller and Paul Siegel, *Loving: A Psychological Approach*, p. 140.

30. John Money, *Love and Lovesickness*, p. 157.

31. William Glasser, *Reality Therapy: A New Approach to Psychiatry* (New York, Harper & Row, 1975), p. 11.

32. Otto Kernberg, "Barriers to Falling and Remaining in Love," *Journal of the American Psychoanalytic Association* (1974): p. 486.

33. Harry Harlow, "Lust, Latency and Love: Simian Secrets of Successful Love," *The Journal of Sex Research* 11 (1975): pp. 79–90.

34. Lawrence Casler, "Toward a Re-evaluation of Love," in *Symposium on Love*, ed. M. Curtin (New York: Behavioral Publications, 1973), p. 13.

35. Richard Restak, *The Brain: The Last Frontier* (New York: Warner, 1979), p. 153.

36. J. Davidson, "The Orgasmic Connection," *Psychology Today* (July 1981): p. 91. See also note 39, chapter 9, for preliminary investigation by this author on this topic.

37. Anthony Walsh and Grace Balazs, "Love, Sex, and Self-Esteem," *Free Inquiry in Creative Sociology* 18 (1990): pp. 37–42.

38. Helen Johnson, *How Do I Love Me?* (Salem, Wis.: Sheffield, 1986), p. 103.

Afterword

The discussions in this book merely touch upon the the numerous pathologies wrought by the absence of love and the pleasures elicited by its presence. The tormented empty loneliness of victims of love deprivation and associated afflictions echo together their desperate cry for love. Temporary remission of the symptoms may sometimes be gained from the modern pharmacopoeia of drugs, but they will not be eliminated save through love.

Love cannot be bottled and purchased like Valium; it must be learned by imitating our lovers in an environment pregnant with its essence. If love is not sown in our hearts early in its existence, its bounty will be difficult to reap in later years. But human existence is not blind fate. We owe it to ourselves and to others to strive to become lovable despite negative experiences. We can alter our personal destinies if we remember that to love is to enjoy the fruits of the human condition, and it is the only way to complete the human circle.

Whether the love in our hearts resembles the fertile fields of Iowa or the sterile Sahara depends both on how it was tended in its incipient form and on how we now respond to it and cultivate it. If our love resembles the former we will view the world as a friendly place; we will be able to scratch the earth at any point and place our roots therein. We will flourish mightily, for the soil will welcome our nourishment as we welcome its. If our love more resembles the latter, we will view the world as a hostile place, a place as rejecting of us as we are of it. We may struggle upon a little oasis willing to accommodate us for awhile and to which we will cling jealously, possessively. We will even imagine that we love it. But, knowing no other way, we will use and abuse its resources until the desert takes it back, and we are left alone once again to go mad beneath the blazing sun.

Sometimes the language of science proves inadequate, too bland, too sterile, to fully express a conviction. The eloquent expression of the English Elizabethan poet George Chapman performs the task more admirably:

> I tell thee, Love is Nature's second sun
> Causing a spring of virtues where he shines;

As without the sun, the World's great eye,
All colours, beauties, both of art and nature,
Are given in vain to men; so without love
All beauties bred in women are in vain,
All virtues born in men lie buried;
For love informs them as the Sun doth colours;
And as the sun, reflecting his warm beams
Against the earth, begets all fruits and flowers;
So love, fair shining in the inward man,
Brings forth in him the honourable fruits
Of valour, wit, virtue, and haughty thoughts,
Brave resolution, and divine discourse.

Bibliography

Adler, Robert, and Nicholas Cohen. "CNS-Immune System Interactions: Conditioning Phenomena." *The Behavioral and Brain Sciences* 8 (1985): pp. 379–394.

Akiskal, H., and W. McKinney. "Overview of Recent Research in Depression." *Archives of General Psychiatry* 32 (1975): pp. 285–305.

Allee, Warder. "Where Angels Fear to Tread: A Contribution from General Sociobiology to Human Ethics." In *The Sociobiology Debate*, edited by A. Caplan. New York: Harper and Row, 1978.

Allen, Allen. "Does Matter Exist?" *Intellectual Digest* 4 (1974): p. 60.

Anastasiow, N. *Development and Disability*. Baltimore: Paul H. Brooks, 1986.

Andrew, June. "Delinquency: Intellectual Imbalance?" *Criminal Justice and Behavior* 4 (1977): pp. 99–104.

Applewhite, Philip. *Molecular Gods: How Molecules Determine our Behavior*. Englewood Cliffs, N.J.: Prentice-Hall, 1981.

AP News Service. "Wanted: Someone to Love Babies, If Only for an Hour." *Idaho Press-Tribune*, Caldwell, Idaho: September 18, 1988, p. D1.

Arluke, A., L. Kutakoff, and J. Levin. "Are the Times Changing? An Analysis of Gender Differences in Sexual Graffiti." *Sex Roles* 16 (1987): pp. 1–7.

Arrington, Carl. "A Generation of Men Grows Up," *Men's Life* 1 (1990): pp. 64–70.

Aslin, R. "Experimental Influences and Sensitive Periods in Development: A Unified Model." In *Development of Perception* (vol. 2), edited by R. Aslin and M. Peterson. New York: Academic Press, 1981.

Asso, D. *The Real Menstrual Cycle*. New York: John Wiley, 1983.

Bailey, William, Clyde Hendrick, and Susan Hendrick. "Relation of Sex and Gender Role to Love, Sexual Attitudes, and Self-Esteem." *Sex Roles* 16 (1987): pp. 637–647.

Balazs, Grace. "The Elderly Offender: Literature Review and Field Interviews." Paper presented at the Second Annual Idaho Conference for Students in the Social Sciences and Public Affairs, 1990.

Barnaby, J. *Amor Dei, A Study of the Religion of St. Augustine.* London: Hodder and Stoughton, 1938.

Barnett, C., P. Lederman, R. Crobstein, and M. Klaus. "Neonatal Separation: The Maternal Side of Interactional Deprivation." *Pediatrics* 45 (1970): pp. 197–204.

Bartop, R., L. Lazarus, E. Luckhurst, L. Kiloh, and R. Penny. "Depressed Lymphocyte Function after Bereavement." *Lancet* 1 (1977): pp. 834–836.

Baskin, Yvonne. "The Way We Act: More Than We Thought, Our Biochemistry Helps Determine Our Behavior." *Science* 85 (November 1985): pp. 94–101.

Bayart, F., K. Hayashi, K. Faull, J. Barchas, and S. Levine. "Influence of Maternal Proximity on Behavioral and Physiological Responses to Separation in Infant Rhesus Monkeys (*Macaca mulatta*)." *Behavioral Neuroscience* 104 (1990): pp. 98–107.

Becker, Carl. *Modern Democracy.* New Haven: Yale University Press, 1941.

Bell, Allen, and Martin Weinberg. *Homosexualities.* New York: Simon and Schuster, 1978.

Bell, I. "The Double Standard: Age." In *Women: A Feminist Perspective*, edited by J. Freeman. Palo Alto, Calif.: Mayfield, 1984.

Bennett, L., T. Rosenbaum, and W. McCullough. *Counseling in Correctional Environments.* New York: Human Sciences Press, 1978.

Berde, R. *Recent Progress in Oxytocin Research.* Springfield, Ill.: Charles C. Thomas, 1959.

Bernard, Jesse. *The Future of Motherhood.* New York: Penguin, 1974.

Berne, Eric. *Games People Play.* New York: Grove Press, 1964.

Blain, Michael. "Fighting Words: What We Can Learn from Hitler's Hyperbole." *Symbolic Interaction* 11 (1988): pp. 257–276.

Blanton, Smiley. *Love or Perish.* New York: Simon and Schuster, 1956.

Blumstein, P., and P. Schwartz. "Bisexuality: Some Social Psychological Issues." *Proceedings of the American Sociological Institute* (New York, 1976).

Bouras, M., H. Bourneuf, and G. Raimbault. "La relation mere-enfant dans le nanism dit d'origine psycho-social." *Archives Francaises de Pediatric* 39 (1982): pp. 263–265.

Bowlby, John. *Child Care and the Growth of Love.* Hamonsworth, England: Penguin, 1977.

Branden, Nathaniel. *The Psychology of Romantic Love.* New York: Bantam, 1980.

Breese, G., R. Smith, R. Mueller, J. Howard, A. Prange, M. Lipton, L. Young, J. McKinney, and L. Lewis. "Induction of Adrenal Catecholamine Synthesizing Enzymes following Mother-Infant Separation." *Nature (New Biology)* 246 (1973): pp. 94–96.

Bringle, R., and L. Williams. "Parental Offspring Similarity on Jealousy and Related Personality Dimensions." *Motivation and Emotion* 3 (1979): pp. 265–285.

Buikhuisen, Wouter. "Aggressive Behavior and Cognitive Disorders." *International Journal of Law and Psychiatry* 5 (1982): pp. 205–217.

Bullough, Vern. *Sexual Variance in Society and History.* Chicago: University of Chicago Press, 1976.

Buri, John, Peggy Kirchner, and Jane Walsh. "Familial Correlates of Self-Esteem in Young American Adults." *The Journal of Social Psychology* 127 (1987): pp. 583–588.

Buss, Arnold. *Psychopathology.* New York: John Wiley, 1966.

Buss, David. "Sex Differences in Human Mate Preferences: Evolutionary Hypotheses Tested in 37 Cultures." *Behavioral and Brain Sciences* 12 (1989): pp. 1–49.

Cairns, Grace. *Philosophies of History.* New York: Citadel Press, 1962.

Cameron, P., and P. Fleming. "Self-Reported Degree of Pleasure Associated with Sexual Activity across the Adult Life-Span." St. Mary's College of Maryland mimeographed research report, 1975.

Campbell, Joseph. *Myths to Live By.* New York: Bantam, 1972.

Capellanus, Andreas. *The Art of Courtly Love,* translated by J. Parry. New York: Unger, 1959.

Casler, Lawrence. "Toward a Re-evaluation of Love." In *Symposium on Love,* edited by M. Curtin. New York: Behavioral Publications, 1973.

Chase, T., P. Fedio, N. Foster, R. Brooks, G. Di Chiro, L. Mansi. "Wechsler Adult Intelligence Scale Performance: Cortical Localization by Fluorodeoxyglucose F 18 Positron Emission Tomography."*Archives of Neurology* 41 (1984): pp. 244–247.

Chauchard, Paul. *Our Need of Love.* New York: P.J. Kennedy & Sons, 1968.

Chein, I., G. Gerhard, R. Lee, and E. Rosenfeld. *The Road to H: Narcotics, Delinquency and Social Policy.* New York: Basic Books, 1964.

Clare, Anthony. *Lovelaw: Love, Sex & Marriage Around the World.* London, England: BBC Publications, 1986.

Clark, Matt, and David Gellman. "A User's Guide to Hormones." *Newsweek* (12 January 1987): pp. 50–59.

Cleckley, Harvey. *The Mask of Sanity.* St. Louis: Mosby, 1964.

Coleman, James, and Donald Cressey. *Social Problems.* 3rd ed. New York: Harper & Row, 1987.

Collins, Randall. *Sociology of Marriage & the Family: Gender, Love, and Property.* Chicago: Nelson-Hall, 1986.

Combs, Arthur, Donald Avila, and William Purkey. *Helping Relationships: Basic Concepts for the Helping Professions.* Boston: Allyn and Bacon, 1971.

Cummins, Mark, and Stephen Suomi. "Long-Term Effects of Social Rehabilitation in Rhesus Monkeys." *Primates* 17 (1976): pp. 43–51.

Davidson, J. "The Orgasmic Connection." *Psychology Today* (July 1981):
p. 91.

de Lacoste-Utamsing, Christine, and Ralph Holloway. "Sexual Dimorphism
in the Human Corpus Callosum." *Science* 216 (1982): pp. 1431–1432.

de Rougemont, Denis. "Love." In *Dictionary of the History of Ideas*, edited
by P. Weiner. New York: Charles Scribner's Sons, 1973.

de Tocqueville, Alexis. *Democracy in America*. New York: Mentor, 1956.

DeLozier, P. "Attachment Theory and Child Abuse." In *The Place of Attachment in Human Behavior*, edited by C. Parks and J. Stevenson-Hinde.
New York: Basic Books, 1982.

Denenberg, Victor. "Hemispheric Laterality in Animals and the Effects of
Early Experience." *Behavioral and Brain Sciences* 4 (1981): 1–49.

Denworth, L. "Why We Want Sex: The Differences between Men and
Women." *Psychology Today* (December 1981): p. 12.

Deykin, Eva, Joel Alpert, and John McNamara. "A Pilot Study of the Effect
of Exposure to Child Abuse or Neglect on Adolescent Suicidal Behavior." *American Journal of Psychiatry* 142 (1985): pp. 1299–1303.

DiCara, L. "Learning in the Autonomic Nervous System." *Scientific American* 222 (1970): pp. 30–39.

Dillingham, S. "Manual on Catching Ones Who Kill and Kill." *Insight*
(February 1988): p. 24.

Dixon, Bernard. "Dangerous Thoughts: How We Think and Feel Can Make
Us Sick." *Science* 86 (April 1986): pp. 63–66.

Dörner, Gunter. *Hormones and Brain Differentiation*. Amsterdam: Elsevier/
North-Holland Biomedical Press, 1976.

———. "Hormone Dependent Differentiation, Maturation and Function of
the Brain and Sexual Behavior." *Endokrinologie* 69 (1977): pp. 306–320.

Dörner, G., W. Rohde, and D. Schnorr. "Evocability of a Slight Positive
Oestrogen Feedback Action on LH Secretion in Castrated and Oestrogen-primed Men." *Endokrinologie* 66 (1975): pp. 373–376.

Doudna, Christine, and Fern McBride. "Where are the Men for the Wom-
en at the Top?" In *Single Life: Unmarried Adults in Social Context*, edited
by P. Stein. New York: St. Martin's Press, 1981.

Dreschner, V., and W. Gantt. "Tactile Stimulation of Several Body Areas
(Effect of Person)." *Pavlovian Journal of Biological Sciences* 14 (1979):
p. 2.

Dreschner, V., W. Whitehead, E. Morrill-Corbin, and F. Cataldo. "Physiological and Subjective Reactions to Being Touched." *Psychophysiology* 22
(1985): pp. 96–100.

Duke, Marshall, and Stephen Nowicki. *Abnormal Psychology: Perspectives on Being Different*. Monterey, Calif.: Brooks/Cole, 1979.

Durant, Will. *The Life of Greece*. New York: Simon & Schuster, 1939.

Durant, Will, and Ariel Durant. *The Lessons of History*. New York: Simon and Schuster, 1968.

Durden-Smith, Jo, and Diane deSimone. *Sex and the Brain*. New York: Arbor House, 1983.

Durkheim, Émile. *Suicide*. Glencoe, Ill.: Free Press, 1951.

Ehrhardt, Anke, and Heino Meyer-Bahlburg. "Effects of Prenatal Hormones on Gender-related Behavior." *Science* 211 (1981): pp. 1312–1318.

Ellis, Albert, and Robert Harper. *A New Guide to Rational Living*. Hollywood, Calif.: Wiltshire, 1975.

Eshleman, J. Ross. *The Family*. 5th ed. Boston: Allyn and Bacon, 1988.

Faia, M. "Discrimination and Exchange: The Double Burden of the Female Academic." *Pacific Sociological Review* 20 (1977): pp. 3–20.

Farb, Peter. *Man's Rise to Civilization*. New York, Avon, 1969.

Fincher, Jack. *The Human Brain: Mystery of Matter and Mind*. Washington, D.C.: U.S. News Books, 1982.

Fine, Reuben. *The Meaning of Love in Human Experience*. New York: John Wiley, 1985.

Flaherty, Joseph, and Judith Richmond. "Effects of Childhood Relationships on the Adult's Capacity to Form Social Supports." *American Journal of Psychiatry* 143 (1986): pp. 851–855.

Flor-Henry, Pierre. "Gender, Hemispheric Specialization and Psychopathology." *Social Science and Medicine* 12b (1978): pp. 155–162.

Ford, Clellan, and Frank Beach. *Patterns of Sexual Behavior*. New York: Harper & Row, 1951.

Freedman, D. *Human Infancy: An Evolutionary Perspective*. Hillsdale, N.J.: Lawrence Erlbaum Associates, 1974.

Freud, Anna. *Normality and Pathology in Childhood*. New York: International Universities Press, 1965.

Freud, Sigmund. "On Narcissism." In *Collected Papers of Sigmund Freud*. Vol. 4. New York: International Psychoanalytic Press, 1924.

———. *Collected Papers*. London: International Psychoanalytic Press, 1950.

———. "Inhibitions, Symptoms and Anxiety." In *The Works of Sigmund Freud*. Standard Edition. London: Hogarth, 1955.

———. *Civilization and its Discontents*. New York: Norton, 1961.

Friedman, Milton. *Free to Choose*. New York: Avon, 1978.

Fromm, Erich. *The Sane Society*. New York: Fawcett, 1955.

———. *The Art of Loving*. New York: Bantam, 1956.

Fry, William, and M. Langeth. *Crying: The Mystery of Tears*. New York: Winston Press, 1885.

Gandhi, Mahatma. *Self-Restraint Versus Self-Indulgence.* Ahmedabad, 1928.

Gardner, Lytt. "Deprivation Dwarfism." In *The Nature and Nurture of Behavior: Developmental Psychobiology,* edited by W. Greenough. Readings from *Scientific American.* San Francisco: W.H. Freeman, 1973.

Gaylin, Wilard. *Rediscovering Love.* New York: Penguin, 1986.

Giallombardo, Rose. *Society of Women: A Study of a Women's Prison.* New York: Wiley, 1966.

Gladue, Brian, Ricard Green, and Ronald Hellman. "Neuroendocrine Response to Estrogen and Sexual Orientation." *Science* 225 (1984): pp. 1496–1499.

Glass, Shirley, and Thomas Wright. "The Relationship of Extramarital Sex, Length of Marriage and Sex Differences on Marital Satisfaction and Romanticism: Athanasio's Data Reanalyzed." *Journal of Marriage and the Family* 39 (1977): pp. 691–703.

Glasser, William. *Reality Therapy: A New Approach to Psychiatry.* New York: Harper & Row, 1975.

———. *The Identity Society.* New York: Harper & Row, 1976.

Goode, William. "The Theoretical Importance of Love." *American Sociological Review* 24 (1959): pp. 38–47.

Gove, Walter. "The Relationship between Sex Roles, Mental Illness, and Marital Status." *Social Forces* 51 (1972): pp. 34–44.

Goy, Robert, and Bruce McEwen. *Sexual Differentiation of the Brain.* Cambridge, Mass.: MIT Press, 1980.

Grant, V. *Falling in Love: The Psychology of the Romantic Emotion.* New York: Springer, 1976.

Green, Wayne, Magda Campbell, and Raphael David. "Psychosocial Dwarfism: A Critical Review of the Evidence." *Journal of the American Academy of Child Psychiatry* 23 (1984): pp. 39–48.

Greenough, William, James Black, and Christopher Wallace. "Experience and Brain Development." *Child Development* 58 (1987): pp. 539–559.

Hamburg, D. "Evolution of Emotional Responses: Evidence from Recent Research on Non-Human Primates." *Science and Psychoanalysis* 12 (1968): pp. 39–54.

Hare, Robert. *Psychopathy: Theory and Research.* New York: Wiley, 1970.

Hare, Robert, and Michael Quinn. "Psychopathy and Autonomic Conditioning." *Journal of Abnormal Psychology* 77 (1971): pp. 223–235.

Harlow, Harry. "The Nature of Love." *American Psychologist* 13 (1958): pp. 673–685.

———. "Lust, Latency and Love: Simian Secrets of Successful Love." *The Journal of Sex Research* 11 (1975): pp. 79–90.

Harlow, Harry, and Margaret Harlow. "Social Deprivation in Monkeys." *Scientific American* 206 (1962): pp. 137–144.

Harrison, Albert, and Laila Saeed. "Let's Make a Deal: An Analysis of Revelations and Stipulations in Lonely Hearts Advertisements." *Journal of Personality and Social Psychology* 35 (1977): pp. 257–264.

Harrison, George. *The Role of Science in Our Modern World*. New York: William Morrow, 1956.

Heilbrun, Alfred, and Mark Heilbrun. "Psychopathy and Dangerousness: A Comparison, Integration and Extension of Two Psychopathic Typologies." *British Journal of Clinical Psychology* 24 (1985): pp. 181–195.

Henderson, Scot. "The Significance of Social Relationships in the Etiology of Neurosis." In *The Place of Attachment in Human Behavior*, edited by C. Parkes and J. Stevenson-Hinde. New York: Basic Books, 1982.

Hendrick, C., S. Hendrick Foote, and M. Slapion-Foote. "Do Men and Women Love Differently?" *Journal of Social and Personal Relationships* 1 (1984): pp. 177–195.

Herberle, R. "The Sociological System of Ferdinand Tönnies: 'Community' and 'Society.' " In *An Introduction to the History of Sociology*, edited by E. Barnes. Chicago: University of Chicago Press, 1948.

Hite, Shere. *The Hite Report*. MacMillan Publishing, 1976.

Hoebel, E. *The Cheyennes: Indians of the Great Plains*. New York: Holt, Rinehart and Winston, 1960.

Hoeffer, C., and M. Hardy. "Later Development of Breast Fed and Artificially Fed Infants." *Journal of the American Medical Association* 96 (1929): pp. 615–619.

Hull, Diana. "Migration, Adaptation, and Illness: A Review." *Social Science and Medicine* 13a (1979): pp. 25–36.

Hofer, Myron. "Early Social Relationships: A Psychobiologist's View." *Child Development* 58 (1987): pp. 633–647.

Holmes, T., and R. Rahe. "The Social Readjustment Rating Scale." *Journal of Psychosomatic Research* 11 (1967): pp. 213–218.

Holtzman, D. "Intensive Care Nurses: A Vital Sign." *Insight* 1 (1986): p. 56.

Humphreys, Laud. *Tearoom Trade, Impersonal Sex in Public Places*. Chicago: Aldine, 1970.

Hunt, Morton. *Sexual Behavior in the 1970s*. Chicago: Playboy Press, 1974.

Irwin, M., M. Daniels, E. Bloom, T. Smith, and H. Weiner. "Life Events, Depressive Symptoms, and Immune Function." *American Journal of Psychiatry* 144 (1987): pp. 437–441.

Jeffery, C. Ray. "Punishment and Deterrence: A Psychobiological Statement." In *Biology and Crime*, edited by C. Jeffery. Beverly Hills, Calif.: Sage, 1979.

Johnson, Helen. *How Do I Love Me?* Salem, Wis.: Sheffield, 1986.

Joseph, Rhawn. "The Neuropsychology of Development: Hemispheric Laterality, Limbic Language, and the Origin of Thought." *Journal of Clinical Psychology* 38 (1982): pp. 4–33.

Kalil, Ronald. "Synapse Formation in the Developing Brain." *Scientific American* 76 (December 1989): pp. 85f.

Kallman, F. "Twins and Susceptibility to Overt Male Sexuality." *American Journal of Human Genetics* 4 (1952): pp. 136–146.

Kandel, Eric. "From Metapsychology to Molecular Biology: Explorations into the Nature of Anxiety." *American Journal of Psychiatry* 140 (1983): pp. 1277–1293.

Kanin, Eugene, Karen Davidson, and Sonia Scheck. "A Research Note on Male-Female Differentials in the Experience of Heterosexual Love." *Journal of Sex Research* 6 (1970): pp. 64–72.

Kaufman, Alan. "Verbal-Performance IQ Discrepancies on the WISC-R." *Journal of Consulting and Clinical Psychology* 5 (1976): pp. 739–744.

Keiser, Thomas. "Schizotype and the Wechsler Digit Span Test." *Journal of Clinical Psychology* 31 (1975): pp. 303–306.

Kephart, William. "Some Correlates of Romantic Love." *Journal of Marriage and the Family* 29 (1967): pp. 470–474.

Kernberg, Otto. "Barriers to Falling and Remaining in Love." *Journal of the American Psychoanalytic Association* 22 (1974): pp. 486–511.

Kiecolt-Glasser, J., D. Ricker, J. George, C. Messick, C. Speicher, W. Garner, and R. Glasser. "Urinary Cortisol Levels, Cellular Immunocompetency, and Loneliness in Psychiatric Inpatients." *Psychosomatic Medicine* 46 (1984): pp. 15–23.

Klopfer, Peter. "Mother Love: What Turns It On?" *American Scientist* 59 (1971): pp. 404–407.

Konnor, Melvin. *The Tangled Wing: Biological Constraints on the Human Spirit.* New York: Holt, Rinehart and Winston, 1982.

Kozlov, A. "Woman of the Year: The Old Girl Network." *Discover* (January 1988): pp. 30–31.

Kozol, Harry, Richard Boucher, and Ralph Garofalo. "The Diagnosis and Treatment of Dangerousness." *Crime and Delinquency* 18 (1972): pp. 371–392.

Lawson, Anette. *Adultery: An Analysis of Love and Betrayal.* New York: Basic Books, 1988.

LaRosa, R., and M. LaRosa. *Transition to Parenthood.* Beverly Hills, Calif.: Sage, 1981.

Lasswell, Marcia, and Norman Lobsenz. *Styles of Loving: Why You Love the Way You Do.* Garden City, N. Y.: Doubleday, 1980.

Lee, John. *The Colours of Love: An Exploration of the Ways of Loving.* Don Mills, Ontario: New Press, 1973.

Lee, John. "The Styles of Loving." *Psychology Today* (October 1974): pp. 44–50.

LeFrancois, Guy. *The Lifespan*. Belmont, Calif.: Wadsworth, 1990.

Lester, D., and J. Philbrick. "Correlates of Styles of Loving." *Personality and Individual Differences* 9 (1988): pp. 689–690.

Levin, R. "The Female Orgasm: A Current Appraisal." *Journal of Psychosomatic Research* 25 (1981): pp. 119–133.

Levinger, George, and James Breedlove. "Interpersonal Attraction and Agreement: A Study of Marriage Partners." *Journal of Personality and Social Psychology* 3 (1969): pp. 367–372.

Lewin, Roger. "Starved Brains." *Psychology Today* 9 (1975): 29–33.

———. "Africa: Cradle of Modern Humans" *Science* 237 (1987): pp. 1292–1295.

———. "The Unmasking of the Mitochondrial Eve." *Science* 238 (1987): pp. 24–26.

Lewis, David. *In and Out of Love: The Mystery of Personal Attraction*. London: Methuen, 1985.

Lidberg, Lars, Ingrid Modin, Lars Oreland, Richard Tuck, and Anders Gilner. "Platelet Monoamine Oxydase Activity and Psychopathy." *Psychiatry Research* 16 (1985): pp. 339–343.

Liebowitz, Michael. *The Chemistry of Love*. New York: Berkley Books, 1983.

Lipsett, Seymour. *Political Man*. New York: Doubleday, 1963.

Lipsitt, Lewis. "Critical Conditions in Infancy: A Psychological Perspective." *American Psychologist* 34 (1979): pp. 973–980.

Long, Mary. "Visions of a New Faith." *Science Digest* 89 (1981): pp. 36–42.

Lorenz, Konrad. *On Aggression*. New York: Oxford University Press, 1973.

Lynch, James. *The Broken Heart: The Medical Consequences of Loneliness*. New York: Basic Books, 1977.

MacLean, Paul. *A Triune Concept of the Brain and Behavior*. Toronto, Canada: University of Toronto Press, 1973.

———. "Brain Evolution: The Origins of Social and Cognitive Behaviors." In *A Child's Brain*, edited by M. Frank. New York: Haworth Books, 1984.

Malinowski, Bronislaw. *The Sexual Life of Savages*. New York: Eugenics Press, 1929.

———. *Sex, Culture, and Myth*. New York: Harcourt, Brace & World, 1962.

Marx, Karl. *Writings of the Young Karl Marx on Philosophy and Society*. Translated and edited by L. Easton and K. Guddat. Garden City, N.Y.: Doubleday, 1967.

Marx, Karl, and Friedrich Engels. *The Holy Family, or Critique of Critical Critique*. London: Foreign Language Publishing House, 1956.

Maslow, Abraham. "Deficiency Motivation and Growth Motivation." In *Personality Dynamics and Effective Behavior*, edited by J. Coleman. Chicago: Scott Foresman, 1960.

Masters, William, and Virginia Johnson. *The Pleasure Bond*. New York: Bantam, 1975.

Matson, R., and N. Brooks. "Adjusting to Multiple Sclerosis: An Exploratory Study." *Social Science and Medicine* 11 (1977): pp. 245–250.

Mawson, A., and Carol Mawson. "Psychopathy and Arousal: A New Interpretation of the Psychophysiological Literature." *Biological Psychiatry* 12 (1977): pp. 49–74.

Mayr, Ernst. "Sexual Selection and Natural Selection." In *Sexual Selection and the Descent of Man 1871–1971*, edited by B. Campbell. London: Heineman, 1972.

McCormac, Earl. *Metaphor and Myth in Science and Religion*. Durham, N.C.: Duke University Press, 1976.

McCord, Joan. "The Psychopath and Moral Development." In *Personality Theory, Moral Development, and Criminal Behavior*, edited by W. Laufer and J. Day. Lexington, Mass.: D.C. Heath, 1983.

McIvor, G., M. Riklan, and M. Reznikoff. "Depression in Multiple Sclerosis Patients as a Function of Length and Severity of Illness, Age, Remissions, and Perceived Social Support." *Journal of Clinical Psychology* 40 (1984): pp. 1028–1033.

Mednick, Sarnoff, and Karen Finello. "Biological Factors and Crime: Implications for Forensic Psychiatry." *International Journal of Law and Psychiatry* 6 (1983): pp. 1–15.

Mei-tel, V., M. Meyerowitz, and G. Engel. "The Role of Psychological Process in a Somatic Disorder: Multiple Sclerosis." *Psychosomatic Medicine* 32 (1970): pp. 67–85.

Mellen, Sydney. *The Evolution of Love*. San Francisco: W.H. Freeman, 1981.

Menninger, Karl. *Love against Hate*. New York: Harcourt, Brace and World, 1942.

Miller, Howard, and Paul Siegel. *Loving: A Psychological Approach*. New York: John Wiley, 1972.

Money, John. *Love and Lovesickness: The Science of Sex, Gender Difference, and Pair Bonding*. Baltimore: Johns Hopkins University Press, 1980.

Money, John, and Anke Ehrhardt. *Man and Woman, Boy and Girl: The Differentiation and Dimorphism of Gender Identity from Conception to Maturity*. Baltimore: Johns Hopkins University Press, 1972.

Montagu, Ashley. "A Scientist Looks at Love." *Phi Beta Kappan* 51 (1970): pp. 463–467.

Montagu, Ashley. *Touching: The Human Significance of the Skin.* New York: Harper & Row, 1978.

——. "My Conception of Human Nature." In *Explorers of Humankind,* edited by T. Hanna. New York: Harper & Row, 1979.

——. *Growing Young.* New York: McGraw-Hill, 1981.

Morgan, Douglas. *Love, Plato, the Bible, and Freud.* Englewood Cliffs, N.J.: Prentice-Hall, 1964.

Morris, Desmond. *The Naked Ape.* New York: Dell, 1967.

Morris, Richard. *Evolution and Human Nature.* New York: Avon, 1983.

Morsbach, G., and C. Bunting. "Maternal Recognition of Their Neonate's Cries." *Developmental Medicine and Child Neurology* 21 (1979): pp. 178–185.

Mullen, P., and L. Maack. "Jealousy, Pathological Jealousy and Aggression." In *Aggression and Dangerousness,* edited by D. Farrington and P. Gunn. New York: John Wiley, 1985.

Murchie, Guy. *The Seven Mysteries of Life.* Boston: Houghton Mifflin, 1978.

Murray, Linda. "Sexual Destinies." *Omni* 9 (1987): pp. 100–128.

Naftolin, Fredrick. "Understanding the Bases of Sex Differences." *Science* 211 (1981): pp. 1263–1264.

Nelson, Niles. "Trebly Sensuous Woman." *Psychology Today* 68 (July 1971): p. 99.

Ornstein, R., and D. Sobel. "The Healing Brain." *Psychology Today* (March 1987): pp. 48–52.

Osborn, Reuben. *Marxism and Psychoanalysis* (New York: Dell, 1965).

Pardes, Herbert. "Neuroscience and Psychiatry: Marriage or Coexistence?" *American Journal of Psychiatry* 143 (1986): pp. 1205–1212.

Patton, R., and L. Gardner. "Deprivation Dwarfism (Psychosocial Deprivation): Disordered Family Environment as a Cause of So-Called Ideopathic Hypopituitarism." In *Endocrine and Genetic Diseases of Childhood and Adolescence,* edited by L. Gardner. Philadelphia: W. B. Saunders, 1975.

Pearsall, Paul. *Superimmunity.* New York: Fawcett, 1987.

Peel, Stanton. "Addiction: The Analgesic Experience." *Human Nature* 1 (1978): pp. 61–66.

Peel, Stanton, and Archie Brodsky. *Love and Addiction.* New York: Taplinger, 1975.

Peterson, Gail, and Lewis Mehl. "Some Determinants of Maternal Attachment." *American Journal of Psychiatry* 135 (1978): pp. 1168–1173.

Philippoulos, G., E. Wittkower, and A. Cousineau. "The Etiological Significance of Emotional Factors in Onset and Exacerbations of Multiple Sclerosis." *Psychosomatic Medicine* 20 (1958): pp. 458–474.

Phillips, Kathryn. "Why Can't a Man Be More Like a Woman . . . and Vice Versa?" *Omni* 13 (1990): pp. 42–68.

Phipps, W., B. Long, and N. Woods. *Medical Surgical Nursing.* St. Louis: C. V. Mosby, 1983.

Pietropinto, Anthony. "Current Thinking on Selecting a Marriage Partner." *Medical Aspects of Human Sexuality* 14 (1980): pp. 81–83.

Powell, G., J. Brasel, and R. Blizzard. "Emotional Deprivation and Growth Retardation Simulating Ideopathic Hypopituitarism. I. Clinical Evaluation of the Syndrome." *New England Journal of Medicine* 276 (1967): pp. 1271–1278.

Powell, G., S. Raiti, and R. Blizzard. "Emotional Deprivation and Growth Retardation Simulating Ideopathic Hypopituitarism. II. Endocrinologic Evaluation of the Syndrome." *New England Journal of Medicine* 276 (1967): pp. 1279–1283.

Plato. *The Symposium.* In *The Republic and Other Works,* translated by B. Jowett. Garden City, N.Y.: Dolphin, 1960.

Prescott, James. "Body Pleasure and the Origins of Violence." *Bulletin of the Atomic Scientists* 31 (1975): pp. 10–20.

President's Commission on Law Enforcement and Administration of Justice. *Task Force Report on Drunkenness.* Washington, D.C.: U.S. Government Printing Office, 1967.

Provence, S., and R. Lipton. *Infants in Institutions.* New York: International Universities Press, 1962.

Rand, Ayn. *For the New Intellectual.* New York: Random House, 1961.

Reik, Theodore. *Listening with the Third Ear.* New York: Pyramid, 1964.

Reinisch, June. "Prenatal Exposure of Human Foetuses to Synthetic Progestin and Oestrogen Affects Personality." *Nature* 266 (1977): pp. 561–562.

Reiss, Ira, and Gary Lee. *Family Systems in America.* New York: Holt, Rinehart and Winston, 1988.

Restak, Richard. *The Brain: The Last Frontier.* New York: Warner, 1979.

———. *The Infant Mind.* Garden City, N.Y.: Doubleday, 1986.

Rice, Ruth. "Neurological Development in Premature Infants Following Stimulation." *Developmental Psychology* 13 (1977): pp. 69–76.

Rohner, Ronald. *They Love Me, They Love Me Not: A Worldwide Study of the Effects of Parental Acceptance and Rejection.* New York: Hraf Press, 1975.

Rose, Steven. *The Conscious Brain.* New York: Vintage, 1978.

Rosenfeld, A. "Tippling Enzymes." *Science* 81/2 (1981): pp. 24–25.

Rosenthal, P., and S. Rosenthal. "Suicidal Behavior by Preschool Children." *American Journal of Psychiatry* 141 (1984): pp. 520–524.

Rosenzweig, M., E. Bennett, and M. Diamond. "Brain Changes in Response to Experience." In *The Nature and Nurture of Behavior: Developmental Psychobiology.* Readings from *Scientific American,* edited by W. Greenough. San Francisco: W.H. Freeman, 1973.

Rossi, Alice. "A Biosocial Perspective on Parenting." *Daedalus* 106 (1977): pp. 1–31.

———. "Gender and Parenthood: American Sociological Association, 1983 Presidential Address." *American Sociological Review* 49 (1984): pp. 1–19.

Ruben, R., J. Reinisch, and R. Haskett. "Postnatal Gonadalsteroid Effects on Human Behavior." *Science* 211 (1981): pp. 1318–1324.

Rushton, J. Philippe, and Anthony Bogaert. "Race Differences in Sexual Behavior: Testing an Evolutionary Hypothesis." *Journal of Research in Personality* 21 (1987): pp. 529–551.

Rushton, J. Philippe, David Falker, Michael Neale, David Nias, and Hans Eysenck. "Altruism and Aggression: The Heritability of Individual Differences." *Journal of Personality and Individual Differences* 6 (1986): pp. 1192–1198.

Rutter, Michael. "Maternal Deprivation, 1972–1978: New Findings, New Concepts, New Approaches." *Child Development* 50 (1979): pp. 283–305.

———. *Maternal Deprivation Reassessed.* Middlesex, England: Penguin, 1972.

Sack, William, Robert Mason, and James Higgins. "The Single-Parent Family and Abusive Child Punishment." *American Journal of Orthopsychiatry* 55 (1985): pp. 252–259.

Safilios-Rothschild, Constantina. *Love, Sex, and Sex Roles.* Englewood Cliffs, N.J.: Prentice-Hall, 1977.

Seeman, P., and T. Lee. "Chemical Clues to Schizophrenia." *Science News* (November 1981): p. 112.

Selye, Hans. "The Evolution of the Stress Concept." *American Journal of Cardiology* 26 (1970): pp. 289–299.

Shalling, Daisy. "Psychopathy-related Personality Variables and the Psychophysiology of Socialization." In *Psychopathic Behavior*, edited by R. Hare and D. Shalling. New York: Wiley, 1978.

Shapiro, E. *Transition to Parenthood in Adult and Family Development.* Ph.D. dissertation. Ann Arbor, Mich.: University Microfilms International, 1979.

Shreeve, J. "Argument over a Woman: Science Searches for the Mother of Us All." *Discover* (August 1990): pp. 52–59.

Simon, R., and N. Sharma. "Women and Crime: Does the American Experience Generalize?" In *Criminology of Deviant Women*, edited by F. Adler and R. Simon. Boston: Houghton Mifflin, 1979.

Singer, Irving. *The Nature of Love: Plato to Luther.* Chicago: University of Chicago Press, 1984.

Sisca, Sam, Anthony Walsh, and Patricia Walsh. "Love Deprivation and Blood Pressure Levels among a College Population: A Preliminary Investigation." *Psychology* 22 (1985): pp. 63–70.

Skeels, Harold. "Adult Status of Children with Contrasting Early Life Experiences." *Monographs of the Society for Research in Child Development* (1966).

Smelser, Neil. *Theory of Collective Behavior.* New York: The Free Press, 1962.

Snyder, S. *Biological Aspects of Mental Disorder.* New York: Oxford University Press, 1980.

Solomon, Richard. "The Opponent-Process Theory of Acquired Motivation." *American Psychologist* 35 (1980): pp. 691–712.

Sorokin, Pitirim. *The Ways and Power of Love.* Boston: Beacon Press, 1954.

Sorokin, P., and R. Hanson. "The Power of Creative Love." In *The Meaning of Love*, edited by A. Montagu. Westport, Conn.: Greenwood, 1953.

Sperry, Roger. "Some Effects of Disconnecting the Cerebral Hemispheres." *Science* 217 (1982): pp. 1223–1226.

Spitz, Rene. "Hospitalism." In *The Psychoanalytic Study of the Child.* International Universities Press, 1945.

Staff Writer. "Human Milk Aids in Health, Fosters Love." *Science Digest* (Winter, 1979): p. 99.

Stendhal. *On Love.* New York: Liveright, 1947.

Strange, Mark. *The Durable Fig Leaf.* New York: William Morrow, 1980.

Stringer, C., and P. Andrews. "Genetic and Fossil Evidence for the Origin of Modern Humans." *Science* 238 (1988): pp. 1263–1268.

Suomi, Stephen. *A Touch of Sensitivity.* Boston: WGBH Educational Foundation, 1980.

———. "Sibling Relationships in Nonhuman Primates." In *Sibling Relationships: Their Nature and Significance Across the Lifespan*, edited by M. Lamg and B. Sutton-Smith. Hillsdale, N.J.: Lawrence Erlbaum, 1982.

Suomi, Stephen, and Harry Harlow. "Social Rehabilitation of Isolate-reared Monkeys." *Developmental Psychology* 6 (1972): pp. 487–496.

Szasz, Thomas. *Psychiatric Slavery.* Garden City, N.Y.: Doubleday, 1977.

Tapp, J., and H. Markowitz. "Infant Handling: Effects on Avoidance Learning, Brain Weight, and Cholinesterase Activity." *Science* 140 (1963): pp. 486–487.

Tavris, Carol, and Carole Offir. *The Longest War: Sex Differences in Perspective.* New York: Harcourt Brace Jovanovich, 1977.

Tavris, Carol, and Susan Sadd. *The Redbook Report on Female Sexuality.* New York: Delacorte, 1977.

Taylor, Gordon. *The Natural History of the Mind.* New York: E. P. Dutton, 1979.

Taylor, Lawrence. *Born to Crime*. Westport, Conn.: Greenwood Press, 1984.

Taylor, P., and N. Glenn. "The Utility of Education and Attractiveness for Female Status Attainment through Marriage." *American Sociological Review* 41 (1976): pp. 484–497.

Tecoma, Evelyn, and Leighton Huey. "Minireview: Psychic Distress and the Immune Response." *Life Sciences* 36 (1985): pp. 1799–1812.

Teilhard de Chardin. *How I Believe*. New York: Harper & Row, 1969.

Terkel, Joseph, and Jay Rosenblatt. "Hormonal Factors Underlying Maternal Behavior at Parturition: Cross Transfusion between Freely Moving Rats." *Journal of Comparative and Physiological Psychology* 80 (1972): pp. 365–371.

Terris, Milton. "Approaches to the Epidemiology of Health." *American Journal of Public Health* 65 (1973): pp. 1037–1045.

Thompson, A. "Emotional and Sexual Components of Extramarital Affairs." *Journal of Marriage and the Family* 46 (1984): pp. 35–42.

Tierney, John, Lynda Wright, and Karen Springen. "In Search of Adam and Eve." *Newsweek* (January 11, 1988): pp. 46–52.

Toynbee, Arnold. *A Study of History*. Vol. 7. London: Oxford University Press, 1955.

Tracy, Paul, Marvin Wolfgang, and Robert Figlio. *Delinquency in Two Birth Cohorts*. Chicago: University of Chicago Press, 1985.

Trotter, Robert. "Schizophrenia: A Cruel Chain of Events." In *Psychology 79/80: Annual Editions*, edited by C. Borg. Guilford, Conn.: Dushkin Publishers, 1979.

Turgenev, Ivan. *Spring Torrents*. Translated by L. Schapiro. New York: Penguin, 1980.

Turnbull, Colin. *The Mountain People*. In *Anthropology 82/83*, edited by E. Angeloni. Guilford, Conn.: Dushkin, 1982.

Tweedie, Jill. *In the Name of Love*. New York: Pantheon, 1979.

United Nations. *U.N. Demographic Yearbook*. New York: U.N., 1986.

Vickers, Geoffrey. "Mental Health and Spiritual Values." *Lancet* (March 1955): p. 524.

Vaillant, George. *Adaptation in Life*. Boston: Little, Brown, 1977.

Wadsworth, Michael. "Delinquency, Pulse Rates and Early Emotional Deprivation." *British Journal of Criminology* 16 (1976): pp. 245–256.

Wagenwood, James, and Peyton Bailey. *Women: A Book for Men*. New York: Avon, 1979.

Waite, Robert. *The Psychopathic God: Adolf Hitler*. New York: Basic Books, 1977.

Walsh, Anthony. "The Prophylactic Effect of Religion on Blood Pressure Levels among a Sample of Immigrants." *Social Science and Medicine* 14b (1980): pp. 59–63.

Walsh, Anthony. *Human Nature and Love: Biological, Intrapsychic and Social-Behavioral Perspective.* Lanham, Md.: University Press of America, 1981.

———. "Neurophysiology, Motherhood, and the Growth of Love." *Human Mosaic* 17 (1983): pp. 51–62.

———. "Love and Human Authenticity in the Works of Freud, Marx, and Maslow." *Free Inquiry in Creative Sociology* 14 (1986): pp. 21–26.

———. "Cognitive Functioning and Delinquency: Property Versus Violent Crime." *International Journal of Offender Therapy and Comparative Criminology* 31 (1987): pp. 285–289.

———. " 'The People Who Own the Country Ought to Govern It': The Supreme Court, Hegemony, and Its Consequences." *Law and Inequality* 5 (1988): pp. 431–451.

———. *Understanding, Assessing, and Counseling the Criminal Justice Client.* Pacific Grove, Calif.: Brooks/Cole, 1988.

Walsh, Anthony, and Grace Balazs. "Love, Sex, and Self-Esteem." *Free Inquiry in Creative Sociology* 18 (1990): pp. 37–42.

Walsh, Anthony, and Patricia Walsh. "Social Support, Assimilation, and Biological Effective Blood Pressure Levels." *International Migration Review* 21 (1987): pp. 577–591.

———. "Love, Self-Esteem, and Multiple Sclerosis." *Social Science and Medicine* 29 (1989): pp. 793–798.

Walsh, Anthony, J. Arthur Beyer, and Thomas Petee. "Violent Delinquency: An Examination of Psycopathic Typologies." *Journal of Genetic Psychology* 148 (1987): pp. 385–392.

Walsh, Anthony, Thomas Petee, and J. Arthur Beyer. "Intellectual Imbalance: Comparing High Verbal and High Performance IQ Delinquents." *Criminal Justice and Behavior* 14 (1987): pp. 370–379.

Warren, Sharon, S. Greenhill, and K. Warren. "Emotional Stress and the Development of Multiple Sclerosis: Case Control Evidence of a Relationship." *Journal of Chronic Disease* 35 (1982): pp. 821–831.

Wax, Douglas, and Victor Haddox. "Enuresis, Fire Setting and Cruelty to Animals in Male Adolescent Delinquents: A Triad Predictive of Violent Behavior. *Journal of Psychiatry and Law* 2 (1972): pp. 45–71.

Wechsler, David. *The Measure and Appraisal of Adult Intelligence.* Baltimore: Williams and Williams, 1958.

Weisenfeld, Alan, Carol Malatesta, Patricia Whitman, Cherlyn Granrose, and Robin Uili. "Psychophysiological Response to Breast- and Bottle-Feeding Mothers to Their Infant's Signals." *Psychophysiology* 22 (1985): pp. 79–86.

Weisner, T. "Sibling Interdependence and Child Caretaking: A Cross-Cultural View." In *Sibling Relationships: Their Nature and Significance Across* the Lifespan, edited by M. Lamg and B. Sutton-Smith. Hillsdale, N.J.: Lawrence Erlbaum, 1982.

Whitman, Howard. "The Amazing New Science of Love." Journal of Lifetime Living (August 1955): pp. 76–84.

Wilson, Colin. A Criminal History of Mankind. London: Panther, 1984.

Wilson, Edward. On Human Nature. Cambridge, Mass.: Harvard University Press, 1978.

Wilson, Glen. Love and Instinct. New York: Quill, 1983.

Wilson, Peter. Man, The Promising Primate. Yale University Press, 1980.

Wilson, H., and C. Kneisl. Psychiatric Nursing. Menlo Park, Calif.: Addison-Wesley, 1983.

Winter, Ruth, and Kathleen McAuliffe. "Hooked on Love." Omni 6 (1984): pp. 81–104.

Witelson, Sandra. "Sex and the Single Hemisphere: Specialization of the Right Hemisphere for Spatial Processing." Science 193 (1976): pp. 425–426.

Wolfgang, Marvin, Robert Figlio, and Thorsten Sellin. Delinquency in a Birth Cohort. Chicago: University of Chicago Press, 1972.

Wolkind, S. "The Components of 'Affectionless Psychopathy' in Institutionalized Children." Journal of Child Psychology and Psychiatry 15 (1974): pp. 215–220.

Wyatt, R., D. Murphy, R. Belmaker, C. Donnelly, S. Cohen, and W. Pollin. "Reduced Monoamine Oxydase Activity in Platelets: A Possible Genetic Marker for Vulnerability to Schizophrenia." Science 179 (1973): pp. 916–918.

Young, Michael. The Rise of the Meritocracy. Middlesex, England: Penguin, 1975.

Zarrow, M., V. Denenberg, and B. Sachs. "Hormones and Maternal Behavior in Mammals." In Hormones and Behavior, edited by S. Levine. New York: Academic Press, 1972.

Zuckerman, Marvin, Monte Buchsbaum, and Dennis Murphy. "Sensation Seeking and Its Biological Correlates." Psychological Bulletin 88 (1980): pp. 187–214.

Index